Lyme Disease

Lyme
Disease

Patricia K. Coyle, MD
Associate Professor of Neurology
State University of New York at Stony Brook
School of Medicine
Stony Brook, New York

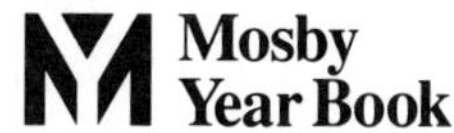

Mosby
Year Book

St. Louis Baltimore Boston Chicago London Philadelphia Sydney Toronto

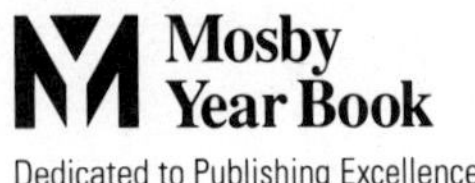

Publisher: George Stamathis
Editor: Stephanie Manning
Developmental Editor: Leslie Fenton
Project Supervisor: Arofan Gregory

Printed in the United States of America

Mosby–Year Book, Inc.
11830 Westline Industrial Drive
St. Louis, Missouri 63146

Library of Congress Cataloging in Publication Data

Lyme disease / [edited by] Patricia K. Coyle.
     p.   cm.
    Includes bibliographical references and index.
    ISBN 1-55664-365-9
    1. Lyme disease.   I. Coyle, Patricia K.
    [DNLM: 1. Lyme Disease.   WC 406 L9857]
RC155.5.L94   1992
616.9'2—dc20
DNLM/DLC
for Library of Congress   92-49259
                                     CIP

92 93 94 95 96 GW/MY 9 8 7 6 5 4 3 2 1

ACKNOWLEDGMENTS

This book was made possible only through the hard work and efforts of a number of people. On a personal level, I want to acknowledge Dr. Richard T. Johnson. He is an important mentor who fostered my early interest in infectious diseases, and he has continued to be supportive and kind. I also want to acknowledge my parents, Eileen and Daniel, for their unfailing support and inspiration.

Contributors

DAVID ALLAN BAKER, M.D.
Associate Professor of Obstetrics and Gynecology, and Director, Division of Infectious Diseases, Department of Obstetrics and Gynecology, State University of New York at Stony Brook School of Medicine, Stony Brook, New York

ANITA L. BELMAN, M.D.
Associate Professor of Neurology and Pediatrics, State University of New York at Stony Brook School of Medicine, Stony Brook, New York

JORGE L. BENACH, Ph.D.
Professor of Pathology, State University of New York at Stony Brook School of Medicine, Stony Brook, New York

RONALD S. BENNETT, M.D., F.A.C.P.
Clinical Assistant Professor of Medicine, State University of New York at Stony Brook School of Medicine, Stony Brook, New York

BERNARD W. BERGER, M.D.
Assistant Clinical Professor of Dermatology, State University of New York at Stony Brook School of Medicine, Stony Brook, New York

EDWARD M. BOSLER, Ph.D.
Research Scientist, Department of Health, Health Science Center, State University of New York at Stony Brook School of Medicine, Stony Brook, New York

WILLY BURGDORFER, Ph.D., M.D. (hon.)
Medical Research Entomologist, and Scientist Emeritus, Laboratory of Vectors and Pathogens, Rocky Mountain Laboratories, National Institute of Allergy and Infectious Disease, National Institutes of Health, Hamilton, Montana

AVRAHAM CALEV, D.Phil.
Associate Professor of Clinical Psychiatry, Department of Psychiatry, and Clinical Neuropsychologist, State University of New York at Stony Brook School of Medicine, Stony Brook, New York

JAMES L. COLEMAN, M.S.
Research Scientist, New York State Department of Health, State University of New York at Stony Brook School of Medicine, Stony Brook, New York

PATRICIA K. COYLE, M.D.
Associate Professor of Neurology, State University of New York at Stony Brook School of Medicine, Stony Brook, New York

RAYMOND J. DATTWYLER, M.D.
Associate Professor of Medicine, State University of New York at Stony Brook School of Medicine, Stony Brook, New York

DAVID T. DENNIS, M.D.
Chief, Bacterial Zoonoses Branch, Centers for Disease Control, Division of Vector-Born Infectious Diseases, Fort Collins, Colorado

PAUL H. DURAY, M.D.
Associate Professor of Pathology, Harvard Medical School; and Clinical Assistant Professor of Medicine, Tufts University School of Medicine, Boston; Attending Surgical Pathologist, Brigham and Women's Hospital, Boston, Massachusetts; and Visiting Scientist, Department of Biology, Brookhaven National Laboratory, Upton, New York

EDWARD DWYER, M.D.
Assistant Professor of Pediatrics, Columbia University College of Physicians and Surgeons, New York, New York

JUAN CARLOS GARCIA-MONCO, M.D.
Neurologist and Attending Physician, Section of Neurology, Hospital de Galdacano, Vizcaya, Spain

MARC G. GOLIGHTLY, Ph.D.
Associate Professor of Pathology and Head of Immunology, Department of Pathology, State University of New York at Stony Brook School of Medicine, Stony Brook, New York

JESSE L. GOODMAN, M.D.
Associate Professor of Medicine, Section of Infectious Diseases, and Attending Physician, University of Minnesota Hospital and Clinics, University of Minnesota Medical School, Minneapolis, Minnesota

MAX I. HAMBURGER, M.D., F.A.C.P.
Clinical Assistant Professor of Medicine, State University of New York at Stony Brook School of Medicine, Stony Brook, New York

LINA JANDORF, M.A.
Research Scientist II, Department of Neurology, State University of New York at Stony Brook School of Medicine, Stony Brook, New York

ALAN T. KAELL, M.D., F.A.C.P., F.A.C.R., F.A.A.P.
Clinical Associate Professor of Medicine, State University of New York at Stony Brook School of Medicine, Stony Brook, New York

LAUREN B. KRUPP, M.D.
Assistant Professor of Neurology, State University of New York at Stony Brook School of Medicine, Stony Brook, New York

BENJAMIN J. LUFT, M.D.
Associate Professor of Medicine, Department of Medicine, Division of Infectious Diseases, State University of New York at Stony Brook School of Medicine, Stony Brook, New York

JOHN NOWAKOWSKI, M.D.
Assistant Professor of Medicine, New York Medical College, Valhalla; Staff Physician, Division of Infectious Diseases, Westchester County Medical Center, Valhalla; and Director of Lyme Disease Service, St. Agnes Hospital, White Plains, New York

HAROLD L. PASS, Ph.D.
Associate Professor of Clinical Psychiatry, Department of Psychiatry and Behavioral Medicine, and Director of Psychology, University Hospital, State University of New York at Stony Brook School of Medicine, Stony Brook, New York

LOUIS REIK, Jr., M.D.
Associate Professor of Neurology, University of Connecticut School of Medicine; Attending Neurologist, John Dempsey Hospital, Farmington, Connecticut

PATRICIA A. ROSA, Ph.D.
Senior Staff Fellow, Laboratory of Microbial Structure and Function, Rocky Mountain Laboratories, National Institute of Allergy and Infectious Disease, National Institutes of Health, Hamilton, Montana

STEVEN E. SCHUTZER, M.D.
Associate Professor of Medicine, Department of Medicine, Division of Allergy and Immunology, University of Medicine and Dentistry of New Jersey, Newark, New Jersey

TOM G. SCHWAN, Ph.D.
Acting Head, Arthropod-Borne Diseases Section, Laboratory of Vectors and Pathogens, Rocky Mountain Laboratories, National Institute of Allergy and Infectious Disease, National Institutes of Health, Hamilton, Montana

JOSEPH E. SCHWARTZ, Ph.D.
Research Associate Professor of Psychiatry and Behavioral Sciences, State University of New York at Stony Brook School of Medicine, Stony Brook, New York

PATRICK A. SIBONY, M.D.
Associate Professor, Ophthalmology and Neurology, Department of Ophthalmology, State University of New York at Stony Brook School of Medicine, Stony Brook, New York

GENEVIEVE SICURANZA, M.D.
Fellow, Maternal-Fetal Medicine, Department of Obstetrics and Gynecology, State University of New York at Stony Brook School of Medicine, Stony Brook, New York

LEONARD H. SIGAL, M.D.
Associate Professor of Medicine, Department of Medicine, and Adjunct Assistant Professor, Department of Molecular Genetics and Microbiology, and Acting Chief, Division of Rheumatology, and Director, Lyme Disease Center, University of Medicine and Dentistry of New Jersey, Robert Wood Johnson Medical School, New Brunswick, New Jersey

CARL URBAN, Ph.D.
Assistant Professor of Microbiology, New York University School of Medicine, New York City; Director, Infectious Disease Research, Department of Medicine, Booth Memorial Medical Center, Flushing, New York

STEPHEN C. VLAY, M.D.
Professor of Medicine, State University of New York at Stony Brook School of Medicine; Director, The Stony Brook Arrhythmia Study and Sudden Death Prevention Center; and Director, Coronary Unit, University Hospital at Stony Brook, Stony Brook, New York

DAVID J. VOLKMAN, Ph.D., M.D.
Associate Professor of Medicine, Division of Allergy, Rheumatology and Clinical Immunology, State University of New York at Stony Brook School of Medicine, Stony Brook, New York

ROBERT WINCHESTER, M.D.
Professor of Pediatrics and Director, Division of Autoimmune and Molecular Diseases, Department of Pediatrics, College of Physicians and Surgeons, Columbia University, New York

JOHN R. WITTPENN, M.D.
Assistant Professor of Ophthalmology, Department of Ophthalmology, State University of New York at Stony Brook School of Medicine, Stony Brook, New York

GARY P. WORMSER, M.D.
Professor of Medicine and Pharmacology, New York Medical College; Chief, Division of Infectious Diseases, Westchester County Medical Center and New York Medical College; and Director, Lyme Diagnostic Center, Westchester County Medical Center, Valhalla, New York

Preface

In the United States Lyme disease has become the second leading new infection after AIDS. Although it is somewhat geographically restricted, it is clear from the phone calls I receive that interest in this infection is nationwide. Because Lyme disease can involve a number of major organ systems to produce a variety of medical problems, it enters into the differential diagnosis of many medical and neurologic disorders. For this reason, every modern clinician needs to be familiar with Lyme disease.

We are in a relatively early period of our understanding of this infection. There are current problems in diagnosis and treatment, and controversy surrounds the pathogenesis and management of postinfectious problems. This book highlights the questions we still need to ask about Lyme disease, as well as the answers we already have.

I have assembled a panel of experts to address various aspects of Lyme disease in North America. Half of the authors are from Stony Brook, and half are experts from other leading centers who deal with this infection on a daily basis. The book is written for clinicians of all specialties, as well as basic researchers with a particular interest in Lyme disease. However, the sophisticated layperson will also find most chapters to be easily read and understood.

Section One covers basic aspects of the disease, while Section Two covers clinical aspects referable to the major organ systems involved. Section Three provides a state-of-the-art review on diagnosis, including the latest nucleic acid and antigen assays. Section Four reviews treatment of early and late Lyme disease, and current vaccine development, and previews new antimicrobials that are likely to be employed in the next few years. Section Five addresses special topics of particular interest, including the pregnant patient, treated patients with persistent symptoms, the seronegative patient, and pediatric Lyme disease. The book is written so that each chapter stands on its own, and can be referred to when a specific problem arises. However, my goal was to provide in one source the best current overview of North American Lyme disease available. I hope I have succeeded.

P. K. Coyle

Contents

SECTION ONE
BASIC ASPECTS

1   Discovery of *Borrelia burgdorferi*, 3
    Willy Burgdorfer

2   Molecular Biology of *Borrelia burgdorferi*, 8
    Patricia A. Rosa
    Tom G. Schwan

3   Tick Vectors and Hosts, 18
    Edward M. Bosler

4   Epidemiology, 27
    David T. Dennis

5   Genetic Basis of Chronic Lyme Disease, 38
    Edward Dwyer
    Robert Winchester

6   Immune Response and Clinical Lyme Disease, 46
    Steven E. Schutzer

7   Histopathology of Human Borreliosis, 49
    Paul H. Duray

SECTION TWO
CLINICAL ASPECTS

8   Overview of Spirochetal Infections, 61
    Jorge L. Benach
    James L. Coleman

9   Dermatologic Aspects, 69
    Bernard W. Berger

10 Rheumatic Manifestations, 73
    Alan T. Kaell
    Ronald S. Bennett
    Max I. Hamburger

11 Cardiac Manifestations, 86
    Stephen C. Vlay

12 Ophthalmic Manifestations, 93
    John R. Wittpenn
    Patrick A. Sibony

13 Neurologic Aspects of North American Lyme Disease, 101
    Louis Reik, Jr.

SECTION THREE
DIAGNOSIS

14 Antibody Assays, 115
    Marc G. Golightly

15 Cellular Immune Assays, 121
    David J. Volkman

16 Nucleic Acid Detection of *Borrelia burgdorferi* Infection, 127
    Jesse L. Goodman

17 Antigen Detection and Cerebrospinal Fluid Studies, 136
    P. K. Coyle

SECTION FOUR
THERAPY

18 Treatment of Early Lyme Disease: Infection Associated with Erythema Migrans, 149
    John Nowakowski
    Gary P. Wormser

19 Treatment of *Borrelia burgdorferi* Infection: Acute and Chronic Disease, 163
    Raymond J. Dattwyler

20 New Antibiotic Agents, 167
    Carl Urban
    Benjamin J. Luft

21 Vaccine Development, 172
    P. K. Coyle

SECTION FIVE
SPECIAL TOPICS

22 Pathogenesis of Lyme Disease, 179
    James L. Coleman
    Jorge L. Benach

23 Lyme Disease in Pregnancy, 184
    Genevieve Sicuranza
    David Allan Baker

24 Persisting Symptoms, 187
    Leonard H. Sigal

25 Seronegative Lyme Disease, 192
Steven E. Schutzer

26 Fatigue, 196
Lauren B. Krupp
Joseph E. Schwartz
Lina Jandorf

27 Cognitive and Psychiatric Aspects, 204
Harold L. Pass
Avraham Calev

28 Pediatric Lyme Disease, 210
Anita L. Belman

29 European Lyme Disease, 219
Juan Carlos Garcia-Monco

Lyme Disease

SECTION ONE

Basic Aspects

1 Discovery of *Borrelia burgdorferi*

Willy Burgdorfer

For Americans, a discussion of the history of Lyme borreliosis usually begins with the story of two persistent women, Polly Murray and Judith Mensch of Old Lyme, Connecticut. In the early 1970s, they were concerned about the occurrence of arthritis in members of their families and in families of the neighboring towns of Lyme and East Haddam. Severe headaches, skin lesions, and subsequent recurring arthritic and neurologic symptoms suggested to them that the physicians' diagnosis of "juvenile rheumatoid arthritis" was wrong. Their suspicion that something unusual was happening was made known to the Connecticut State Health Department, which sought help from Dr. Allen Steere of the Rheumatology Department at Yale University Medical School. In October 1975, he started a retrospective study that eventually led to the description of Lyme arthritis,[39] which was later changed to Lyme disease,[38] a new complex multisystem disorder of unknown cause.

Unknown to most Americans, however, is the earliest reference to manifestations of what today is known as Lyme borreliosis. In 1883, the German physician, Dr. A. Buchwald,[12] described a diffuse idiopathic skin atrophy that in 1902 was named *acrodermatitis chronica atrophicans* (ACA)[24,25]— a skin disorder of unknown cause.

ERYTHEMA CHRONICUM MIGRANS

A few years later in 1909, the Swedish physician, Dr. Arvid Afzelius, demonstrated to the Swedish Society of Dermatology in Stockholm an elderly woman who had a ringlike skin lesion measuring 1/2 to 2/0 cm where she had been bitten by the sheep tick, *Ixodes ricinus*.[4] Because the lesion migrated by expanding its peripheral borders and was accompanied by central clearing, Afzelius, who had noted a similar case in 1908, referred to it as erythema migrans. In 1913, Dr. B. Lipschütz from the Dermatology Section of the Hospital Wieden in Vienna, Austria, introduced the term *erythema chronicum migrans* (ECM) because the lesions on his patient lasted for as long as 7 months.[29]

Afzelius, whose cases were associated with tick bites, speculated that the condition was produced either by a virus transmitted by the tick or by a toxic substance originating from the tick. Lipschütz, on the other hand, rejected the toxin hypothesis because of the affliction's long duration. He speculated that ECM is caused by a tickborne pathogen and suggested microscopic-bacteriologic investigations of the intestinal tract and of the salivary gland secretions of the tick.[29] Regrettably, no one followed his advice.

The first evidence of nervous system involvement with ECM was provided in 1922 by the French neurologists, Drs. Ch. Garin and Ch. Bujadoux.[17] They reported the development of a reddish skin lesion followed by a painful meningoradiculitis in a patient bitten by the hedgehog tick, *I. hexagonus*. Unfortunately, Garin and Bujadoux misdiagnosed their case as tick paralysis. It was not until 1930 that Dr. S. Hellerström[22] from the Karolinska Institute in Stockholm recognized the condition as ECM with nervous system involvement—a condition later referred to as Bannwarth's syndrome. Interestingly, Garin and Bujadoux suggested that a spirochete may have been the cause of their patient's ailment.

In 1936, Dr. H. Askani from the Dermatology Clinic of the University of Heidelberg reviewed the significance of ticks as vectors of human and animal pathogens and concluded that ECM was caused either by a toxin or by a living pathogen from the tick's salivary glands—a conclusion shared by many physicians investigating the disease.[6]

The cause of ECM continued to remain elusive until 1948 when Dr. Carl Lennhoff[28] from the Dermatology Clinic at the Karolinska Institute claimed to have developed a staining technique that permitted him to identify spirochetal elements in at least 27 diseases, including psoriasis, zoster, varicella, rubella, lymphadenosis benigna cutis, various erythemas and lymphogranulomas, endocarditis, leukemia, and erythema migrans. Lennhoff used the interaction of mercuric chloride with spirochetes made visible by ammonium sulfide, resulting in a deposit of mercuric sulfide. Although his staining method appeared suitable for demonstrating spirochetes in cultures, it was not suitable for identifying these microorganisms in smears or in tissue sections of ECM lesions; too often, spirochetes could not be distinguished from spirochete-like elements or tissue fibers. Also, the technique was nonspecific, because it also stained other organisms and fungi.[35]

In 1949, Hellerström addressed the 43rd Annual Meeting of the Southern Medical Association in Cincinnati, Ohio, with a talk entitled "ECM Afzelius with Meningitis."[23] He reviewed several cases in which both erythemas and subsequent meningocerebrospinal symptoms occurred after tick bite, and reported on the successful use of penicillin by his colleague, Dr. E. Hollström, in treating ECM. He also discussed the still unsolved cause of ECM and wondered whether the sheep tick, *I. ricinus*, could be a vector of spirochetes. Spirochetes, he pointed out, have been known to cause circular erythemas that subside in the center and advance peripherally, and to affect the nervous system. Again, no one was interested in collecting and dissecting ticks to search for spirochetes, possibly because spirochetes had never been found associated with ticks of the genus *Ixodes*. Thus, the cause of ECM remained as obscure as ever.

In 1955, Dr. E. Binder and co-workers[11] succeeded in transmitting ECM from human to human by transplanting among themselves pieces of skin taken from the peripheral zone of a lesion of a patient with ECM. In each of the three volunteers, typical lesions developed within 1 to 3 weeks, and a subpassage was equally successful. In each case, treatment with penicillin caused the lesions to disappear within a few days. These experiments clearly established that the cause of ECM is an infectious agent susceptible to penicillin.

The work of Dr. G. Schaltenbrand from the Neurological Clinic of the University of Würzburg also should be mentioned because he showed that the nervous system disorders associated with ECM were not identical to those of the Central European tickborne encephalitis.[34] He assumed that ECM meningitis was caused by an unidentified viral agent associated with *I. ricinus*. But, in 1974, Dr. Klaus Weber,[44] a practicing allergologist from Munich, successfully treated a patient with ECM meningitis with antibiotics (penicillin and chloramphenicol) and concluded that this nervous disorder was a bacterial and not a viral illness. He ruled out spirochetes as the causative agent because "[these microorganisms] are transmitted by argasid and not ixodid ticks." He also referred to the negative results of S. Hard[21] who attempted to infect larval, nymphal, and adult *I. ricinus* by allowing them to feed on the erythematous ring of an ECM lesion. Subsequent darkfield examination of tick tissues showed no spirochetes, and transmission experiments with nymphal ticks that had fed on the lesion as larvae proved negative.

A rickettsial cause of ECM was suggested as early as 1962 by French scientists.[16] Based on results obtained by Giroud's slide agglutination test, they reported six of seven patients with significant titers against the epidemic typhus agent, *Rickettsia prowazekii*, the murine typhus rickettsia, *R. mooseri,* and the boutonneuse fever agent, *R. conorii.* Although these results could not be confirmed, the notion that ECM is caused by a rickettsia was kept alive by the electron microscopic demonstration of rickettsia-like microorganisms in macrophages of two ECM patients.[33] This induced Weber[45] to have sera of 13 ECM patients evaluated by two different laboratories using complement fixation, microagglutination, or immunofluorescence tests for the detection of antibodies to 14 different rickettsial antigens. Excepting nondiagnostic low titers, all tests were negative.

In the United States, the first case of ECM was recorded in 1969[36] in a physician who had been bitten by a tick while hunting grouse in north central Wisconsin. The attending physician, Dr. Rudolf Scrimenty—familiar with ECM lesions described in Europe—accurately diagnosed the manifestations and effectively treated his patient with penicillin. A cluster of four additional cases occurred in midsummer 1975 in southeastern Connecticut.[31] Although these patients did not recall a specific tick or insect bite, they all experienced centrifugally spreading skin lesions with central clearing.

Thus, by the beginning of the 1980s, the causative agent of Lyme disease in the United States and of ECM in Europe still remained elusive.

ACRODERMATITIS CHRONICA ATROPHICANS

Also unsolved was the cause of acrodermatitis chronica atrophicans (ACA), which had been considered a distinct clinical entity in Europe since its description in 1883.[12] Many patients suffering from ACA remembered having been bitten by the sheep tick, *I. ricinus*, and some reported subsequent development of ECM-like skin lesions.

Two major hypotheses had been put forward about the cause of ACA: (1) It resulted from an infection, and (2) it resulted from hormonal-vegetative defects initiated by traumatic and hypothermal factors.

An important observation about the cause of ACA was reported in 1942 by R. H. Kahle[27] of the Dermatological Clinic of the Martin Luther University in Halle, Wittenberg, Germany. He noted that six of seven ACA patients had a positive serologic reaction against *Treponema pallidum*. Ten years later, his superior, Dr. Grüneberg,[20] confirmed these results and speculated that the reactions must have been caused by a group-specific spirochete as the causative agent of ACA.

With the discovery in 1946 that penicillin was effective in the treatment of ACA,[42] all research efforts were directed toward identifying a "living" agent. In 1954 and 1955, Dr. H. Götz[18,19] from the Dermatological Clinic of the University of Munich showed that ACA was indeed an infectious disease. He successfully transplanted affected skin of a patient into four volunteers, including himself, and recorded a clinical picture similar to ACA (i.e., inflammation that lasted for as long as 312 days and promptly disappeared after treatment with penicillin). Götz speculated the etiologic agent to be a large virus, but, lacking evidence, he concluded that the cause of ACA would continue to be an open question.

In 1955, Lohel[30] claimed the production of antibodies against spirochetes in mice inoculated with blood from ACA patients. His observations could not be confirmed, and his claim of ACA being a spirochetosis was rejected.

The next episode leading to the discovery of the causative agent of ECM was the occurrence of arthritis in Old Lyme and Lyme, and the story of Mrs. Murray and Mrs. Mensch referred to at the beginning of this chapter.

Dr. Steere's retrospective study[39] included 51 residents, 39 children, and 12 adults, who had developed recurrent attacks of asymmetric swelling and pain in large joints, particularly the knee. Thirteen remembered an expanding skin lesion that was thought to fit the description of the lesions associated with ECM in Europe. But because arthritis had not been described as part of ECM, Steere and his associates believed that the Lyme patients were suffering from a previously unrecognized clinical entity. Their search for the causative agent concentrated on the serologic evaluation of acute and convalescent sera of patients for antibodies to viral agents, including 216 arboviruses, of which 38 were tickborne.[39] All tests were essentially negative, as were serologic tests against four rickettsial agents, *R. akari, R. rickettsii, R. mooseri,* and *Coxiella burnetii*. Also negative for viruses were 622 *I. dammini*, first considered to be *I. scapularis*, but later redescribed as a new species,[37] that were collected off vegetation in communities east and west of the Connecticut River where the incidence of Lyme disease was high and low, respectively.[43]

DISCOVERY OF THE CAUSATIVE AGENT

The discovery of the causative agent of Lyme disease, ECM, and ACA came unexpectedly and serendipitously in the fall of 1981 during ecologic investigations of Rocky Mountain spotted fever in Long Island, New York. From 1971 to 1976, a total of 124 cases with 8 deaths had occurred there.[8] My colleague, Dr. Jorge Benach from the New York State Health Department and I were particularly interested in obtaining strains of *R. rickettsii* from the vector tick, *Dermacentor variabilis*, in areas where the deaths had occurred. Although almost 6% of ticks were hemolymph test–positive for rickettsiae, all isolates proved to be *R. montana,* a rickettsia nonpathogenic for humans. This caused us to speculate that perhaps other species of ticks, such as the deer tick, *I. dammini,* which occurs abundantly on Long Island, particularly on offshore islands, may play a role in the natural history of *R. rickettsii*. Several hundred *I. dammini,* collected by flagging, were examined for rickettsiae by the hemolymph test; all were negative.

In late September and early October 1981, Benach provided collections of *I. dammini* from Shelter Island, New York, where Lyme disease was known to be endemic. Again, none of 44 male and female ticks had rickettsiae, but the hemolymph of two females contained microfilariae* that appeared similar to a deer microfilaria *(Dipetalonema [Wehrdickmannia] rugosicauda)* associated with *I. ricinus* in Europe.[3] To determine whether this nematode was present also in the digestive system, I dissected both female ticks and prepared Giemsa-stained smears from individual midgut diverticula for microscopic examination. No more microfilariae were found. Instead, I saw poorly stained, rather large, irregularly coiled spirochetes. Darkfield microscopy of midgut tissues confirmed the spirochetal nature of the organisms, which had a rather sluggish and slow movement. Additional tissue, including salivary glands, malpighian tubules, ovary, and central ganglion, of either tick was free of spirochetes. Of 124 additional ticks examined similarly, 75 (60%) contained spirochetes that were limited to the ticks' midgut.

I remembered some of the European literature on ECM, particularly Hellerström's paper given in Cincinnati in 1949, and wondered whether the discovered spirochete could indeed be the long-sought-after cause of this illness and possibly also of Lyme disease. Initial evidence for this, I obtained by indirect immunofluorescence with sera of convalescent Lyme disease patients seen by Dr. E. Grunwaldt, a practicing physician on Shelter Island, New York. Dr. A. Barbour, a molecular

---

*A detailed description of the microfilaria appeared in Beaver PC, Burgdorfer W: *J Parasitol* 70:963, 1984. It has since been suggested that the microfilaria represents the larval stage of a muspiceoid nematode that parasitizes deer or rodents, or both.

biologist at Rocky Mountain Laboratories who at the time was studying the variable proteins of the relapsing fever borrelia, *Borrelia hermsii,* offered his expertise in culturing the *I. dammini* spirochete. On November 13, 1981, I gave him spirochete-containing midgut diverticula of four infected ticks. These tissues were triturated in Stoenner's fortified Kelly medium,[41] and tenfold dilutions of the preparation were inoculated into tubes containing the same medium. After 5 days of incubation at 35° C, several tubes yielded spirochetes that could be subcultured regularly. This original Shelter Island isolate from *I. dammini* was subsequently cloned from the 10^6 dilution culture by limiting dilution and was designated B31.[7]

Shortly after I found the spirochetes in *I. dammini,* I was anxious to learn whether they could also be demonstrated in *I. ricinus,* the incriminated vector of ECM in Europe. This was first confirmed by detecting spirochetes in midgut smears of ticks I had collected during a tick/rickettsiae survey on the Swiss Plateau in 1978. The slides had been stored as reference material and had to be stained with Giemsa for reexamination. Spirochetes similar to those in *I. dammini* were found in 13 (17%) of 135 smears. In the spring of 1982, 112 (29%) of 390 live *I. ricinus* collected near Neuchâtel, Switzerland, were shown infected with spirochetes morphologically identical to those in *I. dammini.*[14]

Spirochetes similar if not identical to those in *I. dammini* and *I. ricinus* were also found in the black-legged western tick, *I. pacificus,* which had been incriminated since 1975 as a possible vector of Lyme disease in California. A tick/spirochete survey in southeastern Oregon and north-central California yielded 2402 ticks of which 39 were infected.[15]

Soon after publication of our discoveries,[13-15] American and European clinicians and dermatologists succeeded in demonstrating spirochetes in ECM lesions[10] and in isolating organisms from blood of ECM patients.[2,9,40] The results of serologic tests also indicated that various clinical manifestations, including lymphocytic meningoradiculitis (Bannwarth's syndrome) and ACA, also have a spirochetal etiology and most likely represent advanced stages of the complex entity now known as Lyme borreliosis. Isolation of spirochetes similar if not identical to the Lyme disease agent have since been reported repeatedly from patients suffering from these diseases.[5,32]

Finally, this story of discovery would be incomplete without reference to investigations by Dr. Rudolf Ackermann from the Virology Department of the Neurologic Clinic in Köln, Germany. Successful treatment of ECM and related disorders with penicillin and tetracyclines, and the prolonged re-

curring clinical manifestations suggested to him a relapsing feverlike spirochetal etiology. His conjecture was strengthened by the demonstration of significant IgM and IgG antibody titers against the African relapsing fever spirochete, *B. duttonii,* in sera and cerebrospinal fluids from patients with ECM or meningopolyneuritis. In addition, by indirect immunofluorescence, he demonstrated spirochetes in *I. ricinus* from two foci of the disease in Germany in June 1982. Although Dr. Ackermann's findings were not reported until 1983,[1] he was the first to confirm the finding in *I. ricinus* of the spirochete now known as *Borrelia burgdorferi.*[26]

REFERENCES

1. Ackermann R: Erythema chronicum migrans und durch Zecken übertragene Meningopolyneuritis (Garin-Bujadoux, Bannwarth) Borrelien-Infektionen? *Dtsch Med Wochenschr* 108:577, 1983.
2. Ackermann R et al: Spirochäten-Aetiologie der Erythema-chronicum-migrans Krankheit, *Dtsch Med Wochenschr* 109:92, 1984.
3. Aeschlimann A et al: Aspects nouveaux du rôle de vecteur joué par *Ixodes ricinus* L. en Suisse, *Acta Trop* 36:181, 1979.
4. Afzelius A: Verhandlungen der Dermatologischen Gesellschaft zu Stockholm, *Arch Derm Syph* 101:404, 1910.
5. Åsbrink E, Hederstedt B, Hovmark A: The spirochetal etiology of acrodermatitis chronica atrophicans, Herxheimer, *Acta Derm Venerol* 64:506, 1984.
6. Askani H: Zur Ätiologie des Erythema chronicum migrans, *Dermatol Wochenschr* 102:125, 1936.
7. Barbour AG: Isolation and cultivation of Lyme disease spirochetes, *Yale J Biol Med* 57:521, 1984.
8. Benach JL et al: Changing patterns in the incidence of Rocky Mountain spotted fever on Long Island (1971-1976), *Am J Epidemiol* 106:380, 1977.
9. Benach JL et al: Spirochetes isolated from the blood of two patients with Lyme disease, *N Engl J Med* 308:740, 1983.
10. Berger BW, Clemmenson OJ, Ackermann AB: Lyme disease is a spirochetosis: a review of the disease and evidence of its cause, *Am J Dermatopathol* 5:111, 1983.
11. Binder E, Doepfmer R, Hornstein O: Experimentelle Übertragung des Erythema chronicum migrans von Mensch zu Mensch, *Hautarzt* 6:494, 1955.
12. Buchwald A: Ein Fall von diffuser idiopathischer Hautatrophie, *Derm Vierteljahresschr* 10:553, 1883.
13. Burgdorfer W et al: Lyme disease—a tick-borne spirochetosis? *Science* 216:1317, 1982.
14. Burgdorfer W et al: Erythema chronicum migrans—a tick borne spirochetosis, *Acta Trop* 40:79, 1983.
15. Burgdorfer W et al: The western black-legged tick, *Ixodes pacificus:* a vector of *Borrelia burgdorferi, Am J Trop Med Hyg* 34:925, 1985.
16. Dégos R, Tourraine R, Arouete J: L'erythema chronicum migrans, *Syph* 89:247, 1962.
17. Garin Ch, Bujadoux Ch: Paralysie par les tiques, *J Med Lyon* 71:765, 1922.
18. Götz H: Die Acrodermatitis chronica atrophicans Herxheimer als Infektionskrankheit, *Hautarzt* 5:491, 1954.
19. Götz H: Die Acrodermatitis chronica atrophicans Herxheimer als Infektionskrankheit—Ergänzung zur 1. Mitteilung, *Hautarzt* 6:249, 1955.

20. Grüneberg T: Auffällige serologische Befunde bei Akrodermatitis chronica atrophicans Herxheimer. *Klin Wochenschr* 32:935, 1954.
21. Hard S: Erythema chronicum migrans (Afzelii) associated with mosquito bite. *Acta Derm Venereol* 46:473, 1966.
22. Hellerström S: Erythema chronicum migrans Afzelii. *Acta Derm Venereol* 11:315, 1930.
23. Hellerström S: Erythema chronicum migrans Afzelius with meningitis. *South Med J* 43:330, 1950.
24. Herxheimer K, Hartman K: Über Acrodermatitis chronica atrophicans. *Arch Derm Syph* 61:57, 1902.
25. Herxheimer K, Hartmann K: Über Acrodermatitis chronica atrophicans. *Arch Derm Syph* 61:255, 1902.
26. Johnson RC et al: *Borrelia burgdorferi* sp. nov.: etiologic agent of Lyme disease. *Int J Syst Bacteriol* 34:496, 1984.
27. Kahle RH: Pallidareaktion bei peripheren Durchblutungsstörungen der Haut, insbesondere bei Akrodermatitis atrophicans, dissertation, Halle, 1942.
28. Lennhoff C: Spirochetes in aetiologically obscure diseases. *Acta Derm Venereol* 28:295, 1948.
29. Lipschütz B: Ueber eine seltene Erythemform (Erythema chronicum migrans). *Arch Derm Syph* 118:349, 1913.
30. Lohel H: Tierexperimentelle Untersuchungen zur Ätiologie der Acrodermatitis chronica atrophicans Herxheimer. *Klin Wochenschr* 33:185, 1955.
31. Mast WE, Burrows WM: Erythema chronicum migrans in the United States, *JAMA* 236:859, 1976.
32. Preac-Mursic V et al: Isolierung einer Spirochäte aus Liquor cerebrospinalis bei Meningoradikulitis-Bannwarth, *Münch Med Wochenschr* 126:275, 1984.
33. Sandbank M, Feuermann EF: Ultrastructural observation of rickettsia-like bodies in erythema chronicum migrans, *J Cutan Pathol* 6:253, 1979.
34. Schaltenbrand G: Durch Arthropoden übertragene Erkrankung der Haut und des Nervensystems, *Verh Dtsch Ges Inn Med* 72:975, 1967.
35. Schuppli R: Zur Frage des Nachweises von Spirochäten bei ätiologisch unabgeklärten Krankheiten, *Dermatol* 101:193, 1950.
36. Scrimenti RJ: Erythema chronicum migrans, *Arch Dermatol* 102:104, 1970.
37. Spielman A et al: Human babesiosis on Nantucket Island, USA: description of the vector, *Ixodes* (Ixodes) *dammini*, n.sp. (Acarina:Ixodidae), *J Med Entomol* 15:218, 1979.
38. Steere AC et al: Erythema chronicum migrans and Lyme arthritis: the enlarging clinical spectrum, *Ann Intern Med* 86:685, 1977.
39. Steere AC et al: Lyme arthritis: an epidemic of oligoarticular arthritis in children and adults in three Connecticut communities, *Arthritis Rheum* 20:7, 1977.
40. Steere AC et al: The spirochetal etiology of Lyme disease, *N Engl J Med* 308:733, 1983.
41. Stoenner HG, Dodd T, Larsen C: Antigenic variation of *Borrelia hermsii*, *J Exp Med* 156:1297, 1982.
42. Svartz N: Penicillinbehandlung vid dermatitis atrophicans Herxheimer, *Nord Med* 32:2783, 1946.
43. Wallis RC et al: Erythema chronicum migrans and Lyme arthritis: field study of ticks, *Am J Epidemiol* 108:322, 1978.
44. Weber K: Erythema chronicum migrans Meningitis—eine bakterielle Infektionskrankheit? *Münch Med Wochenschr* 116:1993, 1974.
45. Weber K: Serological study with rickettsial antigens on erythema chronicum migrans, *Dermatol* 163:460, 1981.

Molecular Biology of *Borrelia burgdorferi*

Patricia A. Rosa and Tom G. Schwan

Borrelia burgdorferi was isolated and identified as the causative agent of Lyme disease approximately one decade ago.[21] Our knowledge of *B. burgdorferi* at the molecular level and our understanding of how that relates to the biology of the organism are, therefore, the products of a relatively brief period of laboratory investigation. Despite the inherently limited nature of this information, significant contributions have been made in the molecular characterization of *B. burgdorferi*. These findings are the subject of this review. We have organized topics on a structural basis, beginning with a brief description of the intact spirochete.

STRUCTURE AND BIOLOGY

The structural components of an organism are not usually included in a discussion of its molecular biology. However, we mention a few basic aspects of the spirochete that are relevant to the molecular features that we describe and that are not discussed elsewhere in this book. Most of this material is covered in greater detail in several review articles.[7,48]

B. burgdorferi grows slowly in vitro, dividing by transverse fission every 8 to 12 hours.[4,40] The outer surface of the spirochete is covered with material of undefined structure and origin, loosely associated with the outer membrane.[7] Surface exposed, acylated proteins are presumably attached to the outer membrane by way of their lipid moiety.[20] The outer membrane of *Borrelia* has a trilaminar structure[48] and is very fluid.[7,10,50] Conflicting reports exist as to the presence of lipopolysaccharide in *B. burgdorferi*.[15,85]

Approximately 7 to 11 flagella are located in the periplasmic space between the outer membrane and the cell wall of *B. burgdorferi*.[40] Only limited information is available regarding the peptidoglycan structure of the *Borrelia* cell wall,[50] but it is presumed to be flexible because the spirochete's helical form is imposed by the flagella. The cytoplasmic membrane is adjacent to the cell wall and also has a trilaminar structure.[40,50]

The organization of chromosomal and plasmid deoxyribonucleic acid (DNA) within the cytoplasm of the spirochete is not well understood. Plasmid DNA has been detected in isolated membrane blebs from *B. burgdorferi*,[26,31] but the biologic role of such blebs is unknown. Bacteriophages have been infrequently observed in *B. burgdorferi* cultures.[7,38] The relationship of viral DNA to the *B. burgdorferi* genome (if any) has not been determined, but bacteriophages are of interest because of their potential utility in genetic studies of *B. burgdorferi*.

GENOME

Fairly basic features of the physical and chemical structure of the *B. burgdorferi* genome have been elucidated. The nucleotide composition of *Borrelia* DNA is approximately 28% guanine plus cytosine (G+C), as determined by thermal denaturation studies of total DNA[44,71] and sequence analysis of cloned segments.* The G+C content of prokaryotic genomes varies from 25% to 75%; phylogenetically related groups of bacteria tend to be similar.[51] Why bacteria have such divergent nucleotide compositions and how they are maintained are unknown. One current theory is that a biased adenine plus thymine (A + T)/G + C mutation pressure, acting on the entire genome during evolution, establishes the nucleotide composition of a particular organism.[60] Candidates for biasing mutation pressure include enzymes involved in DNA synthesis, modification, and repair. A more "biologic" explanation, whereby the temperature of the environment in which a bacteria lives exerts a selective pressure on the G+C content of its DNA (G-C pairs are more thermostable than A-T pairs), cannot be discounted but is inconsistent for many bacteria.

DNA methylation has been found in many different bacteria and may be pertinent to DNA replication and mismatch repair by distinguishing the template strand (methylated) from the newly synthesized DNA strand (unmethylated). Although DNA from a few *B. burgdorferi* strains is partially methylated at GATC sequences, the DNA of most *B. burgdorferi* strains appears to be unmethy-

---

*References 17, 39, 63, 68, 77, 91.

lated.[43] This is in contrast to several other members of the genus *Borrelia* that possess completely methylated DNA.[43,59]

B. burgdorferi appears to contain only single copies of the 16S and 23S ribosomal ribonucleic acid (RNA; rRNA) genes per genome.[66] The rRNA gene copy number ranges from 1 to 10 among other bacteria.[51] In some instances, additional copies of the rRNA genes contribute to a faster growth rate, but there is not a consistent correlation with genome size.[16]

The *Borrelia* genome is composed of DNA elements with distinct sizes and structures. These elements were originally classified as chromosomal and plasmid components, mainly on the basis of size.[44] We have continued to use these terms in this review, but with the caveat discussed below that they may be inappropriate.

Chromosome

Using pulsed field electrophoresis conditions that resolve large DNA molecules, the chromosomes of *B. burgdorferi* and of several other members of the genus *Borrelia* migrate as linear molecules of approximately 10^6 base pairs (bp).[14,29,54,56,69] This linear structure of the *Borrelia* chromosome is unique among characterized bacteria. It is conceivable that the *Borrelia* chromosome is circular in vivo and that it is converted to a linear molecule during cell lysis. Consistent with this possibility, not all molecules of *Borrelia* chromosomal DNA migrate as linear structures; some of the DNA does not enter the gel, characteristic of large circular DNA molecules under these electrophoresis conditions.[14,29,56,69] However, if the *Borrelia* chromosome is not linear in vivo, it is uniquely susceptible to nuclease cleavage or some other linearizing event during the lysis of the bacteria, because identical extraction procedures with other bacteria yield only intact, circular chromosomal DNA.[14,29,69] Isolation and analysis of the ends of the chromosome, and construction of physical and genetic maps, should define the geometry of the *Borrelia* chromosome in vivo. Assuming that the *Borrelia* chromosome is linear, determining the means by which it is replicated, as compared to circular bacterial chromosomes, represents an interesting area of future research.

The *Borrelia* chromosome, at 10^6 bp, is among the smallest of bacterial genomes. *Treponema pallidum*, another pathogenic spirochete, also has a genome of approximately 10^6 bp, but the chromosome is circular.[89] *Leptospira interrogans* has a genome of approximately 3×10^6 bp, but independent studies report different results regarding the structure of the *Leptospira* chromosome.[13,14,86] Genome size is presumed to reflect the complexity

of an organism, ranging from simple bacteria without cell walls and limited metabolic capability (e.g., *Mycoplasma,* $\approx 0.6 \times 10^6$ bp) to developmentally complex fruiting bacteria (e.g., *Myxococcus,* $\approx 9.5 \times 10^6$ bp).[51] Although only a little is known about the chemical nature of the cell wall of *Borrelia*,[50] spirochetal structure has been considered "simple" because it is flexible.[51] Similarly, the metabolic properties of *Borrelia* have not been well-defined, but their nutritional growth requirements are complex.[4,20,57]

The chromosomal copy number per cell varies enormously (from 1 to 80) among different species of bacteria.[51] Ploidy is a pertinent feature when a selectable phenotype, such as antigenic variation, is regulated by gene rearrangement or recombination, as is the case in *B. hermsii*.[59] If the bacterium is not haploid, phenotypic switching requires that all copies of the chromosome undergo rearrangement, or selective expression of only some (rearranged) gene copies, or segregation with cell division until homozygosity is attained. The copy number of the *Borrelia* chromosome has not been directly measured. However, the yield of *B. burgdorferi* DNA per bacterium (0.002 pg)[69] is comparable to the calculated DNA content based on genome size (10^6 bp ≈ 0.001 pg). Although the error in such estimates can be quite large, they are consistent with one or two copies of the *B. burgdorferi* chromosome per cell. *Borrelia burgdorferi* plasmid sequences hybridize to total genomic DNA with comparable intensity as chromosomal fragments,[69] thus, the chromosome and plasmids appear to be present at a roughly equivalent copy number.

Plasmids

Bacterial plasmids are molecules of double-stranded DNA, separate from the larger chromosome, that are capable of independent replication and are not essential to the growth of an organism in its usual environment.[36] These extrachromosomal replicons may contain genes that encode for a wide array of biologic functions in nature.[61] Plasmids have been reported to occur in all three genera of pathogenic spirochetes, *Treponema*,[62] *Leptospira*, and *Borrelia*,[44] and within the latter, plasmids have been identified in *B. burgdorferi*, *B. hermsii*, *B. parkeri*, *B. turicatae*, *B. coriaceae*, *B. duttoni*, and *B. crocidurae*.* Whether these "plasmids" are actually autonomous and expendable in *B. burgdorferi* has not been established in most strains.

Genes that encode for two outer surface proteins (Osps) of *B. burgdorferi* have been identified, sequenced, and found to be on linear plasmids,[6] as

---

*References 5, 37, 44, 45, 54, 75.

have two genes that encode for variable major proteins (Vmps) of *B. hermsii*.[65] No other biologic properties of the Lyme spirochete have been shown conclusively to be encoded by plasmids. However, the diversity, abundance, and wide distribution of such extrachromosomal elements in *B. burgdorferi*, and other circumstantial evidence lead us to suspect that plasmids may encode for spirochetal products important for infection in mammalian and arthropod hosts.

Plasmids in *B. burgdorferi* were first reported in 1984, as demonstrated by relatively faster migrating bands of DNA separate from the larger, slower migrating chromosomal DNA in agarose electrophoresis gels stained with ethidium bromide.[44] Subsequent investigations have demonstrated that *B. burgdorferi* may contain numerous plasmids of different size and structure, including molecules that are composed of either linear, double-stranded DNA with covalently closed ends, or circular double-stranded molecules with a supercoiled structure typical of other bacterial plasmids.[5,46,73,78,83] The linear plasmids of *B. burgdorferi*, and probably *B. hermsii* and other members of the genus, are unique among prokaryotes.[6] Before the discovery of the structural properties of these molecules, linear duplex strands of DNA with covalently closed ends were thought to be restricted to eukaryotes and a few viruses. Recently, the telomeres of a linear plasmid from *B. burgdorferi* were cloned and sequenced.[39] As demonstrated by previous studies, the termini of the linear plasmids are covalently-closed hairpin structures.[6] The sequences from both ends of one plasmid were unique with respect to each other except for an 18-bp inverted terminal repeat. The sequence of one of these telomeres was closely related to a telomere from another plasmid and contained a number of short direct repeats and a palindrome adjacent to an AT-rich sequence. This structure shares features with origins of DNA replication and the termini of other linear replicons, including some viruses.[39] The linear nature of these plasmids poses an interesting question regarding how such extrachromosomal elements replicate.

Although linear plasmids probably occur in all wild type, low-passaged isolates of *B. burgdorferi*, plasmids specifically shown to be linear in structure have been identified in relatively few isolates of *B. burgdorferi*. This is because DNA electrophoresed in agarose gels and stained with ethidium bromide cannot be identified as linear, open circular, or supercoiled molecules without further analysis. In one low-passaged tick isolate (Sh-2-82), agarose gel and electron microscope analysis identified at least seven linear plasmids ranging in size from 16 to 49 kilobase (kb).[73] Linear plasmids with reported sizes ranging between 5 and 58 kb have also been

identified in *B. burgdorferi* isolated from *I. ricinus* in Switzerland.[83]

Circular plasmids also appear to be numerous and widely distributed among North American and Eurasian isolates of *B. burgdorferi*.[5,44,45,78,83] Using agarose gel electrophoresis, cesium chloride density gradient centrifugation, and electron microscopic measurements of open circular molecules, six different-sized circular plasmids were also identified in the strain Sh-2-82 of *B. burgdorferi* mentioned above.[78] Electron microscope analysis also demonstrated concatemers with molecules of different sizes interlocked together. Thus, in the one low-passaged strain (Sh-2-82) examined in detail by various methods, seven linear and six circular plasmids have been identified along with concatemers of various circular plasmids possibly representing intermediates or structures resulting from replication errors.

Very little information is available concerning the genetic relatedness of plasmids among *B. burgdorferi* isolates, although profiles of linear and circular plasmids in agarose gels show considerable variability.[5] One fragment of DNA originating from a 49-kb linear plasmid hybridized with all isolates of *B. burgdorferi* examined but not with other species of *Borrelia*.[75] Two studies have demonstrated that *B. burgdorferi* has circular plasmids of different sizes that share regions with a high degree of DNA sequence similarity. In one study, three distinct fragments of DNA were cloned from circular plasmid DNA of *B. burgdorferi* and used as probes.[79] All three probes hybridized with most of the circular plasmids in seven isolates of Lyme spirochetes, and two of the probes hybridized to each other. None of the cloned sequences hybridized with chromosomal DNA, with linear plasmids (with one exception), or with circular plasmids from five other species of *Borrelia*. In the other study, probes were developed from an entire small circular plasmid, two different linear plasmids, and a cloned fragment from a larger circular plasmid.[83] Again, hybridization studies indicated related sequences among plasmids of different sizes. The nature of these regions of sequence homology is unknown. They may represent structural components shared by all plasmids, such as origins of replication or telomeres of the linear plasmids. They might also represent gene families of related variable proteins.[79]

Both linear and circular plasmids present in wild type isolates of *B. burgdorferi* may be lost after serial cultivation in artificial media.[5,45,73,83] This phenomenon is widespread among other prokaryotes that have circular plasmids known to encode factors important for survival in the wild but that offer no selective advantage when grown in vitro.[61]

In *B. burgdorferi,* some plasmids appear to be relatively unstable in vitro and are lost after the spirochetes have been in cultivation for only a short time. In strain Sh-2-82, for example, two small circular plasmids were lost after only 10 to 15 passages (5 to 8 weeks), whereas other larger plasmids were still present after 202 passages (approximately 2 years) of continuous growth in vitro.[73,78] The relative instability of the smaller circular plasmids during artificial growth is unexplained but may be due to their smaller size, a lower copy number, a peculiar distribution within their bacterial cell, or a selective disadvantage for spirochetes containing them when grown in artificial media. Some linear plasmids were also lost from strain Sh-2-82 during serial cultivation after 5 to 15 passages.[73] The B31 strain of *B. burgdorferi* has also lost linear and circular plasmids resulting from years of continual growth and passage in vitro, and in our laboratory this strain remains viable in artificial media although it contains only the 16-kb and 49-kb linear plasmids and one circular plasmid. It is interesting to note that the 49-kb linear plasmid encodes for the two major outer surface proteins of the spirochete (OspA and OspB, see below), which, if lost, might result in a structurally deficient spirochete that would have difficulty surviving.

Several studies have observed a loss of one or more plasmids and the loss of infectiousness of *B. burgdorferi* during serial passage in vitro.[5,45,73] One study demonstrated a temporal correlation between serial passage, the loss of infectivity in mice, and the loss of plasmids from one uncloned strain of the spirochete.[73] This suggested that either a small circular plasmid or a larger linear plasmid of *B.burgdorferi* may encode for factors important for the spirochetes' ability to colonize and infect mammalian hosts. Subsequent studies, however, demonstrated that whereas many infectious strains from various sources contained the smaller circular plasmids, these plasmids were absent from a few strains that were infectious in either mice or hamsters.[78] Therefore, it appears that these smaller supercoiled plasmids are not essential for infectivity. Yet, other evidence suggests that these small plasmids may offer some advantage during infections in mice. Schwan found that, when DNA was examined from *B. burgdorferi* (Sh-2-82) reisolated from 15 mice that had been infected for 16 months, 14 of 15 reisolates still had the small supercoiled plasmids (unpublished data).

Numerous clones of *B. burgdorferi* have been produced by limiting dilution from the strain Sh-2-82 used in the previous studies. Additionally, a specific probe for detecting the small circular plasmids has been developed to help determine the distribution of these plasmids in numerous isolates from a variety of sources.[78] When Schwan examined clones of Sh-2-82 for plasmids and infectivity in mice, most were infectious, but a few of these cloned populations of *B. burgdorferi* that were infectious lacked the small circular plasmids (unpublished data). The only cloned strain that was not infectious also lacked a plasmid that comigrated with a 22-kb linear molecule, supporting an earlier observation that this plasmid might be important for spirochetal infectivity. Additionally, resolates of the spirochete from mice had a much stronger staining band at about 22 kb in agarose gels, suggesting that, during infection, *B. burgdorferi* containing this linear plasmid had a selective advantage over cells lacking it.

PROTEINS

Considerable effort has been devoted to identifying and characterizing the proteins of Lyme spirochetes from various biologic sources and geographic locations. Initial investigations focused on identifying molecular determinants unique to *B. burgdorferi* that could be used to identify all isolates of this spirochete and distinguish them from other species. Another area of very active investigation concerning *B. burgdorferi* proteins has been to identify specific antigens that improve the specificity and sensitivity of serologic tests for confirming Lyme disease and that elicit a protective immune response for the development of an effective vaccine. As a result of these interests, *B. burgdorferi* proteins that have been characterized to any extent are primarily abundant or immunogenic, or both. Aside from two proteins with homologues of known function in other organisms, the biologic activities of any *B. burgdorferi* proteins are unknown.

OspA and OspB

Most attention has been given to the two major outer surface proteins, OspA and OspB, and the structural protein of the periplasmic flagella, flagellin. First to be described was OspA, a protein of approximately 31 kD that was present in spirochetes isolated from *Ixodes* ticks, wild mammals, and humans with Lyme disease.[11] A monoclonal antibody (H5332) was developed to a conserved epitope of this protein,[10] and reactivity of spirochetes with this antibody by immunoblot or indirect immunofluorescence has become a definitive method to identify *B. burgdorferi.* OspA is surfaced exposed, as demonstrated by protease sensitivity and antibody staining on whole spirochetes.[4,9] The second dominant surface protein to be described, OspB with an estimated size of 34 kD in strain B31, is also apparently unique to *B. burgdorferi.*[9] However, considerable heterogeneity exists in both the apparent sizes and monoclonal reactivities of the Osp proteins among isolates, especially those from throughout Eurasia.[8,92,93] Atypical isolates have been described that apparently lack OspA and OspB, yet by other criteria were presumptively identified as *B. burgdorferi*.[2,3,52,92,93] It is not known if the heterogeneity observed in OspA and OspB among isolates of *B. burgdorferi* reflects a genetic mechanism for antigenic variation.

The genes encoding the Osp proteins have been cloned and sequenced—the first data of its kind available from any gene in *B. burgdorferi*.[17] Through their deduced amino acid sequences, it was demonstrated that OspA and OspB are homologous proteins, sharing approximately 53% identity.[17] It was suggested by the primary sequence of their signal peptides, and subsequently proven, that OspA and OspB are lipoproteins, with fatty acids covalently attached to the amino termini of the mature proteins.[17,20] The lipid moieties could possibly anchor the Osp proteins to the outer membrane. Covalent modification with fatty acid is a feature shared with at least 10 other membrane proteins of *B. burgdorferi*.[20] OspA has a relatively high lysine content (16%)[17] yet is resistant to the protease trypsin.[4,9] This suggests that OspA has a fixed structure that is folded in such a way that tryptic cleavage sites are not exposed.[28] In contrast, OspB is also rich in lysine (14%)[17] but is sensitive to digestion by trypsin.[4,9]

OspA and OspB may be involved with the spirochete's ability to colonize and persistently infect mammalian hosts. These abundant surface components of the spirochete would presumably have direct contact with host tissues during infection and have been detected in the blood and urine of humans with Lyme disease and experimentally infected animals.[27,47] Two studies demonstrated that OspB was lost from an uncloned strain of *B. burgdorferi* during in vitro cultivation, at the same time that the spirochete became noninfectious in mice.[72,73] Conversely, the OspB protein was retained in 15 isolates of the same low-passaged strain after 16 months of infection in mice.[76] Additionally, the ability of *B. burgdorferi* to adhere to monolayers of cultured mammalian endothelial cells was significantly reduced when spirochetes were first incubated with an OspB monoclonal antibody.[87] Monoclonal antibody to OspA has been used to protect severe combined immunodeficiency (scid) mice passively from infection with *B. burgdorferi* and from developing arthritis.[70] Recombinant OspA was used successfully to immunize actively and to protect mice challenged with infectious spirochetes by artificial inoculation.[30] Therefore, evidence from numerous studies demonstrates that OspA and OspB are probably important in the spirochete's interaction with mammalian hosts.

Flagellin

Flagella are potentially important pathogenic features of the spirochete because they are the means of its motility. *B. burgdorferi* is highly motile in extremely viscous fluids that approach the viscosity of skin.[49] The ability to move through such matrixes may be critical in the dissemination and persistence of the spirochete during infection. Much attention has been directed to flagellin because it is believed that this 41-kD antigen is highly immunogenic and promotes one of the earliest antibody responses during human infection with *B. burgdorferi*.[24,34] One monoclonal antibody, H9724, was developed to an epitope of flagellin shared by all species of *Borrelia* tested to date and is used to identify this genus from other spirochetes.[12]

The gene for flagellin has been cloned and sequenced.[32,33,90,91] The deduced *B. burgdorferi* flagellin protein sequence shares considerable similarity to the amino- and carboxy-terminal portions of flagellin proteins from other bacteria.[33] These regions are thought to be important to flagellin export and organelle assembly and are conserved among even distantly related bacteria. The flagellin sequences of *B. burgdorferi* and *B. hermsii* exhibit 95% amino acid identity,[33] thus explaining the cross-reactivity of the monoclonal antibody H9724 within the genus.[12] Additional work is ongoing to identify immunoreactive amino acid sequences of flagellin specific to *B. burgdorferi* that may be used as antigens to improve Lyme serodiagnosis.[18,25,33]

P39

Another protein of approximately the same size as flagellin, a 39-kD protein (P39), has been cloned.[80] Whole-cell lysates of *B. burgdorferi* separated by sodium dodecyl sulfate-polyacrylamide gel electrophoresis (SDS-PAGE) show P39 to be a relatively weak band when compared to OspA, OspB, and flagellin, yet this protein is immunogenic in mice and humans infected with Lyme disease spirochetes.[80,81] It is the first protein to which an antibody response is mounted in rodents after infection by tick bite.[81] P39 is highly conserved among *B. burgdorferi* isolates but not present in other members of the genus. Because this protein migrates closely to flagellin in acrylamide gels, and because P39 is antigenic, we believe that what many investigators have assumed incorrectly to be antibodies to the relatively abundant flagellin are actually antibodies to P39. However, P39 and flagellin clearly represent two distinct proteins that differ in size, antibody reactivity, and species distribution.[80] It has not been possible to determine the location of this protein with immunogold labeling and electron microscope analysis of the spirochete. Sequence information on the P39 gene is not yet available.

Other Proteins

Other proteins of various molecular weight have been identified in whole-cell lysates of *B. burgdorferi* separated by SDS-PAGE. The gene encoding an 83-kD protein from *B. burgdorferi* has been cloned and sequenced.[56,63] The gene is reported to be on the chromosome, and, if this protein is identical to a 93-kD antigen described by others,[88] this protein may be associated with the flagella and firmly anchored in the protoplasmic cylinder of the spirochete. The 83-kD protein is immunogenic and conserved among isolates of *B. burgdorferi* from North America and Europe.[56,88] This protein is probably restricted to *B. burgdorferi,* and its purported presence in *B. anserina*[63] requires confirmation by examining additional isolates of this avian spirochete.

Several investigators have described abundant proteins in the range of 20 to 25 kD that are heterogenous in size and expression among different *B. burgdorferi* isolates. These include protein C (pC) (20 to 24 kD) from various isolates from Europe[92,93] and the 21- to 25-kD protein observed in some North American isolates.[2,19,52] The 21- to 25-kD protein has been shown to be surface-exposed and trypsin-resistant, similar to OspA.[52] Although not established, it is likely that pC and the 21- to 25-kD protein are identical. They both exhibit a similar and very interesting phenotype: their expression often accompanies the loss of OspA and OspB.[52,93] This variable pattern of reciprocal expression has been described even with subculture of a single cloned isolate.[52] The pC/21- to 25-kD proteins may share sequence homology with the Osp proteins, but they do not appear to represent degradative fragments of OspA or OspB.[52,93]

A periplasmic protein of *B. burgdorferi* ranging in size from 20 to 23 kD has been designated P22A.[82] The relatedness of P22A to the pC/24-kD protein is not known, but they are probably distinct because they differ in expression, antigenicity, and cellular localization.[52,82] The gene encoding P22A was cloned, and Southern blot analysis suggests that the gene is located on the chromosome. Immunogold labeling of serum raised to this protein demonstrated that P22A was concentrated in the periplasmic space,[82] however, the biologic significance of this protein is not known. All isolates of *B. burgdorferi* from North America and Europe that were examined by Western blot analysis contained P22A, whereas other species of *Borrelia* did not. Mice infected with *B. burgdorferi* produced antibodies to recombinant P22A; sera from Lyme disease patients have not been tested for antibodies to this protein.

Role of proteins

Considerable interest exists in the role of *B. burgdorferi* proteins in establishing early and persistent infection in mammalian hosts, and in relation to the pathogenesis of Lyme disease. Heat shock proteins (HSPs) or proteins whose expression is induced after a sudden shift in temperature (or stress) have received considerable attention for two reasons. First, the spirochete is exposed to a dramatic temperature change during transmission from the tick vector to the mammalian host. Thus, induction of spirochetal components essential for infection could be regulated by temperature. Second, homologues of the HSPs also exist in humans, and a cross-reactive immune response could lead to an autoimmune disorder resembling Lyme disease.[25] *B. burgdorferi* does express some proteins in proportionately greater amounts when the spirochete is exposed to higher temperatures, although reports vary regarding the number of proteins that show this response.[22,23] Some *B. burgdorferi* proteins also vary in their reactivity with immune sera when the spirochetes are cultured at various temperatures.[74] The 60-kD HSP (common antigen) of *B. burgdorferi* is immunogenic and promotes a strong antibody response in chronic Lyme disease patients.[35,77] It shares 50% amino acid identity with the human HSP60.[77] The possibility that antibodies produced to the 60-kD HSP of *B. burgdorferi* are cross-reactive with the human HSP60, and that this may lead to an autoimmune inflammatory arthritis in chronic Lyme disease patients, is currently an area of active investigation.[77]

GENE STRUCTURE

The genes encoding the *B. burgdorferi* major outer surface proteins (OspA and OspB),[17,42] flagellin,[32,33,91] 16S rRNA,[1,58,64] HSP60,[35,77] and the 83-kD immunodominant protein[56,63] have been cloned and sequenced. The genes for several other *B. burgdorferi* proteins have been cloned,[80,82] but their nucleotide sequences have not been published. Therefore, this summary of gene structure in *B. burgdorferi* encompasses only a few examples.

The *ospA* and *ospB* genes are located on a large linear plasmid that varies somewhat in size among isolates.[5,6] Genetic analysis of the *osp* locus has shown that it is an operon, the only one described for *B. burgdorferi,* with the two proteins produced from a single transcriptional unit.[41] A similar operon structure exists in strains that have fairly different Osp phenotypes.[67] Sequence analysis of the *osp* genes has identified two open reading frames separated by only 12 nucleotides.[17] The deduced amino acid sequences for OspA and OspB exhibit 53% identity, demonstrating that these genes are homologues and probably the result of a gene duplication.[17]

Flagellin,[32,33,91] 16S rRNA,[1] HSP60,[35] and the 83-kD protein[56] are encoded by chromosomal genes. No information is available regarding the positions of these genes on the *Borrelia* chromosome or the stability of chromosomal gene organization among strains. All *B. burgdorferi* protein-encoding genes contain sequences homologous to consensus ribosome binding sites (Shine-Delgarno sequence), preceding open reading frames that initiate with ATG and terminate with TAA. The putative upstream promoter regions of the *osp* operon,[17] flagellin *(fla)*,[32,33,91] and 83-kD protein[63] genes exhibit homology with consensus sequences of control regions of *Escherichia coli* genes. Primer extension studies of *fla* mRNA have defined the transcriptional start site of the *fla* gene, adjacent to the presumptive RNA polymerase recognition sequences in the -10 and -35 regions.[33] Transcript mapping studies have not been published for any other *B. burgdorferi* genes. These *B. burgdorferi* genes also contain inverted repeats capable of forming stem-loop structures following the open reading frames, homologous to *E. coli* transcriptional terminator sequences. Such sequence comparisons, along with what appears to be utilization of *B. burgdorferi* promoters for expression of recombinant *fla*[33,91] and *osp*[42] genes in *E. coli,* suggest that *B. burgdorferi* uses similar transcriptional and translational control signals as other bacteria.

The codon usage of both the *osp*[17] and *fla*[91] genes is different from that of highly expressed *E. coli* genes. This is consistent with the bias imposed by the distinct G + C contents of *Borrelia* and *E. coli* genomes (30% and 55%, respectively). Both *osp* and *fla* genes exhibit a nonrandom bias in the G + C content of the codons, with the lowest % G + C in the third (wobble) position. Despite the fact that *osp* and *fla* genes use some codons that are rare in *E. coli,* this has not presented a barrier to fairly high levels of recombinant expression of these *B. burgdorferi* genes in *E. coli.*[28,33,91]

MOLECULAR TYPING

Phenotypic and genotypic criteria have been used to type *B. burgdorferi* isolates. The impetus for these studies has been to assess whether a correlation exists between strain type and clinical manifestation. As discussed elsewhere in this book, the manifestations of Lyme disease are diverse and vary among infected individuals. At least in perception, the clinical picture of Lyme disease is not the same in Europe and the United States. Lyme disease appears to progress to neurologic and dermatologic manifestations more frequently in Europe, whereas arthritis is the more common late manifestation in the United States.[84]

Serotyping strategies have been proposed using monoclonal antibodies specific for OspA, OspB, and pC proteins.[8,9,93] Similarly, the size differences of Osp and pC proteins among strains have been used for typing.[1,8,9,93] Although groups can be defined, it is difficult to derive a consensus scheme into which any given strain can be placed. Most difficult to type are those strains for which expression of Osp or pC proteins is absent or unstable.

These analyses have been extended to the genotypic level, using a variety of markers and techniques to classify strains. Quantitative DNA:DNA hybridization studies were used in the original description of the Lyme disease spirochete as a new *Borrelia* species,[44,71] with approximately 50% identity to the relapsing fever spirochete *B. hermsii.* More recently, recognition of the diversity of some European *B. burgdorferi* isolates prompted a similar analysis to assess the relatedness of these isolates to the prototype strain B31.[66] Such measurements of the fraction of total DNA that hybridizes between different isolates may be complicated by the presence of multiple, diverse plasmid species in *B. burgdorferi.*

The *B. burgdorferi* rRNA genes have been used as the targets for specific restriction fragment length polymorphisms (RFLP) studies and sequence comparisons.[1,66] Polymerase chain reaction amplifications with primers from the 16S rRNA gene,[1] the *osp* locus,[1,67] and an undefined chromosomal locus[68] also identify separate classes of *B. burgdorferi.* Plasmid content and total genome RFLP analyses have been used with the least success to type strains[55,83]; in general, these methods are too variable and detailed to be interpreted easily.

The general picture emerging from these varied approaches is surprisingly uniform: there appear to be two or three distinguishable groups of *B. burgdorferi* isolates. Most North American and some European isolates comprise one group, of which the original *B. burgdorferi* isolate, strain B31, is the prototype. Strain Sh-2-82 also belongs to this group. The second group is composed of the remainder of the Eurasian isolates; some typing methods further distinguish between the European and Asian members of this group. Because most of these independent studies were done with different sets of strains, it is not possible to assess how good the agreement is among the various methods for strain assignment. However, where this comparison is possible, the results are mostly consistent. The phylogenetic relationship among the groups, or whether they should be considered as separate *B. burgdorferi* subspecies or distinct genomic species, is a debated issue. Most importantly, whether strain type correlates with disease manifestation has not been determined.

CONCLUSION

B. burgdorferi has received significant research attention since its discovery 10 years ago as the agent of Lyme disease. In this review, we have attempted to present the results of research pertinent to the molecular biology of *B. burgdorferi*. Much of the information at this stage represents a description of molecular components (chromosome, plasmids, proteins, and so forth) rather than insight into the regulation or function of these molecules. This, in part, reflects the necessary progression through which the characterization of an organism occurs, and much remains to be described. The nature of current research on *B. burgdorferi* is also a reflection of the existing limitations to the manipulation of this organism in the laboratory, and features of the infection in humans and animals. *B. burgdorferi* grows slowly in vitro and rarely reaches levels in vivo where it can be directly detected. Plating efficiencies for *B. burgdorferi* on undefined solid media are variable, the procedure is complicated, and colonies are visible only after 1 to 2 weeks.[53] Thus, although colony formation is useful, it cannot be easily used to quickly quantitate and clone bacteria. Most importantly, a means of transforming, or introducing DNA into, *B. burgdorferi* is not available, so genetic studies are severely hampered. Whether these technical impediments to plating and transforming *B. burgdorferi* are overcome will significantly influence the nature and swiftness with which investigations of the molecular biology of this organism proceed in the future.

ACKNOWLEDGMENTS

We thank Susan Smaus, Betty Kester, and Carole Smaus for secretarial assistance, and Dr. Patricia Coyle for her patience and efforts as editor. We are grateful to Drs. John Swanson and Paul Policastro for their comments on the manuscript.

REFERENCES

1. Adam T et al: Phenotypic and genotypic analysis of *Borrelia burgdorferi* isolates from various sources, *Infect Immun* 59:2579, 1991.
2. Anderson JF, Magnarelli LA, McAninch JB: New *Borrelia burgdorferi* antigenic variant isolated from *Ixodes dammini* from upstate New York, *J Clin Microbiol* 26:2209, 1988.
3. Anderson JF et al: Antigenically variable *Borrelia burgdorferi* isolated from cottontail rabbits and *Ixodes dentatus* in rural and urban areas, *J Clin Microbiol* 27:13, 1989.
4. Barbour AG: Isolation and cultivation of Lyme disease spirochetes, *Yale J Biol Med* 57:521, 1984.
5. Barbour AG: Plasmid analysis of *Borrelia burgdorferi*, the Lyme disease agent, *J Clin Microbiol* 26:475, 1988.
6. Barbour AG, Garon CF: Linear plasmids of the bacterium *Borrelia burgdorferi* have covalently closed ends, *Science* 237:409, 1987.
7. Barbour AG, Hayes SF: Biology of *Borrelia* species, *Microbiol Rev* 50:381, 1986.
8. Barbour AG, Heiland RA, Howe TR: Heterogeneity of major proteins in Lyme disease borreliae: a molecular analysis of North American and European isolates, *J Infect Dis* 152:478, 1985.
9. Barbour AG, Tessier SL, Hayes SF: Variation in a major surface protein of Lyme disease spirochetes, *Infect Immun* 45:94, 1984.
10. Barbour AG, Tessier SL, Todd WJ: Lyme disease spirochetes and ixodid tick spirochetes share a common surface antigenic determinant defined by a monoclonal antibody, *Infect Immun* 41:795, 1983.
11. Barbour AG et al: Antibodies of patients with Lyme disease to components of the *Ixodes dammini* spirochete, *J Clin Invest* 72:504, 1983.
12. Barbour AG, et al: A *Borrelia*-specific monoclonal antibody binds to a flagellar epitope, *Infect Immun* 52:549, 1986.
13. Baril C, Saint-Girons I: *FEMS Microbiol Lett* 71:95, 1990.
14. Baril C et al: Linear chromosome of *Borrelia burgdorferi*, *Res Microbiol* 140:507, 1989.
15. Beck G et al: Chemical and biologic characterization of a lipopolysaccharide extracted from the Lyme disease spirochete *(Borrelia burgdorferi)*, *J Infect Dis* 152:108, 1985.
16. Bercovier H, Kafri O, Sela S: *Mycobacteria* possess a surprisingly small number of ribosomal RNA genes in relation to the size of their genome, *Biochem Biophys Res Commun* 136:1136, 1986.
17. Bergstrom S, Bundoc VG, Barbour AG: Molecular analysis of linear plasmid-encoded major surface proteins, OspA and OspB, of the Lyme disease spirochete *Borrelia burgdorferi*, *Mol Microbiol* 3:479, 1989.
18. Berland R et al: Molecular characterization of the humoral response to the 41-kilodalton flagellar antigen of *Borrelia burgdorferi*, the Lyme disease agent, *Infect Immun* 59:3531, 1991.
19. Bissett ML, Hill W: Characterization of *Borrelia burgdorferi* strains isolated from *Ixodes pacificus* ticks in California, *J Clin Microbiol* 25:2296, 1987.
20. Brandt ME et al: Immunogenic integral membrane proteins of *Borrelia burgdorferi* are lipoproteins, *Infect Immun* 58:983, 1990.
21. Burgdorfer W et al: Lyme disease—a tick-borne spirochetosis? *Science* 216:1317, 1982.
22. Carreiro MM, Laux DC, Nelson DR: Characterization of the heat shock response and identification of heat shock protein antigens of *Borrelia burgdorferi*, *Infect Immun* 58:2186, 1990.
23. Cluss RG, Boothby JT: Thermoregulation of protein synthesis in *Borrelia burgdorferi*, *Infect Immun* 58:1038, 1990.
24. Coleman JL, Benach JL: Identification and characterization of an endoflagellar antigen of *Borrelia burgdorferi*, *J Clin Invest* 84:322, 1989.
25. Collins C, Peltz G: Immunoreactive epitopes on an expressed recombinant flagellar protein of *Borrelia burgdorferi*, *Infect Immun* 59:514, 1991.
26. Dorward DW, Garon CF: DNA is packaged within membrane-derived vesicles of gram-negative but not gram-positive bacteria, *Appl Environ Microbiol* 56:1960, 1990.
27. Dorward DW, Schwan TG, Garon CF: Immune capture and detection of *Borrelia burgdorferi* antigens in urine, blood, or tissues from infected ticks, mice, dogs, and humans, *J Clin Microbiol* 29:1162, 1991.

28. Dunn JJ, Lade BN, Barbour AG: Outer surface protein A (OspA) from the Lyme disease spirochete, *Borrelia burgdorferi:* high level expression and purification of a soluble recombinant form of OspA, *Protein Express Purifica* 1:159, 1990.

29. Ferdows MS, Barbour AG: Megabase-sized linear DNA in the bacterium *Borrelia burgdorferia,* the Lyme disease agent, *Proc Natl Acad Sci USA* 86:5969, 1989.

30. Fikrig E et al: Protection of mice against the Lyme disease agent by immunizing with recombinant OspA, *Science* 250:553, 1990.

31. Garon CF, Dorward DW, Corwin MD: Structural features of *Borrelia burgdorferi*—the Lyme disease spirochete: silver staining for nucleic acids, *Scan Microsc* [Suppl] 3:109, 1989.

32. Gassmann GS et al: Nucleotide sequence of a gene encoding the *Borrelia burgdorferi* flagellin, *Nucleic Acids Res* 173:1452, 1989.

33. Gassmann GS et al: Analysis of the *Borrelia burgdorferi* GeHo *fla* gene and antigenic characterization of its gene product, *J Bacteriol* 173:1452, 1991.

34. Hansen K, Asbrink E: Serodiagnosis of erythema migrans and acrodermatitis chronica atrophicans by the *Borrelia burgdorferi* flagellum enzyme-linked immunosorbent assay, *J Clin Microbiol* 27:545, 1989.

35. Hansen K et al: Immunochemical characterization of and isolation of the gene for a *Borrelia burgdorferi* immunodominant 60-kilodalton antigen common to a wide range of bacteria, *Infect Immun* 56:2047, 1988.

36. Hardy K: *Bacterial plasmids,* American Society for Microbiology.

37. Hayes LJ, Wright DJM, Archard LC: Segmented arrangement of *Borrelia duttonii* DNA and location of variant surface antigen genes, *J Gen Microbiol* 134:1785, 1988.

38. Hayes SF, Burgdorfer W, Barbour AG: Bacteriophage in the *Ixodes dammini* spirochete, etiological agent of lyme disease, *J Bacteriol* 154:1436, 1983.

39. Hinnebusch J, Bergstrom S, Barbour AG: Cloning and sequence analysis of linear plasmid telomeres of the bacterium *Borrelia burgdorferi, Mol Microbiol* 4:811, 1990.

40. Hovind-Hougen K: Ultrastructure of spirochetes isolated from *Ixodes ricinus* and *Ixodes dammini, Yale J Biol Med* 93, 1984.

41. Howe TR, LaQuier FW, Barbour AG: Organization of genes encoding two outer membrane proteins of the Lyme disease agent *Borrelia burgdorferi* within a single transcriptional unit, *Infect Immun* 54:207, 1986.

42. Howe TR, Mayer LW, Barbour AG: A single recombinant plasmid expressing two major outer surface proteins of the Lyme disease spirochete, *Science* 227:645, 1985.

43. Hughes CAN, Johnson RC: Methylated DNA in *Borrelia* species, *J Bacteriol* 172:6602, 1990.

44. Hyde FW, Johnson RC: Genetic relationship of Lyme disease spirochetes to *Borrelia, Treponema,* and *Leptospira* spp, *J Clin Microbiol* 20:151, 1984.

45. Hyde FW, Johnson RC: Genetic analysis of *Borrelia, Zentralbl Bakteriol Mikrobiol [A]*263:119, 1986.

46. Hyde FW, Johnson RC: Characterization of a circular plasmid from *Borrelia burgdorferi,* etiologic agent of Lyme disease, *J Clin Microbiol* 26:2203, 1988.

47. Hyde FW et al: Detection of antigens in urine of mice and humans infected with *Borrelia burgdorferi,* etiologic agent of Lyme disease, *J Clin Microbiol* 27:58, 1989.

48. Johnson RC: The spirochetes, *Annu Rev Microbiol* 31:89, 1977.

49. Kimsey RB, Spielman A: Motility of Lyme disease spirochetes in fluids as viscous as the extracellular matrix, *J Infect Dis* 162:1205, 1990.

50. Klaviter EC, Johnson RC: Isolation of the outer envelope, chemical components, and ultrastructure of *Borrelia hermsii* grown in vitro, *Acta Trop* 36:123, 1979.

51. Krawiec S, Riley M: Organization of the bacterial chromosome, *Microbiol Rev* 54:502, 1990.

52. Kurashige S, Bissett M, Oshiro L: Characterization of a tick isolate of *Borrelia burgdorferi* that possesses a major low-molecular-weight surface protein, *J Clin Microbiol* 28:1362, 1990.

53. Kurtti TJ et al: Colony formation and morphology in *Borrelia burgdorferi, J Clin Microbiol* 25:2054, 1987.

54. LeFebvre RB, Perng GC: Genetic and antigenic characterization of *Borrelia coriaceae,* putative agent of epizootic bovine abortion, *J Clin Microbiol* 27:389, 1989.

55. LeFebvre RB, Perng GC, Johnson RC: Characterization of *Borrelia burgdorferi* isolates by restriction endonuclease analysis and DNA hybridization, *J Clin Microbiol* 27:636, 1989.

56. LeFebvre RB, Perng G-C, Johnson RC: The 83-kilodalton antigen of *Borrelia burgdorferi* which stimulates immunoglobulin M (IgM) and IgG responses in infected hosts is expressed by a chromosomal gene, *J Clin Microbiol* 28:1673, 1990.

57. Livermore BP, Bey RF, Johnson RC: Lipid metabolism of *Borrelia hermsii, Infect Immun* 20:215, 1978.

58. Marconi RT, Garon CF: Phylogenetic analysis of the genus *Borrelia:* a comparison of North American and European isolates of *Borrelia burgdorferi, J Bacteriol* in press, 1991.

59. Meier JT, Simon MI, Barbour AG: Antigenic variation is associated with DNA rearrangements in a relapsing fever *Borrelia, Cell* 41:403, 1985.

60. Muto A, Osawa S: The guanine and cytosine content of genomic DNA and bacterial evolution, *Proc Natl Acad Sci USA* 84:166, 1987.

61. Neidhardt FC, Ingraham JL, Schaechter M: *Physiology of the bacterial cell. A molecular approach,* Sunderland, MA, Sinauer Associates.

62. Norgard MV, Miller JN: Plasmid DNA in *Treponema pallidum* (Nichols): potential for antibiotic resistance by syphilis bacteria, *Science* 213:553, 1981.

63. Perng G-C, LeFebvre RB, Johnson RC: Further characterization of a potent immunogen and the chromosomal gene encoding it in the Lyme disease agent, *Borrelia burgdorferi, Infect Immun* 59:2070, 1991.

64. Persing DH et al: Detection of *Borrelia burgdorferi* DNA in museum specimens of *Ixodes dammini* ticks, *Science* 249:1420, 1990.

65. Plasterk RHA, Simon MI, Barbour AG: Transposition of structural genes to an expression sequence on a linear plasmid causes antigenic variation in the bacterium *Borrelia hermsi, Nature* 318:257, 1985.

66. Postic D et al: Two genomic species in *Borrelia burgdorferi, Res Microbiol* 141:465, 1990.

67. Rosa PA, Hogan D, Margolis N: Molecular analysis of the major outer surface protein locus from a divergent *Borrelia burgdorferi* isolate from Europe. In *Banbury Conference— The molecular immunobiology of Lyme disease.* Cold Spring Harbor, NY, 1991 (in press).

68. Rosa P, Hogan D, Schwan T: Polymerase chain reaction analyses identify two distinct classes of *Borrelia burgdorferi, J Clin Microbiol* 29:524, 1991.

69. Rosa PA, Schwan TG: A specific and sensitive assay for the Lyme disease spirochete *Borrelia burgdorferi* using the polymerase chain reaction, *J Infect Dis* 160:1018, 1989.

70. Schaible UE et al: Monoclonal antibodies specific for the outer surface protein A (OspA) of *Borrelia burgdorferi* prevent Lyme borreliosis in severe combined immunodeficiency (scid) mice, *Proc Natl Acad Sci USA* 87:3768, 1990.

71. Schmid GP et al: DNA characterization of the spirochete that causes Lyme disease, *J Clin Microbiol* 20:155, 1984.

72. Schwan TG, Burgdorfer W: Antigenic changes of *Borrelia burgdorferi* as a result of in vitro cultivation, *J Infect Dis* 156:852, 1987.

73. Schwan TG, Burgdorfer W, Garon CF: Changes in infectivity and plasmid profile of the Lyme disease spirochete, *Borrelia burgdorferi*, as a result of in vitro cultivation, *Infect Immun* 56:1831, 1988.

74. Schwan TG, Simpson WJ: Factors influencing the antigenic reactivity of *Borrelia burgdorferi*, the Lyme disease spirochete, *Scand J Infect Dis* [Suppl] 77:94, 1991.

75. Schwan TG et al: Identification of *Borrelia burgdorferi* and *B. hermsii* using DNA hybridization probes, *J Clin Microbiol* 27:1734, 1989.

76. Schwan TG et al: Changes in antigenic reactivity of *Borrelia burgdorferi*, the Lyme disease spirochete, during persistent infection in mice, *Can J Microbiol* 37:450, 1991.

77. Shanafelt M-C et al: T cell and antibody reactivity with the *Borrelia burgdorferi* 60-kDa heat shock protein in lyme arthritis, *J Immunol* 146:3985, 1991.

78. Simpson WJ, Garon CF, Schwan TG: Analysis of supercoiled circular plasmids in infectious and non-infectious *Borrelia burgdorferi*, *Microb Pathog* 8:109, 1990.

79. Simpson WJ, Garon CF, Schwan TG: *Borrelia burgdorferi* contains repeated DNA sequences that are species specific and plasmid associated, *Infect Immun* 58:847, 1990.

80. Simpson WJ, Schrumpf ME, Schwan TG: Reactivity of human Lyme borreliosis sera with a 39-kilodalton antigen specific to *Borrelia burgdorferi*, *J Clin Microbiol* 28:1329, 1990.

81. Simpson WJ et al: Antibody to a 39-kilodalton *Borrelia burgdorferi* antigen (P39) as a marker for infection in experimentally and naturally inoculated animals, *J Clin Microbiol* 29:236, 1991.

82. Simpson WJ et al: Molecular and immunological analysis of a polymorphic periplasmic protein of *Borrelia burgdorferi*, *J Clin Microbiol* 29:1940, 1991.

83. Stalhammar-Carlemalm M et al: Plasmid analysis and restriction fragment length polymorphisms of chromosomal DNA allow a distinction between *Borrelia burgdorferi* strains, *Zentrabl Bakteriol* 274:28, 1990.

84. Steere AC: Lyme disease, *N Engl J Med* 321:586, 1989.

85. Takayama K, Rothenberg RJ, Barbour AG: Absence of lipopolysaccharide in the Lyme disease spirochete, *Borrelia burgdorferi*, *Infect Immun* 55:2311, 1987.

86. Taylor KA, Barbour AG, Thomas DD: Pulsed-field gel electrophoretic analysis of leptospiral DNA, *Infect Immun* 59:323, 1991.

87. Thomas DD, Comstock LE: Interaction of Lyme disease spirochetes with cultured eucaryotic cells. *Infect Immun* 57:1324, 1989.

88. Volkman DJ et al: Characterization of an immunoreactive 93-kDa core protein of *Borrelia burgdorferi* with a human IgG monoclonal antibody, *J Immunol* 146:3177, 1991.

89. Walker EM et al: *Treponema pallidum* subsp. *pallidum* has a single, circular chromosome with a size of ≈900 kilobase pairs, *Infect Immun* 59:2476, 1991.

90. Wallich R et al: Cloning and sequencing of the gene encoding the outer surface protein A (OspA) of a European *Borrelia burgdorferi* isolate, *Nucleic Acids Res* 17:8864, 1989.

91. Wallich R et al: The *Borrelia burgdorferi* flagellum-associated 41-kilodalton antigen (flagellin): molecular cloning, expression, and amplification of the gene, *Infect Immun* 58:1711, 1990.

92. Wilske B et al: Immunochemical and immunological analysis of European *Borrelia burgdorferi* strains, Zentralbl Bakteriol Mikrobiol Hyg [A] 263:92, 1986.

93. Wilske B et al: Antigenic variability of *Borrelia burgdorferi*. In Benach JL, Bosler EM, editors: *Lyme Disease and Related Disorders*, p 126, New York, 1988, New York Academy of Sciences.

3 Tick Vectors and Hosts

Edward M. Bosler

TICK CLASSIFICATION

Taxonomically, ticks are classified in the invertebrate phylum Arthropoda, a large assemblage of bilaterally symmetric animals that possess pairs of jointed appendages and a hard chitinous exoskeleton. Ticks are not insects, but related to spiders, scorpions, and mites and placed in the class Arachnida. They are further grouped with mites into the subclass Acari and separately form the suborder (Ixodida).[44] Ticks differ from insects (Arthropoda, class Hexapoda) in that they lack wings, mandibles, and antennae and have four pairs of legs, instead of three, except in the larval stage.

The generalized tick life cycle involves three successive postembryonic stages or instars: the larva, nymph, and adult. Larvae are six-legged, whereas nymphs and adults possess eight legs. Sexual dimorphism occurs in adults, whereas the genetically predetermined sex of subadults cannot be differentiated morphologically. During each postembryonic instar, ticks feed once as obligate blood and tissue fluid feeding ectoparasites of terrestrial vertebrates. Ticks, however, spend the majority of their life in a free living state either acquiring a host, molting to the next stage after feeding, or in diapause (quiescent resting state) throughout an adverse season, generally winter. Type of life cycle, host availability, and seasonal activity of the tick determine the tenure of each phase. Tick life cycles are divided into several types based on the number of developmental stages and the number of hosts required for completion of the life cycle.

There are two families of ticks, the Ixodidae (hard-bodied ticks) and the Argasidae (soft-bodied ticks), which differ morphologically and behaviorally.

Of the 13 worldwide genera of Ixodidae, 8 occur in the United States: *Haemaphysalis, Boophilus, Rhipicephalus, Dermacentor, Anocentor, Aponomma, Ixodes,* and *Amblyomma.* Ixodidae are grouped into three categories based on the number of hosts required to complete their life cycle. The vast majority of Ixodidae are three-host ticks. Each of the three stages feeds once, each on a different host, and each successive molt occurs off the host on the ground. One-host ticks, such as *Boophilus* and certain *Dermacentor,* engorge and molt in situ on the same animal, whereas in two-host ticks, such as certain *Rhipicephalus,* both subadult stages feed on the same host and the adult feeds on a second host. Hard ticks feed for long periods lasting for many days, and each successively larger instar ordinarily prefers a progressively larger host. Females generally mate on the host while feeding and, when replete, drop to the ground, lay a singular egg mass typically containing several thousand ova, and then die.

Argasid ticks are contained in four genera: *Argas, Otobius, Antricola,* and *Ornithodoros.* Argasids are multihost ticks that are closely associated with the nests, caves, or burrows of birds, bats, and mammals they parasitize. Larvae feed for several days whereas the nymphs and adults are rapid intermittent feeders that quickly leave their host to ensure they are not carried away from the habitat by their host. Unlike hard ticks, argasid nymphs have a variable number of instars, and adult females feed and oviposit smaller egg masses more than once during their lifetime. Because soft ticks have not been implicated in transmission of *Borrelia burgdorferi* they will not be considered in more detail.

BIOLOGY OF VECTOR TICKS
Geographic distribution

Ixodes ricinus ticks are the principal vectors of *B. burgdorferi* worldwide. In the United States, the majority of human cases of Lyme disease are concentrated in three regions: the northeast, the midwest, and along the Pacific coast. Disease transmission is most intense in the northeast and upper plains; approximately 90% of human cases have been reported from seven states contained in these two regions.[31] *I. dammini,* the northern deer or bear tick, and *I. pacificus,* the western black-legged tick, are known vectors in these major foci.[25,27]

I. dammini was described as a new species based on larval, nymphal, and adult specimens collected in Massachusetts by Spielman, Clifford, Piesman, and Corwin in 1979.[78] This tick's range in the

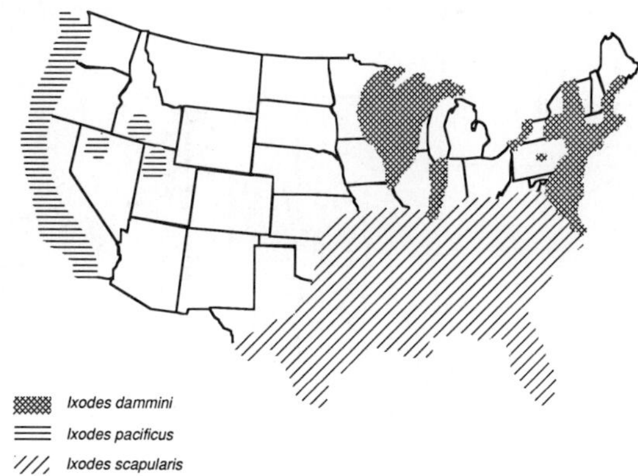

Figure 3–1 Geographic distribution of *Ixodes ricinus* complex vectors in the United States.

northeast and mid-Atlantic states extends from Maryland and Virginia northward along the coast and offshore islands to Massachusetts. It has also been recorded from the New England states of New Hampshire, Vermont, and Maine and has recently expanded its range into upstate New York (Fig. 3–1). *I. dammini* is also found in Nova Scotia and Long Point, Ontario, Canada.* In the upper midwest, *I. dammini* is found in Wisconsin, Minnesota, Iowa, Illinois, the upper peninsula of Michigan, and western Indiana.[20,35,41,63]

I. pacificus has a geographic range west of the Cascade and Sierra Nevada mountain ranges extending from British Columbia south to Baja, California, and Mexico.[39] This species also occurs in Nevada, west of the Wasatch range in Utah, and in Idaho.[15,22]

Although the number of human cases of Lyme disease continues to increase outside the range of either *I. dammini* and *I. pacificus* in the southeastern United States,[31] the vector(s) ticks remain to be identified. *I. scapularis,* also a member of the *I. ricinus* complex, is a putative vector within this area. This species has been shown to be a competent vector experimentally[22,59] and *B. burgdorferi* has been identified in field-derived ticks.[52] Geographically, *I. scapularis* is widely distributed and abundant in the south-central and southeastern portions of the country. The species ranges from Florida westward through the Gulf Coast states and Texas and northward through Oklahoma, Kansas, Missouri, and Iowa. This species has additionally been reported in Ohio, southern Indiana, Tennessee, and Arkansas[22] (Fig. 3–1).

I. ricinus, the castor bean tick or sheep tick, is the most common vector of *B. burgdorferi* in Europe. This species is common in pastures and woodlands in the British Isles, southern Scandinavia to Spain, Portugal, Algeria, Morocco, the majority of southern and central Europe, and the eastern portion of Russia to the Caspian Sea.[21]

The taiga tick, *I. persulcatus,* is responsible for *B. burgdorferi* transmission in a broad geographic band from eastern Europe across Asia to Japan and overlaps the range of *I. ricinus* from its western border in Germany through portions of Russia.[1,43]

Life history and seasonal activity of *I. dammini*

The life cycle of *I. dammini* is a complex process (Fig. 3–2), and it must be taken into consideration when trying to determine seasonal periods when risk of transmission of *B. burgdorferi* is greatest. It is important to understand that the acquisition of the pathogen occurs during the developmental stage preceding the stage in which the tick transmits the organism to a host. Immature ticks demonstrate an inverted pattern of seasonal abundance in which nymphs are abundant in the spring and precede peak larval densities. This pattern permits infectious nymphs from a previous season to infect reservoir animals before larval feeding, thereby perpetuating the cycle of *B. burgdorferi* transmission.

Eggs are generally deposited in June and early July. Larvae do not hatch from the eggs until late July or early August and remain on or around the egg mass for approximately 2 weeks. Unfed larvae disperse, clustering within a range of about 2 m from the hatch site.[79] Larvae employ a strategy of ambush (questing) and await an unsuspecting host to traverse their domain.[79]

Larvae that feed before September usually molt to nymphs before winter and do not feed again until the following spring. Those that fed later in September overwinter engorged and do not molt to a nymph until the following spring. Larvae that are unsuccessful in obtaining a blood meal overwinter and resume questing in the spring. Larvae that feed successfully usually molt within 25 to 30 days after dropping from the host.[45] Larvae that do not feed the following spring die in July, 11 months after hatching.[88]

The nymphal population that quests each spring is composed of two groups: nymphs that molted the previous summer and nymphs that molted during the current season.[88] A nymph that has survived the winter unfed and does not obtain a blood meal during the following spring will die in July, 15 months after molting.[88] Nymphs that successfully feed usually molt to adults in the same season and commence questing in September. However, it has been documented that nymphs possess the capacity to endure the winter engorged and molt in late August of the following season, yet such is believed

---

*References 5, 32, 40, 48, 65, 75, 78, 84.

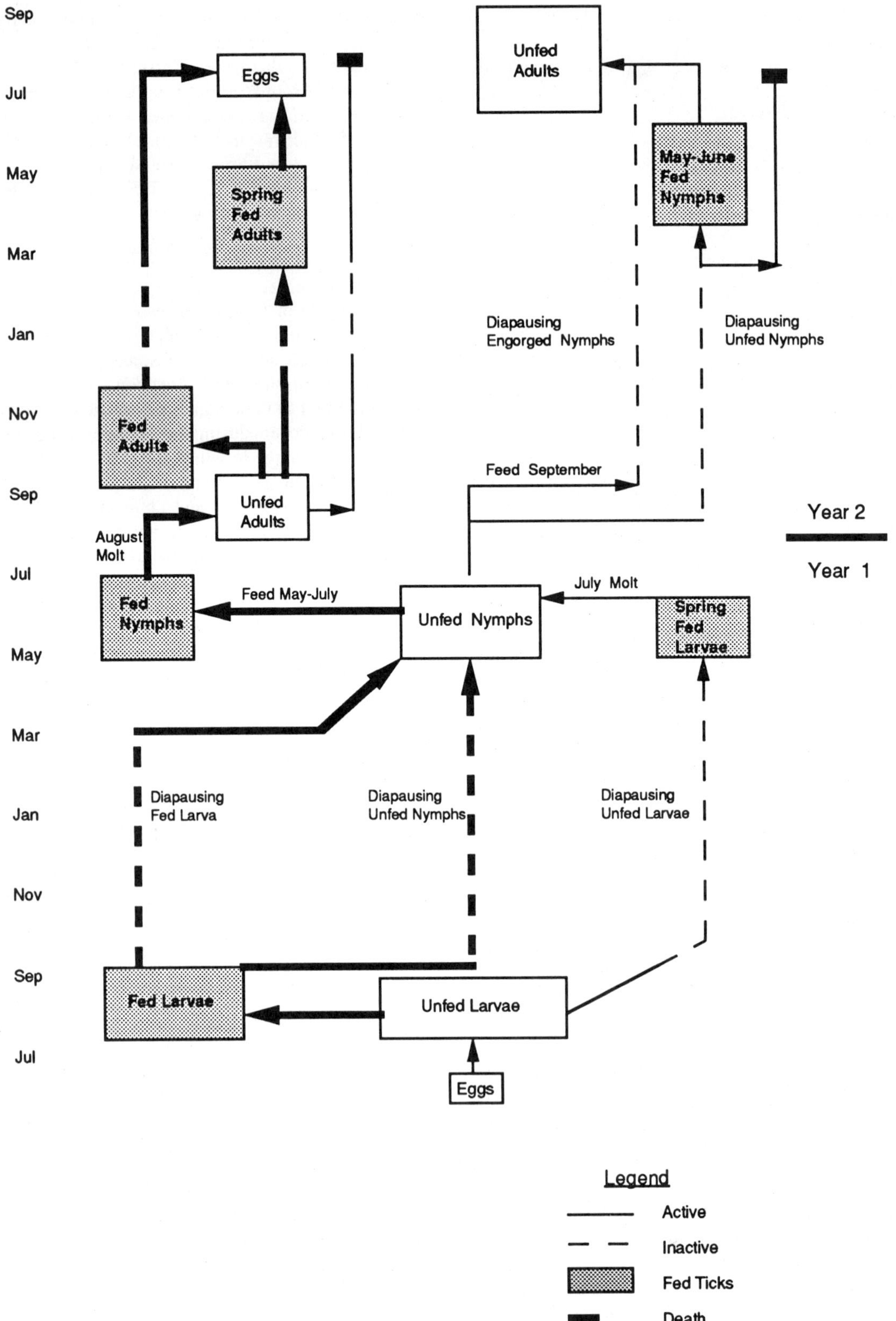

Figure 3–2 Life cycle of *Ixodes dammini*. (Adapted from several sources by Joseph Gebbia.)

to be infrequent and the majority of engorged overwintering nymphs do die.

Adults emerge in late July through early September and, after a prequesting period, begin to seek large vertebrate hosts from October through warm days in December. Adults that do not feed during this period resume questing the following spring. This life stage is the shortest of all active stages if deprived of a blood meal and ticks unfed by May will die during the summer. Females that have successfully fed in either the fall or spring oviposit in June and July. Larvae hatch in late July to August completing the 2-year life cycle.[88] Females attach to large vertebrates to feed and to mate. Females feed to repletion in 8 to 11 days, drop to the ground, and wait for the onset of spring to oviposit, after which they die. Males rarely imbibe blood and primarily seek hosts to mate with engorging females.[21,45,60]

Pathobiology of *B. burgdorferi* in vector ticks

The tickborne *Borrelia, B. duttonii,* the relapsing fever pathogen, and *B. theileri,* the etiologic agent of bovine borreliosis, penetrate and leave the tick midgut to multiply in the hemolymph causing systemic infections within 14 days of feeding. *B. burgdorferi* demonstrates a unique behavior in *Ixodes* ticks in that it persists in the midgut where it accumulates at the microvillar brush border and in the interstitial spaces of the epithelium.[21] Additionally, the pathogen survives in the digestive tract between feedings, and it may be that such residence is necessary for long-term survival in the tick.[70] *B. burgdorferi* was initially discovered and most frequently is detected in the lumen of the digestive tract of *I. dammini, I. pacificus,* and *I. ricinus.*[18,27] In fact, midgut infection in the absence of concurrent systemic infection has been observed in most unfed female *I. dammini* examined.[16,25,70] Systemic infection has been detected in slightly less than 5% of unfed *I. dammini* and *I. ricinus,* suggesting the *Borrelia* is capable of penetrating the midgut.

A higher percentage of systemically infected ticks have been observed after feeding in both natural and experimentally infected *I. dammini.*[23] In these studies, the percentage of ticks demonstrating generalized infections increased over time after engorgement to as high as 78%. Systemic infection involved all tissues, especially the central ganglion, malpighian tubules, salivary glands, and ovaries. Penetration of *B. burgdorferi* through the gut wall appears to be closely linked to tick feeding and histologic changes that occur in the gut epithelium during feeding.[13,16,70]

Histologic evidence demonstrates spirochetal cell division in close association or attached to the epithelial cells of the midgut diverticulae shortly after ingestion of blood. Three to 5 days after attachment, during the midfeeding period, spirochetes were found in clusters deeply between or adhering to the protruding fully pedunculate epithelial cells suggesting a specific organism-cell interaction.[16] At this time, some *B. burgdorferi* are able to penetrate the gut wall to enter the hemolymph and central ganglion while a larger population remains persistent in the gut. Additionally, electron microscope studies show *B. burgdorferi* in pitlike structures between epithelial cells of the midgut and closely associated with the basal plasma membrane.[21] *B. burgdorferi* disseminated from the midgut of 57% of *I. dammini* to the hemolymph 4 days after attachment.[70]

Transmission of *B. burgdorferi* by ticks appears to be through the mouthparts either by salivation, regurgitation, or both. Spirochetes seen in the feeding cavity in host skin indicated transmission by way of the mouthparts, and salivary delivery was hypothesized.[16] *B. burgdorferi* were detected in pilocarpine-induced saliva as early as day three post-attachment and thereafter in continuously increasing numbers.[70] Electron microscopy studies have provided structural evidence in support of salivary transmission of *B. burgdorferi.* Spirochetes are capable of passing both intracellularly and intercellularly through the epithelium without causing damage into the hemocoel. The organism then nonpreferentially invades the type I and granular salivary gland acini as well as salivary ducts.[89] The salivary glands of ixodid ticks perform an osmoregulatory function and excrete copious amounts of excess water and ions in saliva beginning during initial digestion when concentrating the bloodmeal.[62] Because ixodid ticks feed for long periods of time, bloodmeal concentration and concurrent osmoregulation take place while the tick is still attached to the host, and salivary transmission of *B. burgdorferi* could easily occur.

Experimental transmission of *B. burgdorferi* by nymphal ticks to hamsters and white-footed mice became more efficient with increased duration of feeding. Accumulated data suggest that systemically infected ticks can transmit *B. burgdorferi* during early salivation, whereas ticks with only gut infections do not transmit for several days after spirochetes have penetrated the gut and invaded the salivary glands. *B. burgdorferi* multiply in the midgut during early feeding, and within 3 to 5 days a percentage penetrate the gut wall into the hemocoel to invade tissues including the salivary glands. Transmission of spirochetes to a host occurs during the late stages of feeding by way of the saliva. Regurgitation has been suggested as another mode of transmission.[24]

Transovarial transmission

In *I. dammini,* disseminated spirochetes have occasionally caused massive infections in ovarian tissues resulting in either production of small egg masses, which generally fail to develop, or in complete lack of oviposition. Numerous spirochetes have been detected in oocytes between the vitelline and oocyte membranes where they destroy the microvillar processes, which prevents formation of the egg's chitinous cuticle, subsequent egg maturation, and oviposition.[23]

Evidence suggests that normal oogenesis can occur under certain, as yet undetermined, conditions to result in a highly variable rate of transovarially infected ticks. Field-collected, unfed larval ticks have been shown to contain *B. burgdorferi* in New York and Massachusetts.[18,62] F_1 filial infections from 3.3% to 15% have been documented in a small sample of *I. dammini* removed from deer and in 25% to 27% of the progeny from two ticks removed from a dog.[50] Although as many as 100% of the eggs from experimentally infected *I. dammini* contained at least a few spirochetes, a decreased rate of infection in resultant larval ticks and loss of infection in the nymphal stage suggested a gradual diminution of organisms. In general, the prevalence of infection in unfed *I. dammini* larvae is less than 2%[50,62] and transovarial transmission is considered insignificant epidemiologically.

Transovarial transmission has also been documented for *I. pacificus,*[46] *I. scapularis,*[52] and *I. ricinus.*[80] *I. scapularis* experimentally is susceptible to the agent and able to maintain it transtadially,[22] and evidence exists that a low percentage of filial ticks may be ovarially infected.[52]

ANIMAL HOSTS OF VECTOR TICKS

The *Ixodes* vectors of *B. burgdorferi* that feed on humans as incidental hosts also parasitize a large number of different small, medium, and large wild and domestic animals.

I. dammini subadults feed on at least 31 different mammals and 49 species of birds.[3] Small rodents, in particular *Peromyscus leucopus* (white-footed mouse), are important hosts for both larvae and nymphs. Numerous larvae have been reported to parasitize gray squirrels *(Sciurus carolinensis),* short-tailed shrews *(Blarina brevicauda),* raccoons *(Procyon lotor),* woodland jumping mice *(Napaeozapus insignis),* and white-tailed deer *(Odocoileus virginianus).* Although adult ticks appear to have a narrower host range and a predilection for white-tailed deer,[4] they have been removed from 13 mammal species including dogs and large domestic animals.[4]

In addition to parasitizing rodents and birds, larvae and nymphs of *I. scapularis* commonly feed on skinks *(Sceloporus* species) in the southeastern United States.[71] Adults feed on large mammals including deer, cows, bobcats *(Lynx* species), bears, and hogs *(Sus* species).[4]

Approximately 80 species of mammals, reptiles, and birds serve as hosts for *I. pacificus.* Inland (Idaho, Utah, and Nevada) subadult populations feed principally on rodents, whereas in coastal populations, lizards, birds, rabbits, and deer *(Cervus* species) are more frequently parasitized than are rodents. Adults commonly feed on dogs, deer, and cattle.*

I. ricinus is a somewhat more indiscriminate feeder and has been recorded from 148, 149, and 20 species of mammals, birds, and reptiles, respectively.[4] The subadult stages feed on a variety of small rodents. Larvae feed primarily on *Apodemus* species, namely *A. sylvaticus* (woodmouse) and *A. flavicollis* (yellow-necked mouse), and bank voles *(Clethrionomys glareolus).* Nymphs feed on a narrower range of hosts and much less frequently on common rodents than does the larval stage. Nymphs are abundant on squirrels, hares, birds, and sand lizards. Nymphs also feed on *Apodemus agrarius* (black-striped mouse), which may be abundant in local situations where habitat has been disturbed generally by humans.[56] Deer, sheep, cattle, dogs, and hares are favored hosts of the adult stage.[4]

I. persulcatus is associated with small deciduous woodland areas close to coniferous forests and has been recovered from 241 different species of host animals. Subadults feed on a variety of small mammals and birds associated with the woodland habitat, whereas adults feed on deer, cattle, hares, and hedgehogs.[4,13]

Transmission of *B. burgdorferi* depends on a complex interaction of properties of the pathogen, tick vector, and vertebrate host as well as environmental and behavioral factors such as seasonal activity and population densities of the vector and host. Many animals and birds found to be infected with *B. burgdorferi,* to possess specific borrelia antibodies, and/or to be infested with infected ticks have been indirectly incriminated as reservoir hosts. Although various host species may contribute to the maintenance of tick and spirochete populations, the relative contributions of each species may differ greatly. For an animal to serve as an efficient reservoir of infection to ticks it must be capable of maintaining spirochetes for extended periods of time in sites accessible to feeding ticks and have a high degree of repeated contact with competent vector ticks.

Within the geographic range of *I. dammini,*

---

*References 12, 17, 27, 33, 36, 42.

white-footed mice are considered the most important natural host in maintaining *B. burgdorferi* transmission. In these areas *Peromyscus leucopus* is the most prevalent and ubiquitously distributed small rodent, is more frequently parasitized by immature *I. dammini* than are other rodents, and appears to contribute the most to infection of natural tick populations.[55] *Peromyscus leucopus* appears tolerant to repeated and prolonged tick feeding, accounting for the high degree of feeding success of *I. dammini*. The ability to overcome host defenses might be due to the salivary components of the tick that are able to antagonize the inflammatory response of the rodent.[67-69]

B. burgdorferi was first isolated from the blood of a low percentage of white-footed mice by in vitro cultivation. The low percentage of spirochetemic mice suggested an intermittent blood phase and that timing of sample acquisition was critical to determine blood infection.[18] Additional observations indicated that both field- and laboratory-infected individuals appear to be virtually aspirochetemic. In contrast, *B. burgdorferi* can routinely be cultured from various organs including the spleen, kidney, and urinary bladder. Spirochetes appear to be collected more efficiently by ticks than by blood cultivation. Such findings suggest that utilization of a xenodiagnostic procedure may provide a more precise simultaneous measurement of host infection and infectivity. The superiority of *Peromyscus leucopus* to serve as a competent reservoir of *B. burgdorferi* has been demonstrated.[68] The bite of one nymphal tick is sufficient to infect white-footed mice, and infection prevalence in larval ticks fed on mice previously infected approached 100%. Although infectivity to ticks gradually decreased, persistent spirochetal infection from 200 days to 13 months has been demonstrated.[58,68] Additionally, noninfected larval ticks placed on aspirochetemic yet infected mice progressively accumulated organisms in the midgut in which by day three virtually all ticks were infected. Skin preparation from these animals contained demonstrable *B. burgdorferi*, indicating that the organisms reside in the skin throughout infection where they accumulate and are available to feeding ticks.

A remarkably high percentage of *Peromyscus leucopus* are infected with *B. burgdorferi* in endemic areas. As many as 75% or more of total collected mice were infected in Connecticut, Rhode Island, and Long Island, New York, and infectivity of mice to feeding ticks was considered to be universal in coastal Massachusetts.[4,7,9,10,19] Even though white-footed mice are infected throughout the year, infection rates are twice as high in the summer months and in early fall. Higher infection rates during the early summer may reflect seasonal changes in infection intensity rather than absolute prevalence. Nonetheless, greatest spirochete infection in mice correlates with the seasonal activity of the vector. Amplification of infection in vector ticks and increased risk for zoonotic transmission occur when larval ticks feed on infected mice and pass the infection transtadially to the nymph.[34,58] Infection rates in adult ticks are approximately twice that of nymphs because adults can be transtadially infected from infections acquired as larvae or nymphs. Although most mice are infected by tick bite, alternative routes for *B. burgdorferi* transmission have been suggested including other arthropods,[49,66] by way of infected urine and milk,[28,64] contact with infected animals,[29] and by transplacental transmission.[72,82] Although these alternate routes could serve to increase transmission efficiency and to maintain enzootic foci in areas where infectious nymphal ticks are rare, they do not appear to contribute universally to the force of transmission.

I. dammini appears to provide excellent physiologic conditions for the multiplication of *B. burgdorferi*. The pathogen multiplies rapidly in larval ticks to a mean density of 2735 spirochetes per individual by day 15 after repletion. During the subsequent premolting period, spirochete levels dropped fivefold, which resulted in less than 300 organisms per freshly molted nymph. After nymphal feeding, spirochete multiplication was renewed and a mean level of 61,275 organisms per nymph was reached 75 days after repletion. A tenfold decrease in spirochetes was noted when ticks molted to adults, suggesting that molting hormones adversely affect spirochetal development. Feeding ticks probably inject *B. burgdorferi* intradermally, and the coinoculation of tick salivary components with organisms may play a crucial role in establishment of infection. An inoculum of 10,000 spirochetes is necessary to infect hamsters uniformly by an intraperitoneal route. Likewise, inocula derived from unfed nymphs failed to produce infection, whereas inocula from replete nymphs did prove to be infectious to hamsters.[58]

The duration of feeding by larval ticks is directly correlated with the proportion of individuals acquiring infection. Only 1.4% of ticks attached for 8 hours were infected, whereas 87.5% that fed to repletion were infected. *B. burgdorferi* infection has been detected in partially fed larval ticks that have dropped from a dead host. These partially fed ticks successfully reattach to other rodents, renew feeding, and successfully molt to nymphs. During refeeding, larvae were not capable of transmitting spirochetes, whereas the resultant transtadially infected nymphs were capable of transmitting *B*.

24 Basic Aspects

burgdorferi. These data suggest that infected host-seeking larvae in nature cannot be judged a priori to have acquired infection transovarially and that transovarial infection rates may actually be lower than currently thought.[57]

Medium-sized mammalian hosts of *I. dammini*

Medium-sized mammals have been shown to be significant hosts of adults as well as immature *I. dammini.*[30,38,51,54] Raccoons, opossums *(Didelphis virginiana),* and skunks *(Mephitis mephitis)* have been implicated indirectly as reservoir hosts of *B. burgdorferi* based on either spirochetal isolation from blood or serology.[6,9] Direct evidence using xenodiagnostic methods has shown that skunks and raccoons, although less efficient than white-footed mice, are indeed competent reservoir hosts and may possibly be more important in suburban residential areas where their density may exceed that of *Peromyscus leucopus.*[37] The role of medium-sized mammals in the epizootiology of Lyme borreliosis in varying geographic regions requires further clarification.

White-tailed deer

White-tailed deer, in addition to immatures stages, are more commonly infested by adult *I. dammini,* suggesting they serve as an important blood meal source necessary for tick reproduction and maintenance of *I. dammini* populations.[61,74,87] Although it is generally accepted that deer are a major host for robust populations of *I. dammini,* tick distribution and abundance may be influenced by complex interactions involving climate and physical and biotic factors that vary in different physiographic regions.[2] Tick abundance was positively correlated with deer density,[85] and sharp reduction in tick abundance and in human Lyme disease was noted in an area where deer were virtually eliminated.[86] Infestations of ticks were not sustained unless deer were abundant in one study,[10] and, in another, the vast majority of eggs resulted from female ticks that had fed on deer.[87] In New Jersey and Maryland, however, tick and deer densities did not correspond.[2,74] *Ixodes dammini* densities were greatest in the coastal plains in both states where deer densities are lower than in areas of higher elevation. The role of deer in the epizootiology of Lyme borreliosis remains unclear.

Deer have been implicated as reservoirs of infection based on detection of spirochetes in their blood[19] and on serologic evidence of infection.[53] Another study determined that deer are incompetent as reservoirs by examining nymphal ticks derived from engorged larvae that had fed on deer.[81] These authors suggested that such reservoir incompetence may actually exert a zooprophylactic effect and may dilute transmission intensity of *B. burgdorferi.*

Avian hosts and reservoirs

Borrelia burgdorferi is unique in that it can infect both mammalian and avian species. Although birds are naturally infected by the pathogen, duration of spirochetemia is unknown and may be brief when compared to that in mammals. *B. burgdorferi* isolated from the liver of a veery *(Catharus fuscescens)* was infectious to chickens and hamsters under laboratory conditions, indicating that birds can serve as reservoir hosts. Subadult ticks fed to repletion on infected birds successfully transtadially transmitted the spirochete, which, in turn, was infectious to laboratory hamsters.[8] In addition to acting as reservoirs of infection, both resident and migratory birds harbor significant numbers of immature *I. dammini* and may serve to disperse ticks locally during breeding seasons and over long distances during migrations. The distribution pattern of Lyme disease and *I. dammini* parallel existing migration routes and flyways in the eastern and midwestern United States.[14,77,83]

REFERENCES

1. Ai C et al: Clinical manifestation and epidemiological characteristics of Lyme disease in Hailin County, Heilongjiang Province, China, *Ann NY Acad Sci* 539:302, 1988.
2. Amerasinghe FP et al: Distribution, density, and Lyme disease spirochete infection in *Ixodes dammini* (Acari: Ixodidae) on white-tailed deer in Maryland, *J Med Entomol* 29(1):54, 1992.
3. Anderson JF: Mammalian and avian reservoirs for *Borrelia burgdorferi, Ann NY Acad Sci* 539:180, 1988.
4. Anderson JF: Epizootiology of *Borrelia* in *Ixodes* tick vectors and reservoir hosts, *Rev Infect Dis* 2(Suppl 6):S1451, 1989.
5. Anderson JF, Magnarelli LA, McAninch JB: *Ixodes dammini* and *Borrelia burgdorferi* in northern New England and upstate New York, *J Parasitol* 73:419, 1987.
6. Anderson JF et al: Avian and mammalian hosts for spirochete infected ticks and insects in Connecticut, *Yale J Biol Med* 57:627, 1984.
7. Anderson JF et al: Identification of endemic foci of Lyme disease: isolation of *Borrelia burgdorferi* from feral rodents and ticks, *Dermacentor variabilis, J Clin Microbiol* 22:36, 1985.
8. Anderson JF et al: Involvement of birds in the epidemiology of the Lyme disease agent *Borrelia burgdorferi, Infect Immun* 51:394, 1986.
9. Anderson JF et al: *Peromyscus leucopus* and *Microtus pennsylvanicus* simultaneously infected with *Borrelia burgdorferi* and *Babesia microti, J Clin Microbiol* 23:135, 1986.
10. Anderson JF et al: Prevalence of *Borrelia burgdorferi* and *Babesia microti* in mice on islands inhabited by white-tailed deer, *App Environ Microbiol* 52:892, 1987.
11. Anderson JF et al: Antigenically variable *Borrelia burgdorferi* isolated from cottontail rabbits and *Ixodes dentatus* in rural and urban areas, *J Clin Microbiol* 27:13, 1989.
12. Arthur DR, Snow K: *Ixodes pacificus* Cooley and Kohls, 1943, its life history and occurrence, *Parasitology* 58:893, 1968.

13. Balashov YS: Bloodsucking ticks (Ixodoidea)—vectors of diseases of man and animals, *Misc Publ Entomol Soc Am* 8:160, 1972.

14. Battaly GR, Fish D, Dowler RC: The seasonal occurrence of *Ixodes dammini* (Acarina: Ixodidae) and *Ixodes dentatus* on birds in a Lyme disease endemic area of south-eastern New York State, *J NY Entomol Soc* 95:461, 1987.

15. Beck DE, Allred DM, Brinton EP: Ticks of the Nevada test site, *Brigham Young Univ Sci Bull*, Biol Series 4, 1963.

16. Benach JL et al: Adult *Ixodes dammini* on rabbits: a hypothesis for the development and transmission of *Borrelia burgdorferi*, *J Infect Dis* 155(6):1300, 1987.

17. Bishopp FC, Trembley HL: Distribution and hosts of certain North American ticks, *J Parasitol*, 31:1, 1945.

18. Bosler EM et al: Natural distribution of the *Ixodes dammini* spirochete, *Science* 220:321, 1983.

19. Bosler EM et al: Prevalence of the Lyme disease spirochete in populations of white-tailed deer and white-footed mice, *Yale J Biol Med* 57:651,1984.

20. Bouseman JK et al: Status of *Ixodes dammini* (Acari:Ixodidae) in Illinois, *J Med Entomol* 27(4):556, 1990.

21. Burgdorfer W: Vector/host relationship of the Lyme disease spirochete, *Borrelia burgdorferi*, *Rheum Dis Clin North Am* 15(4):775, 1989.

22. Burgdorfer W, Gage KL: Susceptibility of the black-legged tick, *Ixodes scapularis*, to the Lyme disease spirochete, *Borrelia burgdorferi*, Zentralbl Bakteriol Mikrobiol Hyg [A] 263:15, 1986.

23. Burgdorfer W, Hayes SF, Benach JL: Development of *Borrelia burgdorferi* in Ixodid vector ticks, *Ann NY Acad Sci* 539:172, 1988.

24. Burgdorfer W, Hayes SF, Corwin D: Pathophysiology of the Lyme disease spirochete, *Borrelia burgdorferi*, in ixodid ticks, *Rev Infect Dis* 2(Suppl 6):S1442, 1989.

25. Burgdorfer W et al: Lyme disease—A tick-borne spirochetosis? *Science* 216:1317, 1982.

26. Burgdorfer W et al: Erythema chronicum migrans—a tick-borne spirochetosis? *Acta Trop* 40:73, 1983.

27. Burgdorfer W et al: The western black-legged tick, *Ixodes pacificus*: a vector of *Borrelia burgdorferi*, *Am J Trop Med Hyg* 34:925, 1985.

28. Burgess EC: *Borrelia burgdorferi* infection in Wisconsin horses and cows, *Ann NY Acad Sci* 539:235, 1988.

29. Burgess EC et al: Experimental inoculation of *Peromyscus* spp. with *Borrelia burgdorferi*: evidence for contact transmission, *Am J Trop Med Hyg* 35:355, 1986.

30. Carey AB, Krinsky WL, Main AJ: *Ixodes dammini* (Acari: Ixodidae) and associated ixodid ticks in south-central Connecticut, USA, *J Med Entomol* 17:89, 1980.

31. Ciesielski CA et al: Lyme disease surveillance in the United States, 1983-1986, *Rev Infect Dis* 11(suppl 6):S1435, 1989.

32. Coan ME, Stiller DS: *Ixodes dammini* (Acari: Ixodidae) in Maryland, USA, and a preliminary survey for *Babesia microti J Med Entomol* 23:446, 1986.

33. Cooley RA, Kohls GM: The genus *Ixodes* in North America, *Natl Inst Health Bull* 184:1, 1945.

34. Donahue JG, Piesman J, Spielman A: Reservoir competence of white-footed mice for Lyme disease spirochetes, *Am J Trop Med Hyg* 36(1):92, 1987.

35. Drew ML et al: *Ixodes dammini*: Occurrence and prevalence of infection with *Borrelia* spp. in Minnesota, *J Wildl Dis* 24(4):708, 1988.

36. Easton ER et al: The distribution in Oregon of *Ixodes pacificus*, *Dermacentor andersoni* and *Dermacentor occidentalis* with a note on *Dermacentor variabilis* (Acarina: Ixodidac), *J Med Entomol* 13:501, 1977.

37. Fish D, Daniels TJ: The role of medium-sized mammals as reservoirs of *Borrelia burgdorferi* in southern New York, *J Wildl Dis* 26(3):339, 1990.

38. Fish D, Dowler RC: Host associations of ticks (Acari: Ixodidae) parasitizing medium-sized mammals in a Lyme disease endemic area of southern New York, *J Med Entomol* 26:200, 1989.

39. Furman DP, Loomis EC: The ticks of California (Acari: Ixodidae), *Bull Ca Insect Sur 25*, 1984.

40. Ginsberg HS, Ewing CP: Deer ticks, *Ixodes dammini* (Acari: Ixodidae), and Lyme disease spirochetes, *Borrelia burgdorferi*, in Maine, *J Med Entomol* 25(4):303, 1989.

41. Godsey MS Jr et al: Lyme disease ecology in Wisconsin: distribution and host preference of *Ixodes dammini* and prevalence of antibody to *Borrelia burgdorferi* in small mammals, *Am J Trop Med Hyg* 37:180, 1987.

42. Gregson JD: *The Ixodoidea of Canada*, Canada Dept of Agriculture Science Service Entomology Division Publ, 930:1, 1956.

43. Kawabata M et al: Lyme disease in Japan and its possible incriminated tick vector, *Ixodes persulcatus*, *J Infect Dis* 156:854, 1987.

44. Krantz GW: *A Manual of Acarology*, ed 2, Corvallis, 1978, Oregon State University.

45. Krinsky WL: Development of the tick, *Ixodes dammini* (Acarina: Ixodidae) in the laboratory, *J Med Entomol* 16:354, 1979.

46. Lane RS, Burgdorfer W: Transovarial and transtadial passage of *Borrelia burgdorferi* in the western black-legged tick *Ixodes pacificus*, *Am J Trop Med Hyg* 37:188, 1987.

47. Lane RS, Burgdorfer W: Spirochetes in mammals and ticks (Acari: Ixodidae) from a focus of Lyme borreliosis in California, *J Wildl Dis* 24:1, 1988.

48. MacNeil DR: Lyme disease vector, *Ixodes dammini*, identified in Nova Scotia, *Can Dis Wkly Rep* 16(15):69, 1990.

49. Magnarelli LA, Anderson JF: Ticks and biting insects infected with the etiologic agent of Lyme disease, *Borrelia burgdorferi*, *J Clin Microbiol* 26:1482, 1988.

50. Magnarelli LA, Anderson JF, Fish D: Transovarial transmission of *Borrelia burgdorferi* in *Ixodes dammini* (Acari: Ixodidae), *J Infect Dis* 156:234, 1987.

51. Magnarelli LA et al: Parasitism by *Ixodes dammini* (Acari: Ixodidae) and antibodies to spirochetes in mammals at Lyme disease foci in Connecticut, USA, *J Med Entomol* 21:52, 1984.

52. Magnarelli LA et al: Spirochetes in ticks and antibodies to *Borrelia burgdorferi* in white-tailed deer from Connecticut, New York State and North Carolina, *J Wildl Dis* 22:178, 1986.

53. Magnarelli LA et al: Antibodies to *Borrelia burgdorferi* in deer and raccoons, *J Wildl Dis* 27(4):562, 1991.

54. Main AJ et al: Immature *Ixodes dammini* (Acari: Ixodidae) on small mammals in Connecticut, USA, *J Med Entomol* 19:655, 1982.

55. Mather TN et al: Comparing the relative potential of rodents as reservoirs of the Lyme disease spirochete (Borrelia burgdorferi), *Am J Epidemiol* 130(1):143, 1989.

56. Matschka FR et al: Capacity of European animals as reservoir hosts for the Lyme disease spirochete, *J Infect Dis* 165:479, 1992.

57. Piesman J: Experimental acquisition of the Lyme disease spirochete, *Borrelia burgdorferi*, by larval *Ixodes dammini* (Acari: Ixodidae) during partial blood meals, *J Med Entomol* 28(2):259, 1991.

58. Piesman J, Oliver JR, Sinsky RJ: Growth kinetics of the Lyme disease spirochete (*Borrelia burgdorferi*) in vector ticks (*Ixodes dammini*), *Am J Trop Med Hyg* 42(4):352, 1990.

59. Piesman J, Sinsky RJ: Ability of *Ixodes pacificis, Dermacentor variabilis* and *Amblyomma americanum* (Acari: Ixodidae) to acquire, maintain and transmit Lyme disease spirochetes, *Borrelia burgdorferi, J Med Entomol* 25(5):336, 1988.
60. Piesman J, Spielman A: Host associations and seasonal abundance of immature *Ixodes dammini* in southeastern Massachusetts, *Ann Entomol Soc Am* 72:829, 1979.
61. Piesman J et al: Role of deer in the epizootiology of *Babesia microti* in Massachusetts, USA, *J Med Entomol* 15:537, 1979.
62. Piesman J et al: Transovarially acquired Lyme disease spirochetes (*Borrelia burgdorferi*) in field collected larval *Ixodes dammini* (Acari: Ixodidae), *J Med Entomol* 23(2):219, 1986.
63. Pinger RR et al: Collections of adult *Ixodes dammini* in Indiana, 1987-1990, and isolation of *Borrelia burgdorferi, J Med Entomol* 28(5):745, 1991.
64. Post JE, Shaw EE, Wright SD: Suspected borreliosis in cattle, *Ann NY Acad Sci* 539:488, 1988.
65. Rand PW, Smith RP, Lacombe EH: Canine seroprevalence and the distribution of *Ixodes dammini* in an area of emerging disease, *Am J Public Hlth* 81(10):1331, 1991.
66. Rawlings JA: Lyme disease in Texas, *Zentralbl Bakteriol Mikrobiol Hyg [A]* 263:483, 1986.
67. Ribeiro JMC: Role of saliva in blood-feeding by arthropods, *Ann J Rev Entomol* 32:463, 1987.
68. Ribeiro JMC, Spielman A: *Ixodes dammini*: Salivary anaphylatoxin inactivating activity, *Exp Parasitol* 62:292, 1986.
69. Ribeiro JMC et al: Antihemostatic, antiinflammatory and immunosuppressive properties of the saliva of a tick, *Ixodes dammini, J Exp Med* 161:332, 1985.
70. Ribeiro JMC et al: Dissemination and salivary delivery of Lyme disease spirochetes in vector ticks (Acari: Ixodidae), *J Med Entomol* 24(2):201, 1987.
71. Rogers AJ: A study of ixodid ticks of Florida including the biology of *Ixodes scapularis*, PhD dissertation, College Park, 1953, University of Maryland.
72. Schlesinger PA et al: Maternal-fetal transmission of the Lyme disease spirochete, *Borrelia burgdorferi, Ann Intern Med* 103:67, 1985.
73. Schulze TL et al: *Amblyomma americanum*: a potential vector of Lyme disease in New Jersey, *Science* 224:601, 1984.
74. Schulze TL et al: *Ixodes dammini* (Acari: Ixodidae) and other ixodid ticks collected from white-tailed deer from New Jersey, USA. I. Geographical distribution and its relation to selected environmental and physical factors, *J Med Entomol* 21:741, 1984.
75. Schulze TL et al: The role of adult *Ixodes dammini* (Acari: Ixodidae) in the transmission of Lyme disease in New Jersey, USA, *J Med Entomol* 22:88, 1985.
76. Schulze TL et al: Comparison of rates of infection by Lyme disease spirochetes in selected populations of *Ixodes dammini* and *Amblyomma americanum* (Acari: Ixodidae), *Zentrabl Bakteriol Mikrobiol Hyg [A]* 263:72, 1986.
77. Schulze TL et al: Evolution of a focus of Lyme disease, *Zentralbl Bakteriol Mickrobiol Hyg [A]* 263:65, 1986.
78. Spielman A et al: Human babesiosis on Nantucket Island, USA: description of the vector, *Ixodes (Ixodes) dammini*, n. sp. (Acarina: Ixodidae), *J Med Entomol* 15:218, 1979.
79. Stafford III KC: Oviposition and larval dispersal of *Ixodes dammini* (Acari: Ixodidae), *J Med Entomol* 29(1):129, 1992.
80. Stanek G et al: Borrelia transfer by ticks during their life cycle, *Zentralbl Bakteriol Mikrobiol Hyg [A]* 263:29, 1986.
81. Telford III SR et al: Incompetence of deer as reservoirs of the Lyme disease spirochete, *Am J Trop Med Hyg* 39(1):105, 1988.
82. Weber K et al: *Borrelia burgdorferi* in a newborn despite oral penicillin for Lyme borreliosis during pregnancy, *Pediatr Infect Dis* 7:286, 1988.
83. Weisbrod AR, Johnson RC: Lyme disease and migrating birds in the Saint Croix River Valley, *Appl Environ Microbiol* 55:1921, 1989.
84. White DJ et al: The geographic spread and temporal increase of the Lyme disease epidemic, *JAVMA* 266(9):1230, 1991.
85. Wilson ML, Adler GH, Spielman A: Correlation between deer abundance and that of the deer tick, *Ixodes dammini* (Acari: Ixodidae), *Ann Entomol Soc Am* 78:172, 1985.
86. Wilson ML et al: Reduced abundance of *Ixodes dammini* (Acari: Ixodidae) following elimination of deer, *J Med Entomol* 25:224, 1988.
87. Wilson ML et al: Host-dependent differences in feeding and reproduction of *Ixodes dammini* (Acari: Ixodidae), *J Med Entomol* 27(6):945, 1990.
88. Yuval B, Spielman A: Duration and regulation of the developmental cycle of *Ixodes dammini* (Acari: Ixodidae), *J Med Entomol* 27(2):196, 1990.
89. Zung JL et al: Fine structural evidence for penetration of the Lyme disease spirochete *Borrelia burgdorferi* through the gut and salivary tissues of *Ixodes dammini, Can J Zool* 67:1737, 1989.

4 Epidemiology

David T. Dennis

Lyme disease has, in the 15 years since it was first described, been recognized as a worldwide tick-borne borreliosis of public health importance, with endemic foci distributed throughout North America, Europe, and northern Asia. It has become the leading vectorborne infectious disease in the United States, with more than 40,000 cases reported to the Centers for Disease Control (CDC) in the 10-year period 1982 to 1991. The known range of the disease continues to expand—in the United States, enzootic transmission by established tick vectors has now been confirmed in 23 states. The epidemiology and ecology of Lyme disease are complex, there is much about the disease that is unknown, and new information challenges some established concepts.

TRANSMISSION CYCLE

Lyme disease is a zoonosis in which humans are incidental hosts of the causative agent, *Borrelia burgdorferi,* and do not contribute to its maintenance in nature. The basic elements in the life cycle of *B. burgdorferi* in North America, recently reviewed in depth,[29] are the following: (1) small rodents serve as the usual reservoirs of infection for vector ticks; (2) three stages of tick are involved in a 2-year cycle, each stage normally taking a single blood meal; (3) transstadial transmission from larva to nymph helps maintain the infective cycle; (4) the efficiency of the cycle is further enhanced by sequential feeding patterns, in which nymphs, feeding in the spring, infect rodents that then serve as source of infection for larvae, which feed in the summer months; (5) deer, especially the white-tailed deer, *Odocoileus virginianus,* and other large- and medium-sized animals, such as raccoons and canids, serve as mating ground for adult ticks and provide the blood meal required for egg production. Deer are thought to be incompetent reservoirs of *B. burgdorferi.*[71] Humans acquire Lyme disease from infective nymphs, usually in the late spring and early summer, and infrequently from adult ticks, which feed mostly in the fall and winter, but also in early spring. Figure 4–1 is a schematic diagram showing forces of infection involved in the transmission cycle.

DYNAMICS OF INFECTION IN HUMANS

Lyme disease of humans is a multistage, multisystem, acute and chronic, noncontagious inflammatory condition.[63] The causative spirochetal agent is not directly transmitted from one person to another, except, in apparently rare instances, by crossing the placenta to infect the fetus.[48,76] The portal of entry is the skin, at the site of infective tick attachment. Dissemination is cutaneous, lymphatic, and hematogenous, The incubation period is usually days to weeks from infective exposure to earliest signs of illness, such as erythema migrans (EM), localized lymphadenitis, and mild constitutional symptoms.[67] Not all patients remember rash illness or other early symptoms, and weeks or months may elapse before later-stage manifestations are recognized. The latent period also may be several days to weeks or even months: *B. burgdorferi* can be cultured in a high proportion of biopsy specimens taken from EM lesions within days of their appearance[12]; IgM antibodies to *B. burgdorferi* can be detected as early as 1 to 2 weeks after the appearance of earliest symptoms and usually peak between the third and sixth week; IgG responses may be delayed for weeks.[19] The time-course of cell-mediated immune responses is also variable.[56] The duration of infection in humans is not known, although isolation of *B. burgdorferi* from skin, cerebrospinal fluid, myocardium, and synovial fluid months and years after onset of symptoms has been reported.[10,44,58,62] Asymptomatic and subclinical infection is probably common,[27,57] and symptoms may persist or increase in seronegative patients with and without evidence of continuing infection.[21,32,51] It is not known whether humans have genetic differences in susceptibility to infection or can acquire protective immunity; persons with chronic and refractory arthritic manifestations are, however, more likely than controls to have HLA-DR4 markers,[65] and cases of reinfection with *B. burgdorferi* have been reported.[75]

Although morbidity can be severe, chronic, and disabling, the disease is almost never fatal.

GLOBAL DISTRIBUTION

Lyme disease cases have been documented in North America, Europe, and Asia. The distribution of the disease is limited to the range of ticks of the *Ixodes (Ixodes) ricinus* complex in neoarctic and paleoarctic regions (Fig. 4–2).[9,29] Endemic areas in Europe include the British Isles, Scandinavia, western Europe, and states of the former Union of Soviet Socialist Republics, from the Baltic states east through Russia to the Pacific Coast.[23,49] The disease

is endemic in China in forested northeastern regions, particularly in Hailongjiang and Jilin Provinces,[2] and in widely scattered foci elsewhere.[1] More than 40 cases have been described from Japan, mostly from Hokkaido and other eastern parts of the country.[16] *Ixodes ricinus* is the principal vector in western and central Europe,[29] and *I. persulcatus* is the main vector in eastern Russia,[23] China[2] and Japan.[16] There are extensive areas of eastern Europe where these two vectors coexist. Both also transmit the tickborne encephalitis virus.

Lyme disease reported from Africa,[47,49] South America, and Australia[70] has not been confirmed by cultural isolation of *B. burgdorferi* from patients, tick vectors, or vertebrate hosts. *Borrelia* with characteristics distinct from *B. burgdorferi* have been identified in *Ixodes holocyclus* and *Haemaphysalis longicornus* ticks collected in New South Wales.[70,79] In the western hemisphere, Lyme disease has been documented in the United States and Canada, where disease is concentrated in northeastern and north-central states, in northern California counties,[29] and in southeastern Ontario Province.[7] Reported Lyme disease elsewhere in the western hemisphere has not been confirmed by isolation of the causative organism or by documentation of the enzootic cycle.

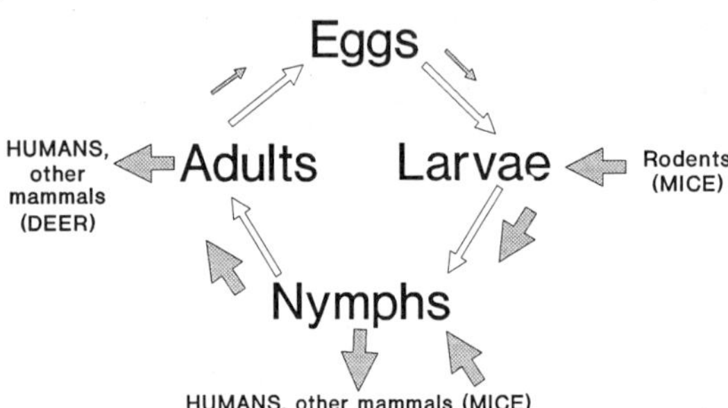

Figure 4–1 Schematic diagram of the tick cycle showing the force of infection *(hatched arrows)* as ticks advance from one stage to another *(open arrows)*. Transovarial transmission is minimal. Infection is from the rodent reservoir to larvae and nymphs, and transtadially from larva to nymph to adult.

DISTRIBUTION IN THE UNITED STATES AND CANADA
Underlying ecologic factors

The original studies of Steere et al[68] on clusters of cases of arthritis in Lyme and surrounding towns in estuarial Connecticut quickly and clearly iden-

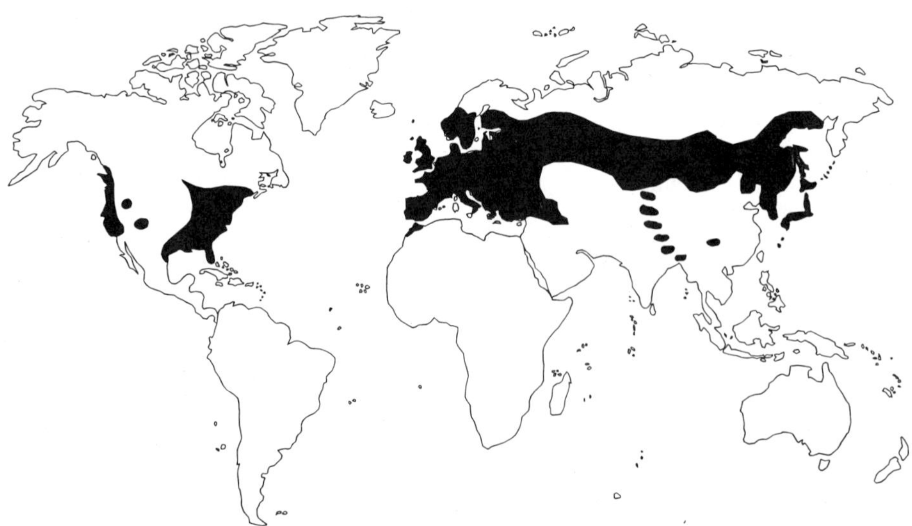

Figure 4–2 The global distribution of *Ixodes* ticks able to transmit the agent of Lyme disease, *Borrelia burgdorferi*. Modified from Filippova NA, editor: Taiga tick, *Ixodes persulcatus* Schulze (Acarina, Ixodidae). Leningrad, 1985, Nauka Publishers.

tified the principal epidemiologic features of Lyme disease as it occurs in the northeastern United States: a disease that affects children and adults of both sexes; clustering of cases within townships and even by road and household, but without apparent contagiousness; onsets of illness mostly occurring in summer months; and association of cases with residence in wooded areas. The studies went on to link the characteristic EM rash with antecedent tick bite and showed that cases were more likely than controls to reside in townships in which tick-infested mice and deer were abundant.[64] These findings supported the hypothesis that the illness was caused by an infectious agent vectored by the deer tick, later described as *Ixodes dammini*.[60] A survey of 512 patients with Lyme disease from across the United States[66] identified three distinct regional foci of disease: northeastern coastal states, Wisconsin, and California and Oregon—the known range of *I. dammini* in the East, and the range of the closely related western black-legged tick, *Ixodes pacificus*, in the West.[26]

Detailed studies had been carried out in the 1970s on the deer tick as a vector of babesiosis on islands off the coast of Massachusetts by Spielman et al.[59] After the isolation of *B. burgdorferi* from the deer tick and from Lyme disease patients, the transmission of *B. burgdorferi* in this northeastern coastal habitat became the model of enzootic Lyme disease in the United States.[61] In this model, the white-footed mouse, *Peromyscus leucopus*, is the most competent amplifying reservoir, demonstrating nearly universal infection in highly endemic foci, maintaining infection without apparent ill-effect, as well as serving as the preferred host for the larval and nymphal stages of the deer tick. Deer are thought to be a prerequisite for the establishment of *I. dammini* populations[80]; the emergence of deer tick populations on the mainland of New England and their extension in a band from Maine to Virginia have been linked to the recent explosive repopulation of these areas by deer. Wherever *I. dammini* are abundant, deer are abundant as well. However, *I. dammini* has been found on at least 33 species of mammals and 49 species of birds,[4] and the experimental removal of deer from selected areas has not resulted in elimination of the tick in these areas.[81]

Several avian species appear to be potential reservoir hosts, and it is possible that migrating birds have established foci of disease in areas previously free of *I. dammini*. The Atlantic coastal strip, from Canada to Florida, is a major flyway, which might partially explain the rapid extension northward and southward from the first described foci of Lyme disease in New England and Long Island. Similarly, there are migrating pathways between On-

tario, Canada, and the Chesapeake Bay, that might account for multiple sites of enzootic Lyme disease along the route not easily explainable by contiguous spread alone.[3,33] Contiguous spread, through movement of cervids (deer) and carnivores, is, however, probably most important in establishing new enzootic foci. Surveillance of humans and animals has shown a slow but steady emergence from known foci outward in states such as Connecticut,[6] New York,[77] and Wisconsin.[22] Combined studies mapping the distribution of ticks, seropositivity of dogs and deer, and human cases over time are providing valuable information on the dynamics of spread of this disease in the United States.[31,45] Seropositivity of dogs appears to be a more sensitive epidemiologic marker of the geographic distribution of Lyme disease than human seropositivity.[25]

Lyme disease outbreaks

A number of outbreaks of Lyme disease have occurred in the eastern United States since 1980, and they provide important information on the emergence of disease in populations newly at risk under differing epidemiologic circumstances. A description of two clusters of cases in New Jersey related risk to residence in new suburban housing developments and to occupational exposures among outdoor workers at a military reservation.[13] A study on Fire Island, a barrier island off the south coast of Long Island, found a cumulative prevalence of 7.5% and a seasonal incidence of 1% to 3% among residents of this summer vacation site.[27] Steere et al, in a longitudinal study of a community of about 160 persons on Great Island, Massachusetts, found a slow build-up of incidence to a peak of 3 per 100 per year, and a total cumulative prevalence of 16% over a 20-year period.[69] The most explosive outbreak described occurred in a community of persons living adjacent to a nature preserve with a large deer population near Ipswich, Massachusetts.[30] The attack rate from 1980 through 1987 was estimated to be 35% for the 190 persons living within 5 km of the preserve, and 66% among those living closest to the preserve. A similar situation was described in Montgomery County, Pennsylvania, on the outskirts of Philadelphia.[5]

State and regional emergence

Of greater importance than the small outbreaks, however, has been the insidious introduction and build-up of transmission to hyperendemic levels within states and regions. This has been most pronounced in suburban residential areas in northeastern states. A review of the situation in Connecticut from 1977 to 1985 suggested a threefold to eightfold increase in incidence in the communities originally described by Steere and an extension of disease to all counties within the state.[17] Lyme disease was first recognized in New York by Suffolk and Nassau counties, Long Island, beginning in 1977.[11] In retrospect, cases had been seen years earlier, and polymerase chain reaction tests of ticks from museum collections document the presence of *B. burgdorferi* in eastern Long Island as early as 1946.[42] By 1982, the disease was known in two other southeastern counties, Putnam and Westchester.[78] The known range of the disease continued to expand, and by 1989 eight counties had been classified as endemic. The numbers of reported cases were doubling annually—by 1989, the incidence in Suffolk County was 150 per 100,000, and 12 towns in the endemic area had rates exceeding 200 per 100,000. The hospital discharge rate of Lyme disease among residents of endemic townships increased dramatically over the same period. Concomitant surveillance for ticks documented a marked spatial and temporal increase of *I. dammini*.[77] Before 1979, *I. dammini* was known only from eastern Long Island; by 1989, the tick was recognized in 22 New York counties and found to be infected with *B. burgdorferi* in 8 contiguous southeastern counties. The Hudson River Valley appears to be a natural avenue of spread. The latest count identifies 34 infested counties, including counties bordering on Canada. Similar patterns of disease emergence have been noted in New Jersey.[53]

A prospective population-based study of two highly endemic neighborhoods in Westchester County in 1990 identified a cumulative prevalence of Lyme disease of 17.6% and an incidence across one transmission season of 2.5% (unpublished data). Infective *I. dammini* ticks were found on 60% of properties surveyed in these neighborhoods—30% of nymphs and 50% of adult ticks were infected.[38] Ticks were most often found on large properties and were found in decreasing order of density in woods, ecotone, ornamental shrubbery areas, and on lawns.

Emergence of Lyme disease in the north-central and Pacific coastal areas has not been so apparent, most probably because transmission is less likely to occur in suburban residential areas. There has, however, been considerable geographic spread. In Wisconsin, the disease has spread throughout most of the state from an original endemic focus in the northwestern counties.[15,22] The disease has also emerged in contiguous areas of Minnesota, Michigan, and Iowa. Extensions down the Mississippi Valley into northern Illinois have been reported.[40] In the western United States, Lyme disease was recognized early in northern California, Utah, Nevada, and Oregon.[18] Although the number of cases reported from the Pacific region has increased significantly since reporting began in 1982, the in-

crease has been limited to California. As compared to the Northeast, the epidemiologic situation is stable. Cases are isolated, infrequent, and sporadic, except in a few northern California counties, where the incidence of reported cases approaches 13 per 100,000 per year. The vector of Lyme disease in the western states, *I. pacificus,* has been found in 53 of 58 California counties,[29] and infected ticks have been reported in 34 of these. In marked contrast to hyperendemic foci in the northeastern and north-cental United States, where *B. burgdorferi* infection rates of vector ticks are frequently 30% to 50%, infection rates of *I. pacificus* are more often 1% to 2%.[29] This is in part due to the preferential feeding of vector nymphs on lizards, rather than on rodent reservoirs, such as the wood rat. Lizards are not reservoirs of *B. burgdorferi* and can, therefore, be considered zooprophylactic hosts. In the West, transmission most often occurs in sparsely populated rural areas and is the result of human intrusion into natural areas.

NATIONAL SURVEILLANCE

A system of Lyme disease surveillance has been in place in the United States since 1982. The national system became fully established only in 1991, when a new, uniform national case definition was adopted for surveillance purposes (see box on p. 31). Laws for mandatory reporting have now been implemented in 46 states. In this system, CDC receives weekly reports of cases from state health departments, publishes totals in the *Morbidity and Mortality Weekly Report*, and analyzes validated national data on an annual basis. In addition, an effort is being made to create a national map of the distribution, by county, of established populations of vector ticks, to identify counties with enzootic transmission, and to describe the various ecologic settings where transmission occurs.

Trends of incidence

Review of national surveillance statistics shows important trends of increase over time.[8,39,50,74] More than 9300 cases were reported by 47 states in 1991. This represents an eighteenfold annual increase over the 497 cases reported by 11 states in 1982, and a 17% increase over the number reported in 1990 (Fig. 4–3). More than 40,000 cases have been reported from 1982 to 1991, and Lyme disease accounted for 91% of all vectorborne infectious disease cases reported in the United States in 1991. The national incidence was 3.97 per 100,000 in 1991, ranging from 0 in several western states and Hawaii to 37.4 in Connecticut. Using surveillance data to determine the incidence of Lyme disease and trends of its occurrence over time has many pitfalls.[8,24] Like syphilis, Lyme disease has been called a "great imitator" and is often difficult to diagnose clinically, particularly when EM is absent. Laboratory tests are not yet standardized, and recent studies have highlighted the poor agreement between test results using various serologic methods.[28,35,54] None of the available tests is highly sensitive in the first few weeks of illness, and the antibody response may be blunted by antibiotic treatment in the early stages of disease. Cross-reactive antibodies occur in persons with other spirochetal diseases.[37] A true measure of the accuracy of serologic tests awaits the development of gold standards for comparison. At present, serologic testing is appropriate only as an adjunct to a careful clinical diagnosis; inappropriate use for screening gives high false-positive rates, leading to misdiagnosis and the reporting of nonexistent cases.

Lyme disease can best be documented in a person by isolating *B. burgdorferi* from clinical material. Cultural isolation rates of 70% and greater have been achieved by inoculating biopsies of EM lesions into BSKII medium,[12] and the expanded use of bacterial isolation for diagnosis is encouraged. To date, *B. burgdorferi* has been isolated from residents of only seven states.

Because of difficulties in establishing clear diagnostic criteria for Lyme disease, case definitions and surveillance practices have varied among states and over time, and surveillance data have been inconsistent. Despite mandatory reporting in most states, Lyme disease is probably greatly underreported, as are most common reportable infectious diseases.[73] Increasing public awareness, which reached a peak in the late 1980s, undoubtedly con-

---

THE NATIONAL SURVEILLANCE CASE DEFINITION ADOPTED FOR USE IN THE UNITED STATES, 1991

Lyme disease

Clinical description

A systemic, tickborne disease with protean manifestations, including dermatologic, rheumatologic, neurologic, and cardiac abnormalities. The best clinical marker for the disease is the initial skin lesion, erythema migrans, that occurs among 60% to 80% of patients.

Clinical case definition

- Erythema migrans or
- At least one late manifestation, as defined below, and laboratory confirmation of infection

Laboratory criteria for diagnosis

- Isolation of *Borrelia burgdorferi* from clinical specimens, or
- Demonstration of diagnostic levels of IgM and IgG antibodies to the spirochete in serum or CSF, or
- Significant change in IgM or IgG antibody response to *B. burgdorferi* in paired acute- and convalescent-phase serum samples.

Case classification

Confirmed: a case that meets one of the clinical case definitions above

Comment

This surveillance case definition was developed for national reporting of Lyme disease; it is *not* appropriate for clinical diagnosis.

Definition of terms used in the clinical description and case definition:

Erythema migrans (EM) For purposes of surveillance, EM is defined as a skin lesion that typically begins as a red macule or papule and expands over a period of days to weeks to form a large round lesion, often with partial central clearing. A solitary lesion must reach at least 5 cm in size. Secondary lesions may also occur. Annular erythematous lesions occurring within several hours of a tick bite represent hypersensitivity reactions and do not qualify as EM. For most patients, the expanding EM lesion is accompanied by other acute symptoms, particularly fatigue, fever, headache, mild stiff neck, arthralgia, or myalgia. These symptoms are typically intermittent. The diagnosis of EM must be made by a physician. Laboratory confirmation is recommended for persons with no known exposure.

Continued.

THE NATIONAL SURVEILLANCE CASE DEFINITION ADOPTED FOR USE IN THE
UNITED STATES, 1991—cont'd

Late manifestations   Late manifestations include any of the following when an alternate explanation is not found:

Musculoskeletal system   Recurrent, brief attacks (weeks or months) of objective joint swelling in one or a few joints, *sometimes* followed by chronic arthritis in one or a few joints. Manifestations not considered as criteria for diagnosis include chronic progressive arthritis not preceded by brief attacks and chronic symmetric polyarthritis. Additionally, arthralgia, myalgia, or fibromyalgia syndromes alone are not criteria for musculoskeletal involvement.

Nervous system   Any of the following, alone or in combination:
Lymphocytic meningitis; cranial neuritis, particularly facial palsy (may be bilateral); radiculoneuropathy; or, rarely, encephalomyelitis. Encephalomyelitis must be confirmed by showing antibody production against *B. burgdorferi* in the cerebrospinal fluid (CSF), demonstrated by a higher titer of antibody in CSF than in serum. Headache, fatigue, paresthesia, or mild stiff neck alone are not criteria for neurologic involvement.

Cardiovascular system   Acute onset, high-grade (2° or 3°) atrioventricular conduction defects that resolve in days to weeks and are sometimes associated with myocarditis. Palpitations, bradycardia, bundle branch block, or myocarditis alone are not criteria for cardiovascular involvement.

Exposure   Exposure is defined as having been in wooded, brushy, or grassy areas (potential tick habitats) in a county in which Lyme disease is endemic no more than 30 days before onset of EM. A history of tick bite is *not* required.

Disease endemic to county   A county in which Lyme disease is endemic is one in which at least two definite cases have been previously acquired or in which a known tick vector has been shown to be infected with *B. burgdorferi*.

Laboratory confirmation   As noted above, laboratory confirmation of infection with *B. burgdorferi* is established when a laboratory isolates the spirochete from tissue or body fluid, detects diagnostic levels of IgM or IgG antibodies to the spirochete in serum or CSF, or detects a significant change in antibody levels in paired acute- and convalescent-phase serum samples. States may determine the criteria for laboratory confirmation and diagnostic levels of antibody. Syphilis and other known causes of biologic false-positive serologic test results should be excluded when laboratory confirmation has been based on serologic testing alone.

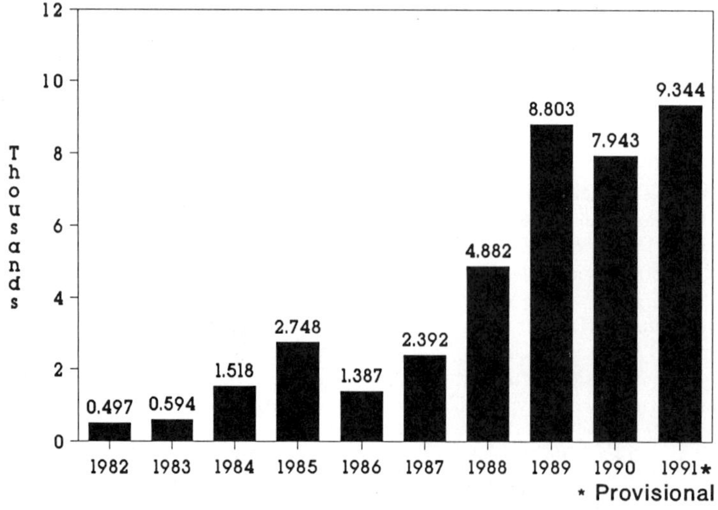

Figure 4–3 Annual totals of Lyme disease cases reported by states to the Centers for Disease Control, United States, 1982–1991.

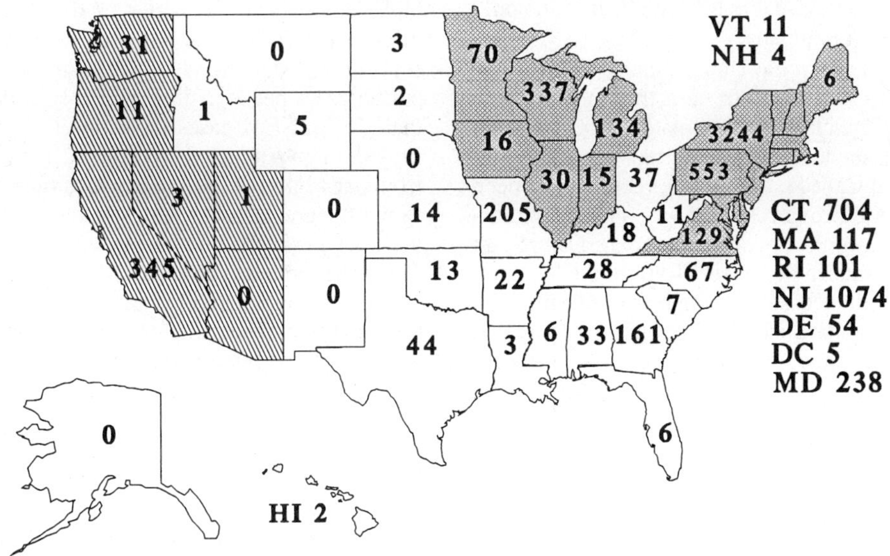

Figure 4–4 Numbers of Lyme disease cases reported by states to the Centers for Disease Control, United States, 1990. Shaded areas show distribution of known tick vectors in the East (deer tick) and in the West (western black-legged tick).

tributed to the sharp rise in reported cases over the past decade.

Geographic distribution

The map of the distribution of cases by state clearly shows the geographic concentration in the northeastern region, the north-central region, and in California (Fig. 4–4). Ten states reported 88% of all cases nationally from 1982 to 1991: 75% were reported from New York, Connecticut, New Jersey, Pennsylvania, Rhode Island, Massachusetts, and Maryland, and 13% were reported from Wisconsin, Minnesota, and California. New York alone reported 40% of cases. This clustering is highly correlated with the abundance of the known vectors, *I. dammini* and *I. pacificus*. Of all cases reported, 90% have been from the 20 states with established populations of these ticks. Incidence rates per 100,000 population range from more than 13 in the northeastern and mid-Atlantic regions to less than 0.2 in the Rocky Mountain region. The rate is about 2 per 100,000 in the north-central region and 0.9 per 100,000 in the Pacific region. Distribution within regions is also focal. Rates in the most endemic counties in Connecticut and New York range from 108 to 150 per 100,000 and are about 13 per 100,000 in endemic counties in northern California. Rates of reported cases by region are crudely related to infection rates of vector ticks with *B. burgdorferi*. Infection rates of nymphal ticks in highly endemic areas of the northeast and mid-Atlantic regions commonly range from 25%

to 50%[60] and were found to be 10% to 16% in one study in the north-central region.[15] Adult *I. pacificus* ticks usually have infection rates of only 1% to 2%.[29] The reporting of cases from areas without known enzootic transmission, such as throughout the southern, midwestern, and Rocky Mountain states, remains enigmatic. Recent unpublished epidemiologic studies in Missouri, a state that reports about 200 cases a year, have validated the occurrence of EM–like lesions with antecedent bites by the lone star tick, *Amblyomma americanum*. Spirochetes detected in *A. americanum* in Missouri differ from *B. burgdorferi*, and a causal association between these organisms and EM is not yet established. *B. burgdorferi* has not been isolated from clinical specimens from any state without known established populations of *I. dammini* or *I. pacificus*, except Texas.[46]

Spirochetes thought to be *B. burgdorferi* have been found in blood-sucking insects, such as fleas, mosquitoes, and horse flies.[36,52,72] Possible transmission of *B. burgdorferi* to humans by *A. americanum* and by horse flies has been reported.[34,52] If hematophagous arthropods other than *Ixodes* ticks do transmit *B. burgdorferi*, such occurrences are likely to be sporadic and infrequent and not to influence significantly the epidemiologic patterns of Lyme disease in the United States. *Ixodes scapularis*, a closely related species to *I. dammini* that is widely distributed in the southern United States, is capable of transmitting *B. burgdorferi* under experimental conditions[43]; however, it has a low infection rate and preferably feeds on lizards and only occasionally on humans.

In Canada, as in the United States, distribution of reported cases may not be a true indication of disease endemicity. Approximately 100 cases of Lyme disease have been reported from 7 of 12 provinces in Canada, and *Ixodes* vectors have been collected in 6 provinces; however, enzootic transmission has been established only in the Long Point peninsula, Ontario Province.[7] To improve the quality of surveillance data, Canada has recently developed a standard case definition similar to that in use in the United States, as well as criteria for identifying established populations of vector ticks.

Temporal distribution

Onsets of illness of Lyme disease in the United States are reported from all months of the year; there is, however, a marked seasonality that corresponds with human outdoor activity and with highest population densities of questing nymphal ticks in the spring and summer months. National surveillance data show that the incidence of reported cases peaks in June and July and that more than 70% of EM cases have onsets in the period May through August. The pattern differs somewhat from one region of the country to another: the curve shows the greatest seasonality in the Northeast, and the least in the Pacific coastal region (Fig. 4–5). These patterns suggest that, in North America, adult ticks are relatively unimportant in transmitting infection. The same may not be true in China, where adult *I. persulcatus* are thought to be important transmitters to humans in spring and summer.[2]

Age, sex, and racial distribution

Lyme disease affects persons in all age groups. The original description by Steere and colleagues showed a high incidence in children[68]; subsequent

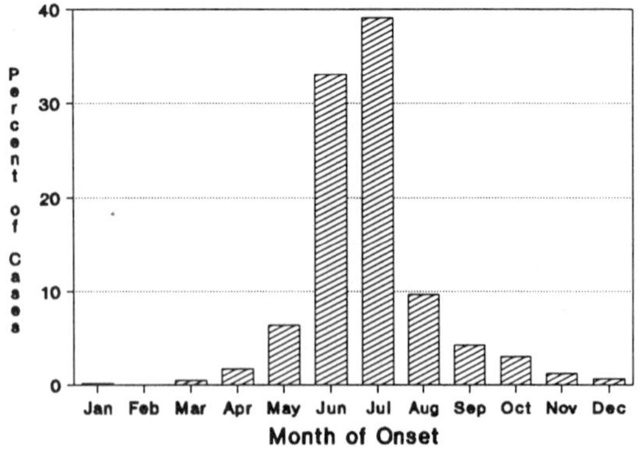

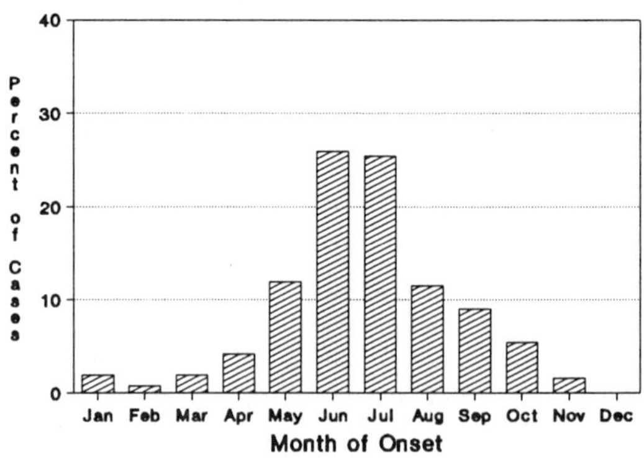

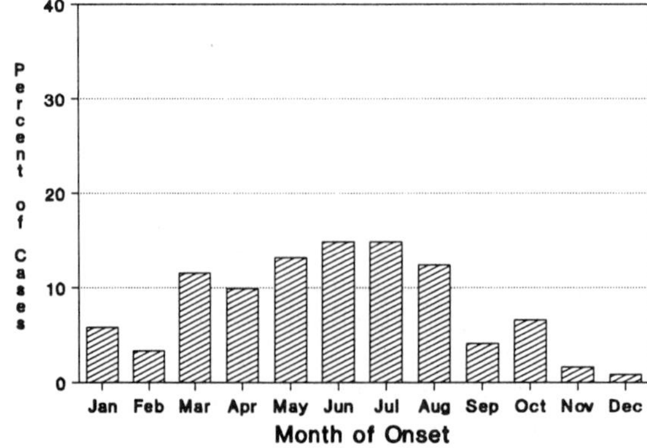

Figure 4–5 Proportional distribution of Lyme disease cases reported to the Centers for Disease Control, by month of onset, by major endemic region, United States, 1990.

Connecticut studies revealed, statewide, a peak incidence of 39 per 100,000 persons in the 5 to 9 year age group, a low of 11 per 100,000 in the age group 20 to 24 years, and a rise to rates of 20 per 100,000 or more in adults 35 years of age and older.[6] National statistics for 1990 demonstrate a similar bimodal pattern (Fig. 4–6). Highest rates for persons with EM reported in the year of disease onset are seen in the age group 0 to 9 years, and lowest rates are in the group 20 to 29 years old. On the other hand, rates for reported cases without EM (mostly arthritis) are, in the national data set, least for the age group 0 to 9, and greatest in the 10-year age groups 30 and above. The highest rates for reported Lyme disease of any clinical presentation are found in adults aged 40 to 70 years. The median age of patients in the national data set was 37 years. Females (53%) made up a greater proportion of cases than males (47%), and this differs from a slight preponderance of males reported in some previous studies. In adults, EM was reported more often in women than men in the Northeast, but, in the north-central and nonendemic regions, EM was more frequently reported in men, suggesting, perhaps, a greater peridomestic risk of infection in the Northeast, and a greater relative risk from recreational exposures in natural, nonresidential areas in the latter two areas. Some outdoor occupations, such as landscaping, forestry, and those involving trail clearing and brush removal might place men at greater risk than women; similarly, leisure activities such as hunting and fishing could bias exposure toward men. National surveillance data for 1990 present the following racial breakdown: white, 95.8%; black, 2.4%; other, 1.8%. This reflects the nonurban nature of risk, and the concentration of cases in areas of the country where minority populations are underrepresented. Recent findings of *I. dammini* in parks in Baltimore[55] and greater Philadelphia[5] raise the possibility of a developing urban risk.

OCCUPATIONAL, RECREATIONAL, AND OTHER BEHAVIORAL RISK FACTORS

A study of employees in New Jersey showed that outdoor workers were more than four times as likely to have had Lyme disease as indoor workers.[13] A comprehensive study of workers in endemic counties of downstate New York showed that persons with a history of outdoor employment were twice as likely to be seropositive than those without such a history.[57] Although this difference was not statistically significant, the seroprevalence rate of outdoor employees was 5.9 times higher than a comparison group of anonymous blood donors from the same region of New York. A study of Bavarian forest workers found serologic evidence

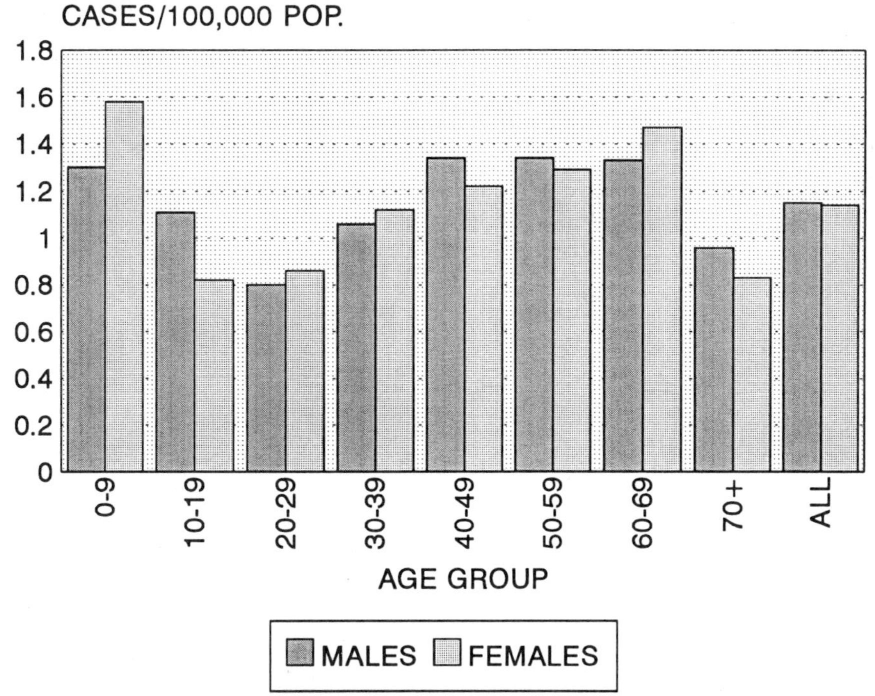

Figure 4–6 Lyme disease case rates per 100,000 reported by states to the Centers for Disease Control, by sex and age grouping, United States, 1990.

of infection in 27% of 414 persons surveyed.[41] Both studies showed associations between age, history of tick bites, a history of EM, and seropositivity. The most important risk factor for Lyme disease was, in the New York study, found to be a history of spending 30 or more hours of leisure a week outdoors, an association that was not seen in some other studies.[27,64]

Direct contact transmission between animals and humans has also been raised as a possible occupational risk factor.[14] Unpublished results of a recent study in an endemic rural area of Wisconsin failed, however, to show a greater risk of Lyme disease in dairy farmers than crop farmers. Ownership of cats was found to be associated with an increased risk of acquiring Lyme disease in early studies by Steere et al in Connecticut,[64] and domestic cats were observed to bring unattached nymphal ticks into the home in an endemic area of New York where 49% of nymphal ticks collected from vegetation were found to be infected with *B. burgdorferi*.[20] A study of dogs and of persons living in the same households in two highly endemic areas of Massachusetts showed that dogs were more likely to have serologic evidence of *B. burgdorferi* infection than their human coresidents. Although methods of selection of controls was not described, the authors noted that there was no difference in the risk of infection between people from the dog-owning households and other residents in the study sites.[25]

REFERENCES

1. Ai CX, WU XM: *Lyme disease in China.* In Stanek, editor: *Lyme borreliosis II, Zentralbl Bakteriol Mikrobiol Hyg [A]* (suppl) 18:76, New York, 1989, Gustav Fischer.
2. Ai CX et al: Epidemiological and aetiological evidence for the transmission of Lyme disease by adult *Ixodes persulcatus* in an endemic area in China, *Int J Epidemiol* 19:1061, 1990.
3. Amerasinghe FP et al: Distribution, density, and Lyme disease spirochete infection in *Ixodes dammini* (Acari: Ixodidae) on white-tailed deer in Maryland, *J Med Entomol* 29:54, 1992.
4. Anderson FJ: Mammalian and avian reservoirs for *Borrelia burgdorferi*, *Ann NY Acad Sci* 539:180, 1985.
5. Anderson JF, Duray PH, Magnarelli LA: *Borrelia burgdorferi* and *Ixodes dammini* prevalent in the greater Philadelphia area, *J Infect Dis* 161:811, 1990.
6. Anonymous: Lyme disease—Connecticut, *MMWR* 37:1, 1988.
7. Anonymous: Lyme disease in Canada, *Can Dis Weekly Rep* 16:141, 1990.
8. Anonymous: Lyme disease surveillance—United States, 1989-1990, *MMWR* 40:417, 1991.
9. Arthur DR: *The ecology of ticks with reference to the transmission of protozoa.* In Soulsby EJL, editor: *Biology of parasites*, New York, 1966, Academic Press.
10. Asbrink E, Hovmark A, Hederstedt B: The spirochetal etiology of acrodermatitis chronica atrophicans Herxheimer, *Acta Derm Venereol (Stockh)* 64:506, 1984.
11. Benach JL et al: Spirochetes isolated from the blood of two patients with Lyme disease, *N Engl J Med* 308:740, 1983.
12. Berger BW et al: Cultivation of *Borrelia burgdorferi* from erythema migrans lesions and perilesional skin, *J Clin Microbiol* 30:359, 1992.
13. Bowen SG et al: A focus of Lyme disease in Monmouth County, New Jersey, *Am J Epidemiol* 120:387, 1984.
14. Burgess EC: *Borrelia burgdorferi* infection in Wisconsin horses and cows, *Ann NY Acad Sci* 539:235, 1988.
15. Callister SM et al: *Borrelia burgdorferi* infection surrounding La Crosse, Wis., *J Clin Microbiol* 26:2632, 1988.
16. Carlberg H, Naito S: Lyme borreliosis—a review and present situation in Japan, *J Dermatol* 18:125, 1991.
17. Cartter ML, Mshar P, Hadler JL: The epidemiology of Lyme disease in Connecticut, *Conn Med* 53:320, 1989.
18. Ciesielski CA et al: The geographic distribution of Lyme disease in the United States, *Ann NY Acad Sci* 539:283, 1988.
19. Craft JE et al: Antigens of *Borrelia burgdorferi* recognized during Lyme disease: appearance of a new immunoglobulin M response and expansion of the immunoglobulin G response late in the illness, *J Clin Invest* 78:934, 1986.
20. Curran KL, Fish D: Increased risk of Lyme disease for cat owners, *N Engl J Med* 320:183, 1989 (letter).
21. Dattwyler RJ et al: Seronegative Lyme disease: dissociation of the specific T- and B-lymphocyte responses to *Borrelia burgdorferi*, *N Engl J Med* 319:1441, 1988.
22. Davis JP et al: Lyme disease in Wisconsin: epidemiologic, clinical, serologic, and entomologic findings, *Yale J Biol Med* 57:685, 1984.
23. Dekonenko EJ et al: Lyme borreliosis in the Soviet Union: a cooperative US-USSR report, *J Infect Dis* 158:748, 1988.
24. Dennis DT: Lyme disease: tracking an epidemic, *JAMA* 266:1269 (editorial).
25. Eng TR et al: Greater risk of *Borrelia burgdorferi* infection in dogs than people, *J Infect Dis* 158:1410, 1988.
26. Furman DP, Loomis EC: The ticks of California (Acari:Ixodidae), *Bull Calif Insect Surv* 25:1, 1984.
27. Hanrahan JP et al: Incidence and cumulative frequency of Lyme disease in a community, *J Infect Dis* 150:489, 1984.
28. Hedberg CW et al: An interlaboratory study of antibody to *Borrelia burgdorferi*, *J Infect Dis* 155:1325, 1987.
29. Lane RS, Piesman J, Burgdorfer W: Lyme borreliosis: relation of its causative agent to its vector and hosts in North America and Europe, *Annu Rev Entomol* 36:587, 1991.
30. Lastavica CC et al: Rapid emergence of a focal epidemic of Lyme disease in coastal Massachusetts, *N Engl J Med* 320:133.
31. Lindenmayer JM, Marshall D, Onderdonk AB: Dogs as sentinels for Lyme disease in Massachusetts, *Am J Public Health* 81:1448, 1991.
32. Logigian EL, Kaplan RF, Steere AC: Chronic neurologic manifestations of Lyme disease, *N Engl J Med* 323:1438, 1990.
33. Lord R: (in press).
34. Luger SW: Lyme disease transmitted by a biting fly, *N Engl J Med* 322:1752, 1990.
35. Luger SW, Krause E: Serologic tests for Lyme disease: interlaboratory variability, *Arch Intern Med* 150:761, 1990.
36. Magnarelli LA, Anderson JF, Barbour AG: The etiologic agent of Lyme disease in deer flies, horse flies and mosquitoes, *J Infect Dis* 154:355, 1986.
37. Magnarelli LA, Anderson JF, Johnson RC: Cross-reactivity in serological tests for Lyme disease and other spirochetal infections, *J Infect Dis* 156:183, 1987.
38. Maupin GO et al: Landscape ecology of Lyme disease in a residential area of Westchester County, New York, *Am J Epidemiol* 133:1105, 1991.
39. Miller SL et al: The epidemiology of Lyme disease in the United States 1987–1988, *Lab Med* 21:285, 1990.

40. Nelson JA et al: Isolation and characterization of *Borrelia burgdorferi* from Illinois *Ixodes dammini*, *J Clin Microbiol* 29:1732, 1991.

41. Neubert U et al: *Borrelia burgdorferi* infections in Bavarian forest workers: a follow-up study, *Ann NY Acad Sci* 539:476, 1988.

42. Persing DH et al: Description of *Borrelia burgdorferi* DNA in museum specimens of *Ixodes dammini* ticks, *Science* 249:1420, 1990.

43. Piesman J, Sinsky RJ: Ability of *Ixodes scapularis, Dermacentor variabilis,* and *Amblyomma americanum* (Acari:Ixodidae) to acquire, maintain, and transmit Lyme disease spirochetes *(Borrelia burgdorferi)*, *J Med Entomol* 25:336, 1988.

44. Preac-Mursic V et al: Survival of *Borrelia burgdorferi* in antibiotically treated patients with Lyme borreliosis, *Infection* 17:355, 1989.

45. Rand PW, Smith RP, Lacombe EH: Canine seroprevalence and the distribution of *Ixodes dammini* in an area of emerging Lyme disease, *Am J Public Health* 81:1331, 1991.

46. Rawlings JA, Fournier PV, Teltow GJ: Isolation of *Borrelia* spirochetes from patients in Texas, *J Clin Microbiol* 25:1148, 1982.

47. Schafrank SN, Kurba AK, Martone G: Lyme disease acquired in South Africa, *Arch Dermatol* 126:685, 1990 (correspondence).

48. Schlesinger PA et al: Maternal-fetal transmission of the Lyme disease spirochete, *Borrelia burgdorferi*, *Ann Intern Med* 103:67, 1985.

49. Schmid GP: The global distribution of Lyme disease, *Rev Infect Dis* 7:41, 1985.

50. Schmid GP et al: Surveillance of Lyme disease in the United States, 1982, *J Infect Dis* 151:1144.

51. Schoen RT et al: Treatment of refractory chronic Lyme arthritis with arthroscopic synovectomy, *Arthritis Rheum* 34:1056, 1991.

52. Schulze TL et al: *Amblyomma americanum:* a potential vector of Lyme disease in New Jersey, *Science* 224:601, 1984.

53. Schulze TL et al: Evolution of a focus of Lyme disease, *Zentralbl Bakteriol Mikrobiol Hyg [A]* 263:65, 1986.

54. Schwartz BS et al: Antibody testing in Lyme disease; a comparison of results in four laboratories, *JAMA* 262:3431, 1989.

55. Schwartz BS et al: Lyme borreliosis in an inner-city park in Baltimore, *Am J Public Health* 81:803, 1991.

56. Sigal LH et al: Proliferative responses of mononuclear cells in Lyme disease: reactivity to *Borrelia burgdorferi* antigens is greater in joint fluid than in blood, *Arthritis Rheum* 19:761, 1986.

57. Smith PF et al: Occupational risk of Lyme disease in endemic areas of New York State, *Ann NY Acad Sci* 539:289, 1988.

58. Snydman DR et al: *Borrelia burgdorferi* in joint fluid in chronic Lyme arthritis, *Ann Intern Med* 104:798, 1986.

59. Spielman A: Human babesiosis on Nantucket Island: transmission by nymphal *Ixodes* ticks, *Am J Trop Med Hyg* 25:784, 1976.

60. Spielman A et al: Human babesiosis on Nantucket Island, USA: description of the vector, *Ixodes dammini,* n. sp. (Acari: Ixodidae), *J Med Entomol* 15:218, 1979.

61. Spielman A et al: *Ixodes dammini*-borne human babesiosis and Lyme disease, *Annu Rev Entomol* 30:439, 1985.

62. Stanek G et al: Isolation of *Borrelia burgdorferi* from the myocardium of a patient with longstanding cardiomyopathy, *N Engl J Med* 322:249, 1990.

63. Steere AC: Lyme disease, *New Engl J Med* 321:586, 1989.

64. Steere AC, Broderick TF, Malawista SE: Erythema chronicum migrans and Lyme arthritis: epidemiologic evidence for a tick vector, *Am J Epidemiol* 108:312, 1978.

65. Steere AC, Dwyer E, Winchester R: Association of chronic Lyme arthritis with HLA-DR4 and HLA-DR2 alleles, *N Engl J Med* 323:219, 1990.

66. Steere AC, Malawista SE: Cases of Lyme disease in the United States: locations correlated with distribution of *Ixodes dammini, Ann Intern Med* 91:730, 1979.

67. Steere AC et al: The early clinical manifestations of Lyme disease, *Ann Intern Med* 99:76, 1983.

68. Steere AC et al: Lyme arthritis: an epidemic of oligoarticular arthritis in children and adults in three Connecticut communities, *Arthritis Rheum* 20:7.

69. Steere AC et al: Longitudinal assessment of the clinical and epidemiologic features of Lyme disease in a defined population, *J Infect Dis* 154:295, 1986.

70. Stewart A et al: Lyme arthritis in the Hunter Valley, *Med J Aust* 1:139, 1982.

71. Telford SR III et al: Incompetence of deer as reservoirs of the Lyme disease spirochete, *Am J Trop Med Hyg* 39:105, 1988.

72. Teltow SJ, Fournier PV, Rawlings JA: Isolation of *Borrelia burgdorferi* from arthropods collected in Texas, *Am J Trop Med Hyg* 44:469, 1991.

73. Thacker SB, Choi K, Brachman PS: The surveillance of infectious diseases, *JAMA* 249:1181, 1983.

74. Tsai TF, Bailey RE, Moore PS: National surveillance of Lyme disease, 1987–1988, *Conn Med* 53:324, 1989.

75. Weber K et al: Reinfection with erythema migrans disease, *Infection* 14:32, 1986.

76. Weber K et al: *Borrelia burgdorferi* in a newborn despite oral penicillin for Lyme borreliosis during pregnancy, *Pediatr Infect Dis J* 7:286, 1988.

77. White DJ et al: The geographic spread and temporal increase of the Lyme disease epidemic, *JAMA* 266:1230, 1991.

78. Williams CL et al: Lyme disease: epidemiologic characteristics of an outbreak in Westchester County, NY, *Am J Public Health* 76:62, 1986.

79. Wills MC, Barry RD: Detecting the cause of Lyme disease in Australia, *Med J Aust* 155:275, 1991 (letter).

80. Wilson ML, Adler GH, Spielman A: Correlation between abundance of deer and that of the deer tick, *Ixodes dammini* (Acari: Ixodidae), *Ann Entomol Soc Am* 78:172, 1985.

81. Wilson ML et al: Reduced abundance of immature *Ixodes dammini* (Acari:Ixodidae) following elimination of deer, *J Med Entomol* 25:224, 1988.

5

Genetic Basis of Chronic Lyme Disease

Edward Dwyer and *Robert Winchester*

Most people do not experience the late manifestations of infection with the tick-borne spirochete, *Borrelia burgdorferi,* which characteristically involve sustained inflammation of the joints, central nervous system, and heart. However, for a subset of approximately 10% of infected patients, a chronic inflammatory disorder develops, which may persist despite appropriate therapeutic intervention. The unremitting involvement of individual organ systems resulting from exposure to *B. burgdorferi* often resembles more familiar chronic inflammatory diseases, especially those thought to have autoimmune components. This discussion centers on the genetic basis for developing arthritis as a late and chronic manifestation of Lyme disease, and contrasts the current understanding of the immunogenetic basis for some people to develop this response with the immunogenetics that predispose to rheumatoid arthritis. The special circumstance of Lyme arthritis is created by knowledge of the inciting agent of a chronic inflammatory arthritis, and an analysis of this may have relevance not only to understanding Lyme disease but may also be pertinent to elucidating the mechanisms responsible for other chronic inflammatory disorders with autoimmune features.

PREDISPOSITION TO RHEUMATOID ARTHRITIS

The histopathologic lesion of the synovium in people with chronic Lyme arthritis is similar to that of rheumatoid arthritis; hyperplasia of the synovial lining layer and a dense lymphocytic infiltration of the underlying stroma are cardinal features of both diseases. Similar to rheumatoid arthritis, the lesion of Lyme arthritis can also result in erosion of bone and cartilage with consequent permanent joint destruction. A genetic predisposition to develop many autoimmune diseases, especially rheumatoid arthritis, has been linked to alleles of certain genomic loci of the major histocompatibility complex (MHC). This was initially detected as correlations between certain human leukocyte antigen (HLA) specificities, such as DR4 and DR1, and rheumatoid disease. Using the results of nucleotide se-

quencing of genetically different reference DR4 individuals, and correlating the ethnic distributions of these DR4 alleles with rheumatoid arthritis in different populations, the data were explained by postulating a "shared epitope" common to several DR4 susceptibility alleles.[2] Subsequent sequences obtained in rheumatoid patients with DR1 and DR10 further substantiated the critical importance of this "shared epitope" in conferring susceptibility. More recently, the alleles have been further defined through the use of sequence-specific oligonucleotide (SSO) typing of MHC molecules.*

The MHC genetic elements responsible for rheumatoid arthritis susceptibility, located on the short arm of chromosome 6, encode proteins that form membrane-bound heterodimers that are responsible for presenting antigenic peptide fragments recognized by T cells in the process of initiating an immune response. These molecules can be classified as either class I, which are expressed on all somatic tissues and are responsible for presenting antigens to CD8+ T cells, or as class II, which are expressed almost exclusively on B cells and monocyte-derived cell lineages such as tissue macrophages, which present antigen to CD4+ T cells. A salient feature of these MHC gene products is the considerable degree of polymorphism, or allelic diversity, that is typified by many of the loci in this gene complex. This polymorphism is a consequence of discrete differences in primary amino acid structure among alleles of a given locus, and these structural differences are generally restricted to three relatively well-defined regions of the molecule, termed the first, second, and third diversity regions. The predicted tertiary structure of the MHC class II molecule is shown in Fig. 5–1. The association of particular autoimmune disorders with certain MHC class I or class II alleles whose structural uniqueness is often restricted to only a few amino acids in one of these three diversity regions suggests the critical importance of definitive molecular interactions in predisposing toward

---

*See Reference 6 for a more complete description on the genetics of rheumatoid arthritis.

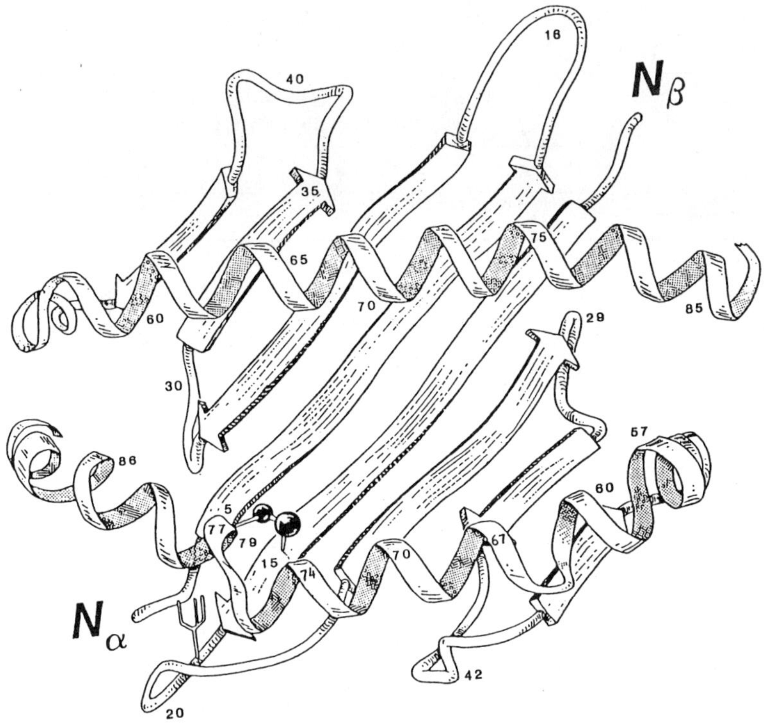

Figure 5–1 MHC class II molecule. The DR heterodimer includes a monomorphic α chain and a polymorphic β chain; the amino acid numbers correspond to those in Table 5–1. The first diversity region (amino acids 9 to 13) and the second diversity region (amino acids 26 to 30) are located on two adjacent strands of the anti-parallel β-pleated sheet. The third diversity region (amino acids 67 to 74) is located on the lower of the two α-helical structures.

susceptibility to these diseases (Table 5–1).

In general, the influence of the expression of MHC gene products in the genesis of an immune response can be conceptualized as originating at two distinct stages of T-cell differentiation and development. First, in the thymus, immature T cells are exposed to the process of "negative selection" whereby T cells reactive to self-peptides associated with MHC molecules are eliminated from the repertoire, thus preventing the population of the periphery with mature autoreactive T cells. Also during thymic maturation, the process of "positive selection" results in the creation of an "MHC-restricted" repertoire whereby foreign antigenic peptides are capable of recognition by T cells strictly in association with self-MHC molecules, and not by other allelic variants. Second, MHC class I and II molecules can be directly involved in determining the characteristics of a tissue-specific mature T cell response by discriminately selecting specific antigenic peptides to be presented to CD4 + or CD8 + T cells. Which foreign peptide is selected may differ in accordance with which MHC allele is involved in the antigen presentation event.

As an example of a chronic inflammatory disease with MHC associations, rheumatoid arthritis sus-

ceptibility has been well-documented to be associated with the expression of certain alleles of the DR loci of the MHC class II region. As the DRα chain monomer is monomorphic, susceptibility has focused on the paired polymorphic β chain whose genomic organization on chromosome 6 is depicted in Fig. 5–2. In particular, it is well-documented that specific DRβ chains associated with the HLA DR4 specificity (e.g., DRB1*0401, DRB1*0404, and DRB1*0405), as well as the β chain of DR1 and the DR6 subtype DRB1*1402 are all associated with increased risk toward developing rheumatoid arthritis. All of these alleles share unique conserved amino acids, L Q K/R A, in the third diversity region at positions 67, 70, 71 and 74, respectively (Table 5–1); these amino acids define the "shared epitope." In contrast, these alleles do not show a similar identity in the structure of the first and second diversity regions of the β chain. This observation strongly implicates the α-helical region of the molecule from residues 67-74 as determining susceptibility to rheumatoid arthritis (see Fig. 5–1). Of course, whether these DRβ alleles are functional in disease pathogenesis at the phase of thymic development or are operative in the periphery at the level of antigen presentation to mature T cells remains to be determined.

Table 5-1 Major sites of sequence polymorphism among DRβ chain alleles illustrating patchwork pattern of developing variability from recombination of a smaller number of antecedent genes*

| | | Amino acid positions in DRβ chain diversity regions† | | | | | | | | | | | | | |
| | | First | | | Second | | | | Third | | | | | | |
Serologic specificity	Determinant	9	11	13	26	28	30	37	57	67	70	71	74	86	DR locus and allele
DR1	Dw1	W	L	F	L	E	C	S	D	L	Q	R	A	G	B1*0101
DR1	Dw20	W	L	F	L	E	C	S	D	L	Q	R	A	V	B1*0102
DR103	DwBON	W	L	F	L	E	C	S	D	I	D	E	A	V	B1*0103
DR2(15)	Dw2	Q	D	Y	F	H	D	D	D	F	D	R	A	G	B1*1501
DR2(15)	Dw12	Q	D	Y	F	H	G	N	D	F	D	R	A	G	B1*1502
DR2(16)	Dw21,AZH	Q	D	Y	F	H	G	N	D	I	Q	R	A	V	B1*1601
DR3(17)	Dw3	E	S	S	Y	D	Y	H	D	L	Q	K	R	V	B1*0301
DR4	Dw4	E	V	H	F	D	Y	Y	D	L	Q	K	A	G	B1*0401
DR4	Dw14	E	V	H	F	D	Y	Y	D	L	Q	R	A	V	B1*0404
DR4	Dw14	E	V	H	F	D	Y	Y	D	L	Q	R	A	G	B1*0408
DR4	Dw15	E	V	H	F	D	Y	Y	S	L	Q	R	A	G	B1*0405
DR4	Dw10	E	V	H	F	D	Y	Y	D	I	D	E	A	V	B1*0402
DR4	Dw13	E	V	H	F	D	Y	Y	D	L	Q	R	E	V	B1*0403
DR4	Dw13	E	V	H	F	D	Y	Y	D	L	Q	R	E	G	B1*0407
DR4	DwKT2	E	V	H	F	D	Y	S	D	L	Q	R	E	V	B1*0406
DR5(11)	Dw5	E	S	S	F	D	Y	Y	D	F	D	R	A	G	B1*11011
DR5(11)	DwJVM	E	S	S	F	D	Y	Y	D	I	D	E	A	V	B1*1102
DR6a(13)	Dw18	E	S	S	F	D	Y	N	D	I	D	E	A	V	B1*1301
DR6b(14)	Dw9	E	S	S	F	D	Y	F	A	L	R	E	E	V	B1*1401
DR6(14)	Amala,Dw16	E	S	S	F	E	Y	N	D	L	Q	R	A	G	B1*1402
DR7	Dw17	W	G	Y	F	E	L	F	V	I	D	R	Q	G	B1*0701
DR8	Dw8.1, MADURA	E	S	G	F	D	Y	Y	S	F	D	R	L	G	B1*0801
DR9	Dw23	K	D	F	Y	H	G	N	V	F	R	R	E	G	B1*09011
DR10		E	V	F	L	E	R	Y	D	L	R	R	A	G	B1*1001
DR52a	Dw24	E	R	S	Y	D	H	F	V	L	Q	K	R	G	B3*0101
DR25b	Dw25	E	R	S	F	E	H	Y	D	L	Q	K	R	V	B3*0201
DR52c	Dw26	E	R	S	F	E	Y	L	V	L	Q	K	R	G	B3*0301
DR53		E	A	C	N	I	Y	Y	D	L	R	R	E	V	B4*0101
DR51	Dw2	W	P	R	F	D	Y	S	D	I	Q	A	A	V	B5*0101
DR51	Dw21,AZH	W	P	R	F	D	Y	S	D	F	D	R	A	G	B5*0201

*Gene conversion or intragenic recombination, methods of lateral gene transfer, appear to be the way in which the current repertoire of alleles was assembled from portions of antecedent genes. The serologic specificities correlate well with the sequence of the first diversity region shown in single letter amino acid code. A family of structurally related sequences include the DR3, 5, and 6 alleles. These share the DRB3 locus, which encodes the DR52 specificity (see Fig. 5-2). In the case of the second diversity region, DR4 shares a sequence with members of this family. The third diversity is of greatest interest because it is completely dissociated from the first two regions. Seven basic patterns are used for the various genes. For example, IDEA is found in DR1 Bon, DR4, Dw10, and DR6a. The sharing of LQ R/K A is found in DR1 Dw1, DR4, Dw4, Dw14, Dw15, and DR6 DRB1 *1402, the presence of which are all associated with susceptibility to rheumatoid arthritis.

† A = alanine, C = cystine, D = asparagine, E = glutamic acid, F = phenylalanine, G = glycine, H = histidine, I = ile, K = lysine, L = leucine, M = methionine, N = asparagine, P = proline, Q = glutamine, R = arginine, S = serine, T = threonine, V = valine, W = tryptophan, Y = tyrosine.

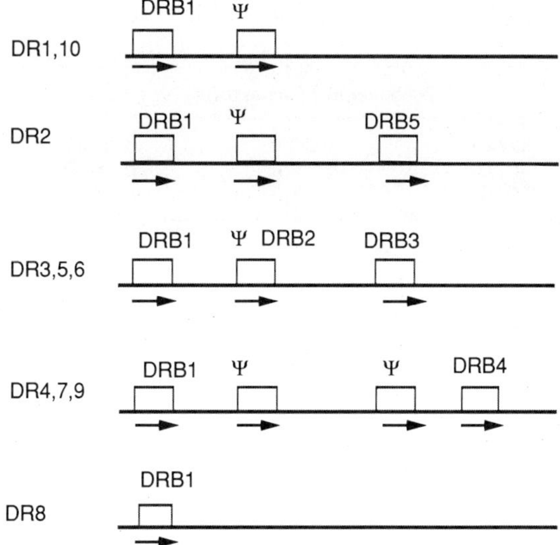

Figure 5–2 Organization of the DRβ region of the MHC class II genes. The allele occupying the DRB1 locus encodes the primary DR specificity (e.g., DR1, DR2, and so forth). The locus with the gene coding the secondary DR specificity varies according to the DR type. In the DR2 haplotype it is the DRB5 locus. In DR4 haplotypes it is the DRB4 locus. The genes at these loci encode, respectively, the DR51 and DR53 specificities. Note these two genes are not true alleles because the locus is different.

PREDISPOSITION TO CHRONIC LYME ARTHRITIS

The similarity of the synovial histopathologic lesions of Lyme arthritis to those of rheumatoid arthritis has prompted an examination of whether the two diseases also demonstrate similar features of genetic susceptibility. As discussed above, the development of an inflammatory arthritis several months after exposure to *B. burgdorferi* is a well-documented sequelae to infection with the organism. However, the duration of the arthritis and response to antibiotic therapy can be quite variable in this subset of patients. Interestingly, a longitudinal study of the relationship between Lyme arthritis and HLA phenotype has revealed a complex relationship whereby certain HLA specificities confer susceptibility not toward the acquisition of inflammatory arthritis once exposed to the spirochete, but rather appear to influence the immunocompetence of the host to resolve successfully the inflammation and prevent the evolution into a chronic arthritic disorder.

Initial examination of an entire cohort of 80 people with Lyme arthritis failed to demonstrate a straightforward relationship between HLA pheno-

type and susceptibility to Lyme arthritis. However, if the group of patients is further subdivided according to whether the arthritis was of brief (1 to 5 months), moderate (6 to 11 months), or chronic (12 to 48 months) duration, a significant relationship emerges correlating HLA specificity with the presence of a chronic arthritis, as shown in Table 5–2.[5] The primary association with a chronic arthritis is with HLA DR4 where 57% of 28 patients with chronic arthritis possess the DR4 specificity as compared to either a frequency of 9% in the group with brief arthritis (relative risk = 13) or to a frequency of 31% in a control population (relative risk = 3; Table 5–2). This observation was of great interest because it superficially appeared to resemble the situation in rheumatoid arthritis. A secondary association can also be demonstrated with the presence of the DR2 specificity, which was present in 43% of those with chronic arthritis as compared to an 18% incidence in the group with short duration (relative risk = 12) or a 26% frequency in a control population (relative risk = 5). Taken together, the data reveal that 89% of people with chronic arthritis exhibit either a DR4 or DR2 specificity as compared to 27% in the group with arthritis of brief duration; this relationship does not appear to be synergistic, however, in that DR2/DR4 heterozygosity does not appear to be increased beyond what would be predicted from the gene frequency of the individual DR specificities.

COMPARISON OF IMMUNOGENETIC PATTERNS IN CHRONIC LYME ARTHRITIS AND RHEUMATOID ARTHRITIS

Although both chronic Lyme arthritis and rheumatoid arthritis exhibit susceptibility patterns that demonstrate an increased frequency of the DR4 phenotype, it appears on closer examination that the molecular bases at the gene level are discordant in that the two disorders encompass partially overlapping yet not at all identical allelic profiles. As discussed above, the DR4 subtypes found to be increased in frequency in rheumatoid arthritis (DRB1*0401, DRB1*0404, and DRB1*0405) all express DRβ chains that share common third diversity region amino acid structure. Conversely, other DR4 subtypes that lack this common third diversity region structure, such as DRB1*0402, DRB1*0403, and DRB1*0407, are not preferentially associated with susceptibility to rheumatoid arthritis.

To examine whether a similar structural relationship exists in conferring susceptibility to chronic Lyme arthritis in the study outlined above, direct nucleotide sequencing of DRβ gene products

Table 5–2 Frequency of HLA-DR specificities in 80 patients with Lyme arthritis and 86 normal subjects[5]

		Duration of Lyme arthritis*		
Specificity	Normal subject ($N = 86$)	Short ($N = 22$) (%)	Moderate ($N = 30$) (%)	Chronic ($N = 28$) (%)
HLA-DR1	29	18	20	21
HLA-DR2	26	18	40	43
HLA-DR3	17	23	13	29
HLA-DR4	31	9	23	57†
HLA-DR5	28	32	20	14
HLA-DR6	10	18	10	0
HLA-DR7	22	18	17	11
HLA-DR2 or HLA-DR4	53	27	63	89‡
HLA-DR52	62	88§	40	37
HLA-DR53	52	31	50	68
HLA-DQ1	56	69	60	53
HLA-DQ2	30	38	20	32
HLA-DQ3	32	63	55	74‖

*For the HLA-DR52, HLA-DR53, and HLA-DQ specificities, the numbers tested were as follows: short duration, $n = 16$; moderate duration, $n = 20$; chronic, $n = 19$.

†$P = 0.003$ for the comparison between patients with chronic arthritis and those with arthritis of short duration; $P = 0.1$ for the comparison between patients with chronic arthritis and normal subjects.

‡$P = 0.00006$ for the comparison between patients with chronic arthritis and those with arthritis of short duration; $P = 0.002$ for the comparison between patients with chronic arthritis and normal subjects.

§$P = 0.003$ for the comparison between patients with arthritis of short duration and those with chronic arthritis; $P = 0.005$ for the comparison between patients with arthritis of short duration and those with arthritis of moderate duration.

‖$P = 0.003$ for the comparison between patients with chronic arthritis and normal subjects.

in selected patients was undertaken (Tables 5–3 and 5–4).[5] Of the four DR4 patients studied, one exhibited the DRB1*0403 allele, which would not be anticipated if the third diversity region "shared epitope" was the critical genetic determinant. This finding suggests that it is the polymorphic β-pleated sheet sequences of the first and second diversity regions, common to all DR4 alleles, that induce susceptibility to chronic Lyme arthritis. Further evidence supporting the contrasting immunogenetic patterns in chronic Lyme arthritis compared to that of rheumatoid arthritis is a recent study using SSO methodology,[3] that revealed the presence of the DRB1*0407 allele in a sample of Lyme disease patients with chronic arthritis. This also encodes the Dw13 determinant found in DRB1*0403 and, similarly, does not express the rheumatoid arthritis "shared epitope." Both of these studies support an immunogenetic basis for chronic Lyme arthritis that is distinct from that of rheumatoid arthritis. Additional observations that further support this interpretation are that the DR1 specificity, which is associated with susceptibility for rheumatoid arthritis, and also expresses the "shared epitope," has not been found to be increased in frequency in any of the groups with Lyme arthritis. Reciprocally,

DR2 is increased in chronic Lyme disease,[5] a specificity not increased in rheumatoid arthritis.

Although the DR4 and DR2 DRB1 alleles associated with Lyme disease susceptibility (DRB1*0401, *0403, *0404, *0407, and *1501) share no extended region of polymorphic sequence in the third diversity region, it is noted that the closely linked DRB5*0101 allele (Table 5–1) of the DRB5 locus present in the DR2 haplotype (Fig. 5–2), shares with the DR4 alleles the amino acid motif of F D Y at positions 26, 28, and 30, in the second diversity region located in the floor of the antigen-binding groove. Furthermore, and possibly of equal significance, the structurally adjacent position 13 of the first diversity region exhibits a positively charged amino acid residue at this position in only the DRB1 alleles of DR4 and the DRB5 alleles of DR2 (e.g., histidine for DR4 DRB1 and arginine for DR2 DRB5). The overlapping, yet distinct, associations of specific amino acid motifs in the three diversity regions with either chronic Lyme arthritis or rheumatoid arthritis are depicted in Table 5–5. This analysis would suggest, to the extent that the first and second diversity regions are structurally distinct from the third diversity region, that the pathogenic mechanisms re-

Table 5–3 Inferred amino acid sequences of DR2 and DR4 haplotype genes determined from patients with Lyme disease

	10	20	30	40
DR4 Dw4 DRB1*0401	G D T R P R F L E Q	V K H E C H F F N G	T E R V R F L D R Y	F Y H Q E E Y V R F
DR4 Dw13 DRB1*0403	G D T R P R F L E Q	V K H E C H F F N G	T E R V R F L D R Y	F Y H Q E E Y V R F
DR4 Dw14 DRB1*0404	G D T R P R F L E Q	V K H E C H F F N G	T E R V R F L D R Y	F Y H Q E E Y V R F
DR2 Dw2 DRB1*1501	G D T R P R F L Q Q	D K Y E C H F F N G	T E R V R F L H R D	Y Y N Q E E D L R F
DR4 Dw53 DRB4*0101	G D T Q E A C L E Q	A K C E C H F L N G	T E R V W N L I R Y	I Y N Q E E Y A R Y
DR2 Dw2 DRB5*0101	G D T Q P R F L W Q	P K R E C H F F N G	T E R V R F L D R Y	F Y H Q E E Y V R F

	50	60	70	80	90
DR4 Dw4 DRB1*0401	D S D V G E Y R A V	T E L G R P D A E Y	W N S Q K D L L E Q	K R A A V D T Y C R	H N Y G V G E S F T V Q R R
DR4 Dw13 DRB1*0403	D S D V G E Y R A V	T E L G R P D A E Y	W N S Q K D L L E Q	R R A E V D T Y C R	H N Y G V V E S F T V Q R R
DR4 Dw14 DRB1*0404	D S D V G E Y R A V	T E L G R P D A E Y	W N S Q K D L L E Q	R R A A V D T Y C R	H N Y G V V E S F T V Q R R
DR2 Dw2 DRB1*1501	D S D V G E Y R A V	T E L G I P D A E Y	W N S Q K D F L E D	A R A A V D T Y C R	H N Y G V G E S F T V Q R R
DR4 Dw53 DRB4*0101	N S D L G E Y Q A V	T E L G R P D A E Y	W N S Q K D L L E R	R R A E V D T Y C R	Y N Y G V V E S F T V Q R R
DR2 Dw2 DRB5*0101	D S D V G E F R A V	T E L G R P D A E Y	W N S Q K D I L E Q	A R A A V D T Y C R	H N Y G V G E S F T V Q R R

Table 5–4 Nucleotide-sequence typing of the HLA-DRβ chain in five representative patients with chronic Lyme arthritis

	Serologic typing	Nucleotide-sequence
1	DR1,DR4	Dw1,Dw4 (DRB1*0401,*0101,DRB4*0101)
2	DR2,DR4	Dw2,Dw14 (DRB1*1501,*0404,DRB4*0101,DRB5*0101)
3	DR3,DR4	Dw3,Dw14 (DRB1*0301,*0404,DRB3*0101,DRB4*0101)
4	DR2,DR4	Dw2,Dw13 (DRB1*1501,*0403,DRB4*0101,DRB5*0101)
5	DR2,DR3	Dw2,DR3 (DRB1*1501,*0301,DRB3*0101,DRB5*0101)

Table 5–5 The molecular basis of susceptibility to rheumatoid arthritis is different from that for Lyme disease

| | Diversity region | | | | | | | | | | | Disease | |
| | First | | | Second | | | | Third | | | | | |
Allele	9	11	13	26	28	30	37	67	70	71	74	Lyme	RA
DRB1*0101	W	L	F	L	E	C	S	L	Q	R	A	−	+
DRB1*1501	Q	D	Y	F	H	D	D	F	D	R	A	+	−
DRB5*0101	W	P	R	F	D	Y	S	F	D	R	A	+	−
DRB4*0401	E	V	H	F	D	Y	Y	L	Q	K	A	+	+
DRB4*0402	E	V	H	F	D	Y	Y	I	D	E	A	(+)	−
DRB4*0403	E	V	H	F	D	Y	Y	L	Q	R	E	+	−
DRB4*0404	E	V	H	F	D	Y	Y	L	Q	R	A	+	+
DRB1*0405	E	V	H	F	D	Y	Y	L	Q	R	A	(+)	+

sponsible for inducing chronic Lyme arthritis may be quite different from those associated with rheumatoid arthritis.

Regardless of the molecular basis of pathogenic mechanisms involved in the heritable susceptibility to chronic Lyme arthritis, the aspect of this inheritance pattern that should be emphasized is that it is the natural history of a sustained inflammatory arthritis, rather than the potential for developing arthritis early in the infection, that appears to be most closely linked with the DR4 and DR2 specificities. In other words, the presence of either DR4 or DR2 in the host in the setting of *B. burgdorferi* infection appears to increase significantly the likelihood that chronic inflammatory synovitis will result. Whether the chronicity is a consequence of a "reactive" arthritis with autoimmune features, or, alternatively, is, in fact, a result of the failure of the host to initiate and maintain an effective immune response to eradicate the organism remains to be determined.

In the first instance, it would be anticipated that people with the DR2 or DR4 specificity exhibit a unique CD4+ T-cell repertoire that when presented with *B. burgdorferi* antigenic peptides by certain self-MHC class II molecules elicits both immune reactivity to the organism as well as simultaneously activating heretofore quiescent autoreactive CD4+ cells, which are responsive to self-antigens. In the second case, it would be predicted that the influence of class II DR molecules during T-cell maturation in the thymus results in a peripheral T-cell repertoire that is at least partially deficient in establishing requisite cell-mediated and humoral immunity toward the spirochete; such an immune constitution with a "hole in the repertoire" would have resulted from the unintended deletion of potential borrelial reactive CD4+ T-cell clones during the thymic process of negative selection, which deletes potentially autoreactive cells.

That the immune response to *B. burgdorferi* may be compromised in some people was suggested by the early finding of a persistence of the organism in synovial tissue obtained from patients with chronic destructive arthritis related to Lyme disease, some of whom had also received appropriate antibiotic therapy.[4] More recent characterizations of the immune response to the organism in patients with chronic Lyme arthritis has revealed a borrelial-reactive CD4+ T-cell compartment entirely populated by clones that exclusively produce and secrete the cytokines γ-interferon and interleukin (IL) 2, both of which are regarded as essential in developing a cell-mediated delayed hypersensitivity response, but may actually inhibit the generation of an effective antibody response to the organism; none of the clones exhibited a capacity to produce IL-4 or IL-5, the CD4 T-cell-derived cytokines that are regarded as crucial for stimulating B-cell immunoglobulin production in the generation of a competent humoral immune response.[7] The potential importance of establishing an antibody response to the spirochete has been demonstrated by the observation that only mice possessing antiborrelial antibodies are protected from infection with the organism.[1] Extrapolating these findings to the genesis of human arthritis, it may be the case that eradicating *B. burgdorferi* from synovial tissue may demand the localized presence of CD4 + T cells that are capable of assisting resident B cells in the generation of an adequate antibody response; the absence of such CD4 + T cells may result in a "nonspecific" inflammatory response to the organism that is ineffective in establishing a "specific" immune response that eventually results in its eradication. Of course, at present, factors responsible for dictating the cytokine profile of individual responsive CD4 + T cells have not been identified. Perhaps the association of specific spirochetal peptides in association with certain DR alleles during antigen presentation, such as DR4 or DR2, may be a determinant in the differentiation of responding CD4 + T cells into clones that exclusively produce γ-interferon and IL-2, and not IL-4 and IL-5.

ACKNOWLEDGMENT

We thank Ms. Modrie Payne for excellent assistance in preparation of the chapter.

REFERENCES

1. Fikrig ES et al: Protection of mice against the Lyme disease agent by immunizing with recombinant OspA, *Science* 250:553, 1990.
2. Gregersen PK, Silver J, Winchester RJ: The shared epitope hypothesis—an approach to understanding the molecular genetics of rheumatoid arthritis susceptibility, *Arthritis Rheum* 30:1205, 1987.
3. Ruberti G et al: Molecular analysis of the role of HLA class II genes DRB1, DQB1, and DPB1 in susceptibility to Lyme arthritis, *Hum Immunol* 31:20, 1991.
4. Steere AC, Duray PH, Butcher EC: Spirochetal antigens and lymphoid cell surface markers in Lyme synovitis. Comparison with rheumatoid synovium and tonsillar lymphoid tissue, *Arthritis Rheum* 31:487, 1988.
5. Steere AC, Dwyer E, Winchester R: Association of chronic Lyme arthritis with increased frequencies of DR4 and DR3, *N Engl J Med* 323:219, 1990.
6. Winchester R, Dwyer E, Rose S: *The genetic basis of rheumatoid arthritis: the shared epitope hypothesis*. In Nepom G, editor: *Rheumatic disease clinics*, New York, 1992.
7. Yssel H et al: *Borrelia burgdorferi* activates a T helper type 1-like T cell subset in Lyme arthritis, *J Exp Med* 174:593, 1991.

6

Immune Response and Clinical Lyme Disease

Steven E. Schutzer

The immune response to *Borrelia burgdorferi* involves coordination of several arms of the immune system including macrophages, T cells, and B cells. Our knowledge of the immune response depends on the state of the art of our techniques to measure such responses. For this reason, much of what is known may later be modified.

As described in the accompanying chapters, *B. burgdorferi* is a multiantigenic organism with different immunogenic potential. Although we are aware of the molecular weights of many of its antigens, others may soon be discovered and consequently new information on the immune response should result.

T CELL RESPONSE

Dattwyler and colleagues[5] have described the dissociation of the T cell and B cell response. By conventional immunology, the T cell is presented by macrophages or other antigen-presenting cells with *B. burgdorferi* antigens in conjunction with major histocompatibility (MHC) components. The T cells often proliferate, as can be measured in a lymphoblastogenic assay.[5] A subset of T cells, CD4 + T helpers, induce B cells to produce antibody and differentiate into plasma cells.

B CELL RESPONSE

In general, the earliest humoral response is IgM directed to various antigenic components.[4,8] The earliest and strongest response detected is frequently against the 41-kD endoflagellar antigen of the spirochete. The peak level of IgM is usually between 3 and 6 weeks.[8] After this IgM response, IgG begins and may peak at 4 to 6 weeks. The IgG response may persist for years. In most cases, the initial response to one or two antigens expands to several others over time. It is common to find antibody directed at antigens of 12, 15, 17, 29, 31, 34, 66, 83, and 93 kD. It should be noted that IgM can persist in chronic cases. In certain instances, a seemingly new IgM response can appear late in the illness.[4] Craft et al described such a response

to the OspB protein of 34 kD.[4] They found that the earliest response was to the 41-kD protein, followed months later by a response to more antigens (15, 27, 66, 83 kD), and months or years later to still others (17, 29, 31, 34, 60, 75). Some recent evidence has shown that reactivity to specific antigens may occur very early but may not be detected in abundant quantities.

The T cell repertoire also includes suppressor cells, which can shut off or tone down the humoral response. The suppressor activity may be specific for particular antigens, or may be more global and limit the response to a number of antigens. By envisioning a dynamic relationship between specific helper and suppressor cells, as well as different temporal exposure of the immune system to particular antigens, one can understand the variable nature of the humoral immune response in different individuals.

In addition to the general isotypes of IgM and IgG subclasses, other isotype responses have been described. Benach noted IgE against the 41-kD protein.[2] Hechemy el al noted prominent IgG1 and IgG3 responses that were not absorbed out by *Treponema phagadenis*.[6] In contrast, the IgG2 response was absorbed out. IgA responses have also been described.

Cross-reactive antibody has been described in Lyme disease. Aberer et al demonstrated cross-reactivity between shared antigenic determinants of the 41-kD antigen and myelinated peripheral nerve fibers, neurons, central nervous system axons, epithelia of the synovium, and cardiac muscles.[1] Sigal also demonstrated reactivity to neural tissue.[11] Other infectious agents, such as *Treponema* and *Borrelia* species, may provoke cross-reactive antibody.

Reactivity to *B. burgdorferi* antigen components in certain instances is also believed to occur from nonspecific polyclonal B cell stimulations. This can occur secondary to infections with viruses including Epstein-Barr virus, a well-known T-independent B cell stimulator.

CYTOKINES

Cytokines are soluble factors produced by immune system cells. They help regulate the immune response, including inflammatory reactions. *Borrelia burgdorferi* can incite cytokine production, and it has been postulated that cytokines such as interleukin-1 and tumor necrosis factor are involved in Lyme disease. Much less is known about the cytokine response to *B. burgdorferi,* compared to the T cell and B cell responses.

CLINICAL APPLICATIONS

The following examples are representative of clinical situations that have been encountered in attempting to determine or exclude the diagnosis of Lyme disease. They serve to illustrate how one can use the existing knowledge of the immune response as an adjunctive aid to clinical diagnosis.

Case 1

A patient living in an endemic area for Lyme disease presents with an expanding annular erythematous lesion on the back that grows from 4 to 10 cm over a 3-day period. The patient does not have any other abnormal signs or symptoms.

If you were to order an Enzyme Linked Immunosorbent Assay (ELISA) or Western blot for antibody to *B. burgdorferi,* the results would likely come back negative because the patient is in the very early stages of Lyme disease and has not yet mounted a detectable antibody response. Your decision to treat should be based on the presence of the almost pathognomonic erythema migrans, regardless of the laboratory result.

Case 2

A patient from an endemic area tells you that he was just bitten by a deer tick, which he shows you. He says that he removed it 4 weeks ago and saw a physician who sent off a Lyme disease test to a commercial laboratory. The result said "nonreactive." He states that a few days after that he felt as if he had the flu. He has now recovered but is concerned that he may have Lyme disease. You order an ELISA test, which comes back borderline positive, and recommend a repeat test in 6 weeks.

The case can easily represent one of the 30–40% or so of people who never develop erythema migrans but who are infected with *B. burgdorferi.*[8] He may be at the threshold of seroreactivity, where he has begun to build up enough specific antibody but the level is still below the laboratory's cutoff for a positive result. This result could happen if the assay measures IgM combined with IgG, or IgG alone. If IgM to *B. burgdorferi* were measured separately, perhaps the assay would have been positive. It would have been helpful if you had a sample of his serum several weeks before. You could send

the new sample with the older one to see if there was a rise in titer of specific antibody under the same laboratory conditions. Even if the result were below the laboratory's cutoff for a positive test but there was a marked rise in titer, you would be more confident in diagnosing recent infection with *B. burgdorferi.* Alternatively, you could try to obtain one of the more experimental assays such as specific immune complex dissociation assay,[10] antigen capture assay, or polymerase chain reaction.[7,9]

Case 3

A young woman presents to you with a story that 1 week ago she spent 2 weeks camping in the woods and brushed many deer ticks off her clothing. She is unsure of whether she has had anything that could be identified as erythema migrans, but does show you a very faint pinkish ring behind her knee. Although you cannot really see a significant difference in symmetry, she thinks the right side of her smile is drooping a bit. You order an ELISA and Western blot for antibody to B. burgdorferi. *The ELISA comes back as nonreactive, and the Western blot shows a faint band of reactivity to the 41-kD antigen. She tells you that 6 months ago she had a routine complete physical that included an ELISA and Western blot for Lyme disease, which were entirely negative; both tests had been performed in the same laboratory.*

This case is likely to represent an early case of Lyme disease with a possible fading erythema migrans and an emerging seventh cranial nerve involvement. Although it would have been more useful to have some of the first blood sample to run in tandem with the current one, the evidence suggests the new appearance of antibody to the flagellar antigen of 41 kD. If the antibody were of the IgM rather than IgG, the case would be stronger for an acute infection. However, IgG antibody would also point toward this diagnosis. Given the history of exposure, the seemingly new antibody response, and the possibility of a Bell's palsy, treatment for Lyme disease would not be inappropriate. You might carry the workup further with nerve conduction study of the facial nerve and look for evidence of bilateral involvement, which would strengthen your diagnosis.[3] By freezing a sample of serum, repeating the tests in 2 to 4 weeks, and comparing the two samples you might see a rise of either IgM or IgG to the *B. burgdorferi* in the ELISA and more intense staining band at 41-kD or even the appearance of new bands on the Western blot.

Case 4

A young man comes to your office, says he pulled a tick off himself 3 months before, and now has persistent headaches. He tells you that he went to the Employee Health Department where he works and they sent off a sample for Lyme disease, which came back positive. He does not know if it was an ELISA or a Western blot. Upon questioning, he admits to you that he was treated for syphilis about 5 months ago. You order a VDRL, which comes back positive, and a Western blot and ELISA for Lyme disease. These are both positive, with the Western blot showing a strong reaction to the 41-kD band.

This patient is likely to have syphilis and possibly even neurosyphilis. His reactivity to the Lyme disease tests is probably based on the cross-reactivity with the shared antigenic determinant of the 41-kD flagellar protein of *B. burgdorferi* and *T. pallidum*. The VDRL is generally negative in Lyme disease. Further workup and history should include questions regarding possible reinfection with syphilis, compliance with his treatment, and a lumbar puncture.

Case 5

A young woman presents to you with a facial palsy on her left side, and she feels that her legs are getting weaker. Last week she felt as if she had the flu. She tells you that 2 years ago she had Lyme meningitis and was treated for 3 weeks with intravenous ceftriaxone. At the time, she had a positive ELISA test for the disease and had intrathecal evidence of antibody synthesis to B. burgdorferi. *She also says that a repeat Lyme disease ELISA test 4 months ago was positive, although she had no symptoms. In a research laboratory, she is tested for* B. burgdorferi *antigen,* B. burgdorferi *specific immune complexes, and PCR for* B. burgdorferi *DNA. All are negative. Nerve conduction studies show bilateral seventh cranial nerve involvement. Within days, her legs become paralyzed.*

This woman has Guillain-Barré syndrome resulting from an antecedent viral infection. The bilateral facial nerve palsy is seen not only with this syndrome, but with sarcoid and Lyme disease.[3] If her legs were not weak and paralysis did not occur, the diagnosis would be more difficult. The detection of either antigen, complexed antibody or antigen, or DNA of *B. burgdorferi* would indicate an active infection with this organism. In such circumstances, antibiotics should be administered. Her persistently positive IgG response to *B. burgdorferi* by the ELISA or Western blot reflect the nature of the response that can last for years. In this sense, it loses its diagnostic ability as a sure measure of active infection.

These cases illustrate some of the complexities involved in using the laboratory measures of the humoral immune response to diagnose the disease. They point out that the clinician can combine his or her knowledge of the immune response with laboratory results to arrive at clinical decisions.

REFERENCES

1. Aberer E et al: Molecular mimicry and Lyme borreliosis, *Ann Neurol* 26:732, 1989.
2. Benach J et al: An IgE response to spirochete antigen in patients with Lyme disease, *Zentralbl Bakteriol Mikrobiol Hyg [A]* 263:127, 1986.
3. Coyle PK, Schutzer SE: Neurologic Lyme disease, *Hosp Pract* 26:55, 1991.
4. Craft JE, Fischer DK, Shimamoto GT, Steere AC: Antigens of *Borrelia burgdorferi* recognized during Lyme disease: appearance of a new immunoglobulin M response and expansion of the immunoglobulin G response late in the illness, *J Clin Invest* 78:934, 1986.
5. Dattwyler RJ et al: Seronegative Lyme disease. Dissociation of specific T- and B-lymphocyte responses to *Borrelia burgdorferi, N Engl J Med* 319:1441, 1988.
6. Hechemy K et al: Immunoglobulin G subclasses of specific antibodies specific to *Borrelia burgdorferi* in patients with Lyme disease, *Ann NY Acad Sci* 539:162, 1988.
7. Persing DH, Telford SR, Spielman A, Barthold SW: Detection of *Borrelia burgdorferi* infection in *Ixodes dammini* ticks using the polymerase chain reaction, *J Clin Microbiol* 28:566, 1990.
8. Rahn DW, Malewista SE: Lyme disease: recommendations for diagnosis and treatment, *Ann Intern Med* 114:472, 1991.
9. Rosa PA, Schwan TG: A specific and sensitive assay for the Lyme disease spirochete *Borrelia burgdorferi* using the polymerase chain reaction, *J Infect Dis* 160:1018, 1989.
10. Schutzer SE et al: Sequestration of antibody to *Borrelia burgdorferi* in immune complexes in seronegative Lyme disease, *Lancet* 335:312, 1990.
11. Sigal LH, Tatum AH: IgM in the sera of patients with Lyme neurologic disease bind to cross-reacting neuronal and *Borrelia burgdorferi* antigens, *Ann NY Acad Sci* 539:422, 1988.

7

Histopathology of Human Borreliosis

Paul H. Duray

Studies on the histopathology of *Borrelia* infections, specifically those due to *Borrelia burgdorferi*, have been slow and painstaking since the intensive drives to study Lyme disease after the initial descriptions of the infectious syndrome by Steere in 1977. One reason for slower progress in identifying the spectrum of pathology in human Lyme disease, compared to great strides, for example, in the cell immune response and in the molecular biology of the agent, is the limited availability of human tissue samples. Tissue availability has hindered knowledge in this area, especially compared to aspects of immunology, cell biology, and genetics of the spirochete. There is recent increasing appreciation among clinicians of the value of tissue biopsy samples and the roles they can play in the management and treatment strategies of an individual case, particularly those with chronic ongoing infections.

The earliest tissue samples came from Connecticut cases studied by the original Yale group of investigators, and consisted of synovial samples from patients with Lyme arthritis. These studies showed the synovial inflammatory changes to be those of a nonspecific, hypertrophic process with lymphoplasmacellular aggregates within the synovial membranes. The changes were reminiscent of rheumatoid arthritis, although necrobiotic granulomas were not seen. These studies were also limited to just a few cases. Increasing numbers of synovial tissue samples in the early 1980s broadened the knowledge of the histopathology of Lyme arthritis.[25] These early studies revealed that there were some unique features to the pathology of this infection not found in rheumatoid arthritis.[25] This information suggested the value of increasing the number of tissue samples, and of expanding investigations into other tissue sites of infection. Several factors have combined to underscore the importance of histopathology investigations in addition to clinical management of patients. There have been isolated clinical cases in which adequate treatment seemed not to have terminated the infection completely.[45] European cases particularly can have diverse neurologic syndromes.[3,4,30] We

have experience with individuals who have ongoing cutaneous and subcutaneous tissue lesions of a chronic infectious nature; other individuals appear to have an autoimmune disease complex after the acute infectious episode. Tissue analysis by limited biopsy plays a major role in identifying selected cases and helps to clarify the underlying basis for ongoing tissue inflammation.

Serologic immune response as measured in general laboratories can sometimes underestimate the extent of *Borrelia* infection. These cases may be considered to be non-Lyme disease, and yet isolated experience has shown that definite and diagnostic *Borrelia* spirochetes can be seen by using the recently developed superior silver impregnation tissue staining methods.[11] This chapter discusses clinical circumstances in which tissue biopsies contribute greatly to the understanding and management of *B. burgdorferi* infection.

HISTOGENESIS

Before covering the histopathology of the systems involvement, it is worthwhile to consider observations on the mechanisms of tissue damage during the course of *B. burgdorferi* infection. It is likely that inflammatory factors, including cytokine release, may be important. For example, production of tumor necrosis factor-alpha (TNF-α) and interleukin-2 (IL-2) could contribute to the cognitive impairment, memory dysfunction, and fatigue syndrome noted in late neurologic involvement (encephalopathy). Similarly, some arthritis patients have shown increased TNF-α and IL-2 levels in synovial fluid. Thus, an important pathway for pathogenesis seems to involve continuing immune stimulation. Cytokines are released from a number of cells, including endothelial cells and macrophages, followed by further lymphocyte recruitment, and with time this process could involve arterial wall smooth muscle cells in a pericrine fashion. Over time, activation of IL-2 receptors, platelet-derived growth factors, complement, and immune complexes could interplay to produce vascular changes including sclerosis, vascular wall hyperplasia, further lymphocyte recruitment, and macrophage hyperplasia. Such interplay would lead to vascular basement membrane damage, edema, and perithelial changes reminiscent of an arthus reaction. Logically this might involve visible fibrinous material in vascular lumina. Such changes have not been noted in the inflammatory lesions of human Lyme infection; however, the basis for the vascular changes in Lyme disease remains to be elucidated.

In vitro studies as well as immunohistochemical results indicate that the T cell is central for recognition of *B. burgdorferi* antigens[10] and is responsible for recruitment of other cells, including mast cells and plasma cells, to the lesional site. In fact, these elements are so persistently present that, if they are absent, the possibility exists that the given inflammatory lesion is not due to *B. burgdorferi*. Lymphocytes, plasma cells, mast cells, macrophages, and vascular changes appear to be the predictable and uniform cell response in a given active Lyme histopathologic lesion,[15,18,20] although exceptions exist in the central nervous system as discussed later. In lesions where the lymphoid infiltrate has been adequate for immunophenotyping, CD4 + and CD8 + lymphocytes have been present in approximately equal ratios.[40] Natural killer (NK) lymphocytes are usually very sparse, if present at all. Plasma cells are present in nearly all sites, with the possible exception of the central nervous system, and form part of an array of precursor plasmacytoid cells including scattered immunoblasts.[15,21] Sometimes the lymphoplasmacellular response is so brisk that lymphoid cell mitoses are easily demonstrated.[15] Mast cells are also present in marked numbers, particularly the synovia,[25] but are also present in various skin manifestations. It is interesting that eosinophils, for the most part, are not significantly present, although a few can be seen in the first stage erythema migrans skin lesions, probably reflecting reaction to the tick or its secretory components.

Practically all human pathologic lesions show few *B. burgdorferi* spirochetes present despite significant inflammatory cell infiltrates. This is a major departure from other spirochetal diseases, including syphilis, yaws, pinta, leptospirosis, and even relapsing fever *Borrelia* infections. This is true for central nervous system, cardiac, joint, and skin lesions in *B. burgdorferi* infection, in both human and animal infections.[18,28] It is possible, however, that this concept could change when wider experience is gained from increasing numbers of biopsies. To date, however, biopsy lesions have shown uniformly very few organism. This does not appear to be a technical problem, because rare spirochetes are visualized by silver staining.[27,28] It is perfectly conceivable that a random spirochete is missed by the pathology laboratory, because they are present in such limited numbers. When spirochetes are seen, they have the typical cytomorphology of an undulating bacterial cell that can extend up to 40 μm in tissue sections, to as small as 10 μm. This spirochete has polymorphic forms ranging from almost straight bacilliform cells, to elbow-shaped spirochetes, to classically undulating corkscrew shapes.[1] At times, there is a hook on the end of an elongated spirochete. This distinguishing hook is highly characteristic of *Borrelia* spirochete. The organisms can be found in the vicinity of inflammatory cells, blood vessels, and epithelial surfaces. They show particular predilection for collagen and collagen sites, such as the interstitium of the heart, kidney, urinary bladder, dermis, and overlying voluntary muscle fibers. Although several *Borrelia* cells can be present in a given microscopic field, *Borrelia* spirochetes in human tissues almost never occur in colonies as occurs in *Treponema* spirochetes. They often align themselves to fit the conformation of collagen fibers, and may be misinterpreted as elastic tissue fibers or procollagen fibrils. They can be distinguished from tissue fibers by their smaller diameter (0.15 to 0.20 μm), with the diameter varying slightly due to membrane folds of the organism.[1] This diameter is less than that expected for procollagen fibrils. Any of the silver impregnation histochemical stains can be used to demonstrate *B. burgdorferi* in tissues or fluids. However, this observer prefers either a modified Steiner or a modified Dieterle stain, both of which yield a light yellow to golden background contrasting with the brown to blue-black spirochetes (Fig. 7–1).[19,27]

CLINICOPATHOLOGIC CORRELATION

The remainder of the chapter deals with the histopathology of the specific lesions encountered during the course of infection. It should be emphasized that this spectrum is not seen in every patient. There is not necessarily a progression from the initial skin manifestations of primary infection to disseminated disease in every clinical circumstance.[26,41] One or more of the following features may be present in a given patient, but it is extremely rare for any individual patient to have most organ systems involved during the course of his or her infection. It is not understood, for example, why one patient will have more intense infection of the spleen, whereas another patient may have severe myocarditis, and yet another may have transient mild hepatitis. It is highly possible that patients do have a comparable clinicopathologic involvement, but that limited clinical investigations simply do not

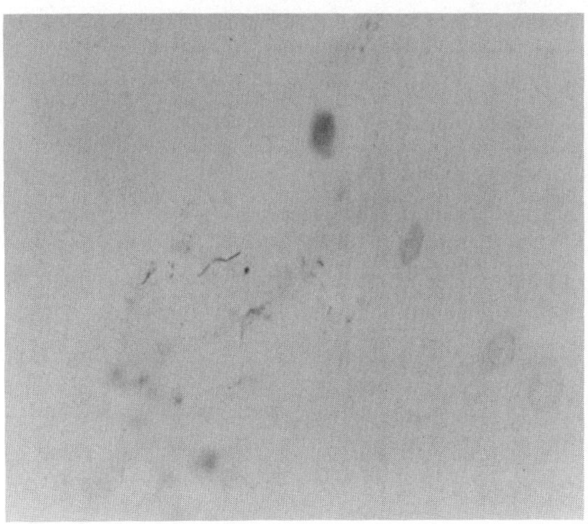

Figure 7–1 Single cell of *B. burgdorferi* in dermal collagen. (Modified Dieterle stain; × 1000.)

uncover mild or asymptomatic multisystem involvement in the average patient. Although variable protein phenotypes of a given strain of *B. burgdorferi* may produce different clinicopathologic lesions, variability is probably tied as well to host factors. Strain differences in major geographic regions do seem to lead to certain types of infections. For example, a predilection for central nervous system (CNS) infections, including radiculopathies, is seen more frequently in northern and central Europe than in North America.[3,4,23,30] Chronic cutaneous and subcutaneous soft tissue inflammatory lesions also seem to be more commonly encountered in cases in Europe than in the United States.[6,7,43] The preinfection immune status and immune function of a patient is likely to be important for the clinical course after infection. However, not enough cases have been studied to draw any firm conclusions on the behavior of *B. burgdorferi* infections in immune compromised human patients.

Multiple pathologic lesions have been postulated to occur in Lyme disease. Before a given tissue derangement can be related to *B. burgdorferi*, either laboratory isolation of the spirochete from such a lesion, or unequivocal demonstration of spirochete in tissue samples is required. Following this, similar cases need to be documented with the same pattern(s) before a real association can be declared. The following discussion includes only those pathologic lesions that have fulfilled these criteria, either from study in the United States, or Europe, or both. Pathologic lesions are described by systems, without regard to time of onset or stage of disease.

SKIN AND SOFT TISSUE
Erythema migrans

The first lesion recognized in human Lyme borreliosis is the rash phase developing as an advancing erythema, usually macular, serpiginous, circinate, and spreading.[11,41,43] There may or may not be a central raised papule where the tick had been attached and feeding. Biopsies are done of the advancing erythema edge, to include the normal skin interface, largely to exclude other similar dermatologic lesions such as erythema multiforme or one of the gyrate erythemas. Clinically, erythema migrans may strongly resemble erythema annulare centrifugum. The epidermis, dermis, and adnexae are all intact in erythema migrans, and usually the only major findings are varying degrees of pericapillary and perivascular dermal lymphocytes and plasma cells with occasional mast cells.[11,15,19] There may be urticarial type edema in certain cases correlating with raised areas seen clinically. The papule of tick attachment shows more inflammation in the dermis with a central infiltrate of macrophages, mast cells, neutrophils, as well as plasma cells and lymphocytes.[20] Eosinophils may be present in the central papule, but they are not the predominant cell of response. At times, chronic arthropod reactions of perivascular aggregates of lymphocytes and eosinophils are present throughout the thickness of the dermis, but this is not a common finding. The epidermis is intact, and there is no interface (dermal-epidermal) dermatitis. Most cases of erythema migrans have plasma cells in a perivascular distribution. The vessels are normal in appearance in this stage as is the appearance of the reticular dermal collagen. Spirochetes are seen in the collagen, either of the papillary dermis or of the reticular dermis (see Fig. 7–1). Rarely, they may be seen in the surface epidermis.

Cutaneous morphea

Morphea, or focal scleroderma, is often reversible in dermatologic practice, and probably has multiple etiologies. They are characterized by firm patches of indurated skin, sometimes surrounded by peripheral hyperpigmentation and palpable firmness. Investigators in both Europe and the United States have encountered such cases in Lyme disease.[19] Sometimes the morphea-form lesions are associated with the chronic form of skin infection described below. Morphea, or linear, localized scleroderma, is characterized pathologically by a widened, expanded dermis by new layers of collagen, accompanied in the early stages by lymphocytic infiltration, at first in a perivascular distribution, followed by patches and layers of lymphocytes in the dermal collagen. These lymphoid aggregates can also involve the underlying fatty subcutaneous tissue. If the lesion is present for any length of time, the lymphocytes diminish, with only a persistent wide zone of collagen as the visible derangement (Fig. 7–2). The eccrine glands are in their usual position with the collagen expansion occurring below them. The Lyme-associated morphea lesions are not distinguishable histopathologically from morphea associated with other causes. *B. burgdorferi* can be demonstrated by appropriate silver stains, and this is what sets this lesion apart from morphea resulting from other causes.

Acrodermatitis chronica atrophicans (ACA)

ACA is more commonly seen in Europe, although I have seen a rare case in the eastern United States (New Jersey). This is a peculiar dermatitis of acral skin of the hands, wrists, feet, ankles, and lower extremities.[2,5,7,16] ACA can occur in other sites as well, but the most common distribution is the hands and feet. These lesions show bilateral symmetry and start as an induration and thickening of the dermis by marked inflammation and dermal edema. This inflammatory hypertrophic stage is characterized by a diffuse dermal infiltration of polymorphic inflammatory cells including macrophages, neutrophils, plasma cells, and lymphocytes (Fig. 7 3).[5] The lesion can go on for years, and, when it does, the dermal collagen, in opposition to morphea, becomes atrophic with overall thinning of the reticular dermis.[5] At all stages, hypertrophy or atrophy, *B. burgdorferi* spirochetes are present and can be demonstrated histochemically as well as cultured. An intermediate stage of ACA demonstrates the presence of characteristic fixed dilatation of the dermal vaculature, a form of lymphatic telangiectasia.[15,16] As stated above, some lesions of ACA have morphealike induration adjacent to the ACA lesions. Additionally, some cases of ACA have subcutaneous fibrotic nodules, which have been referred to as *ulnar fibrous nodules*.[15,16] These arise also in the context of ACA, especially that involving the upper extremities in which the nodules form in the lateral subcutaneous forearm tissues, hence the name ulnar. Clinically, these may resemble gouty tophi or rheumatoid nodules and, therefore, tissue biopsy is especially helpful. Histologically, they are composed of sclerotic nodules with persistent plasma cells and sclerosed small blood vessels. Again, their association has been proven with histologically stainable spirochetes.

Borrelial lymphocytoma

This is a peculiar collection of hyperplastic lymphoid follicles occupying and sometimes replacing the reticular dermis. There are very prominent germinal centers, and a mantle zone of mature lymphocytes with interfollicular plasma cells, macrophages, and other lymphocytes between the lymphoid follicles.[15,16,44] This lesion has the histologic pattern of a pseudolymphoma[9] and is a form of benign cutaneous lymphoid hyperplasia.[13,17] Lymphocytomas show a predilection for the bases of the ear lobes, the axillary skin folds, and the nipples of the breasts. They have not been seen in a bilaterally symmetric distribution. Again, these lesions have yielded spirochetes upon culture, and the organisms have been seen both histochemically and by electron microscopy.

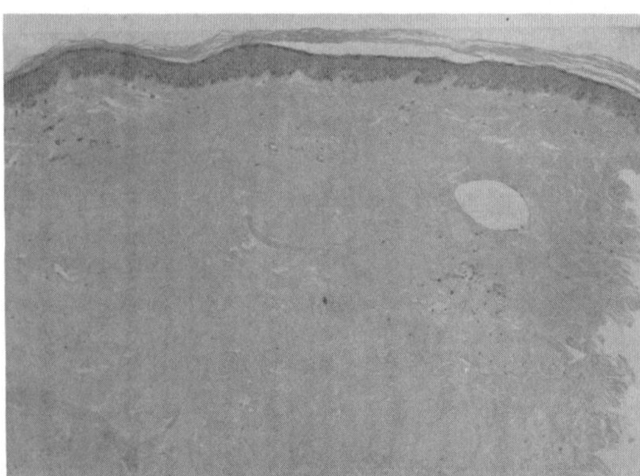

Figure 7–2 *Borrelia* morphea (localized scleroderma) of skin. The histology is indistinguishable from systemic scleroderma with rete ridge effacement, new reticular dermal collagenosis extending deeply, scattered sparse lymphoplasmacytes, and a dilated dermal lymphatic at the upper right. (Hematoxylin-eosin stain; × 100.)

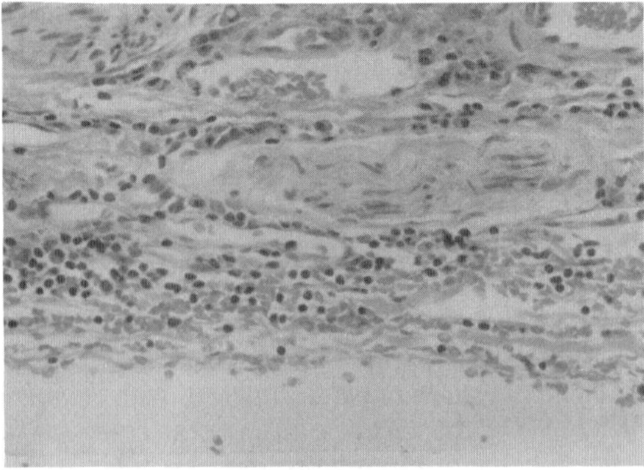

Figure 7–3 Deep dermal perineural plasma cells in ACA at the subcutaneous-fat junction. Transdermal inflammatory infiltrates characterize many cases of ACA. Perineural plasma cells are seen in several pathologic lesions of Lyme borreliosis. (Hematoxylin-eosin stain; ×400.)

Spongiotic dermatitis

This is a recently observed manifestation of skin involvement (unpublished data) in which the epidermis shows mild to moderate acanthosis, focal spongiosis, and perivascular papillary dermal lymphocytes and plasma cells. An occasional spirochete can be demonstrated, and the overall dermatitis histopathologically bears a resemblance to pityriasis rosea. Both of the two clinical examples of this dermatosis have been seen in patients who had begun antimicrobial therapy for their erythema migrans, which then began to evolve into scattered papules. The spongiotic dermatitis was seen on biopsy of these papules.

Panniculitis and fasciitis

Some forms of morphea may have deep dermal lymphocytes and plasma cells in aggregate formation, which can spill over to involve the subcutaneous fat.[21] This defines secondary panniculitis. However, discrete panniculitis with plasma cells located in the lower abdominal subcutaneous tissue and thigh has been seen in several patients. Two of these examples showed a dermis that was only slightly thickened and, therefore, did not constitute true morphea, although there was plasma cell capillaritis in the deep dermis and subcutaneous fat. In some ways, this strongly resembles the histologic picture of lupus profundus. Due to this similarity, the clinical exclusion of systemic lupus erythematosus is necessary. Spirochetes were easily seen in the lower reticular dermal collagen in both our previous examples.

We have seen four examples of subcutaneous fasciitis, one involving the upper extremity and three involving the lower extremity, in which the deep fascial tissue between the subcutaneous soft tissue and underlying skeletal muscle showed infiltration by mononuclear cells and lymphocytes with rare eosinophils. Eosinophils were not as abundant as described in eosinophilic fasciitis. All four cases have also shown moderate edema of the subcutaneous tissues, and where muscle fibers were included in the surgical biopsy, aggregates of lymphocytes in the interstitium of the muscle as well. There is overlap with the myositis, which is described below. Spirochetes were seen with some difficulty in two examples, but were easily demonstrated in two other patients.

Myositis

Large voluntary muscle groups such as in the thigh and shoulder regions can be involved directly by *B. burgdorferi* infections after the primary stages, when pain and induration are seen clinically.[8,36] Histopathologic aggregates of lymphocytes and plasma cells are demonstrated primarily around the interstitial vessels, but also in between muscle fibers.[8,36] *Borrelia burgdorferi* has been found in the interstitium, and spirochetes are sometimes seen overlying individual striated muscle fibers. Occasionally, these myositis foci are juxtaposed to arthritis and synovitis. We have also seen isolated myositis without evidence of arthritis. We have encountered several cases of tenosynovitis of the wrists with palpable induration of the tendon sheaths, which disappeared after antibiotic therapy.

Myocarditis

The heart and pericardium are directly involved in at least 8% of patients, but this prevalence may indeed be higher.[32,37,39] We have seen several examples of pericardial effusion accompanied by hemosiderin deposits and fibrin deposition in the pericardial sac, which regressed after treatment with antibiotics. Of equal importance is the syndrome of infectious carditis heralded by clinical episodes of incomplete or complete heart block. Limited biopsies of the right endocardium by transvenous catheter procedure demonstrate the presence of diffuse interstitial lymphocytes and plasma cells and macrophages. The cells separate the cardiac muscle fibers, but do not appear to invade the fibers directly (Fig. 7–4).[32,37,39] There is a characteristic band-like infiltrate of lymphocytes and plasma cells in the endocardium, which is almost always present in biopsies of Lyme carditis (Fig. 7–5).[15,21] The interstitial infiltrate has been seen also in terminal cases; the myocardial inflammatory infiltrate is transmural and extends out into the epicardial tissue as well. No giant cells or eosinophils as seen in Fiedler's myocarditis are evident, but *B. burgdor-*

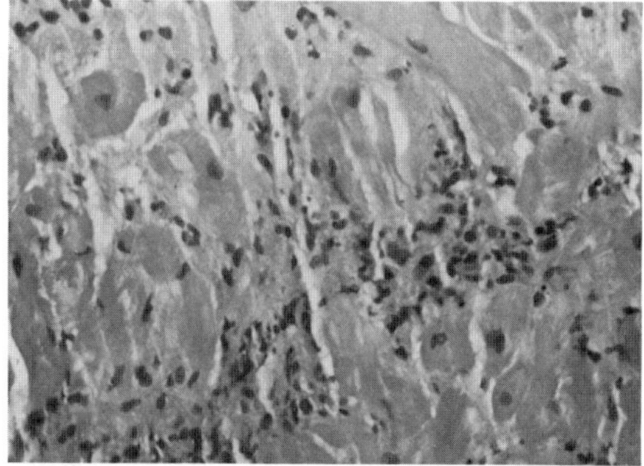

Figure 7–4 Lyme carditis: the inflammatory infiltrate is interstitial without scalloping of the myocardiocyte cytoplasm as seen in cardiac transplant rejection. This biopsy is from a middle-aged Pennsylvania woman who completely recovered with parenteral penicillin. (Hematoxylin-eosin stain; ×400.)

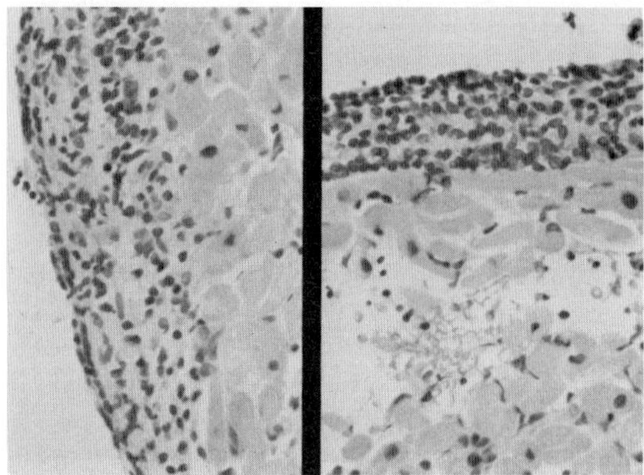

Figure 7–5 Bandlike lymphocytic-plasmocytic endocardial infiltrate seems to characterize Lyme carditis as depicted in this example from a young male with Lyme carditis. (Hematoxylin-eosin stain; ×400.)

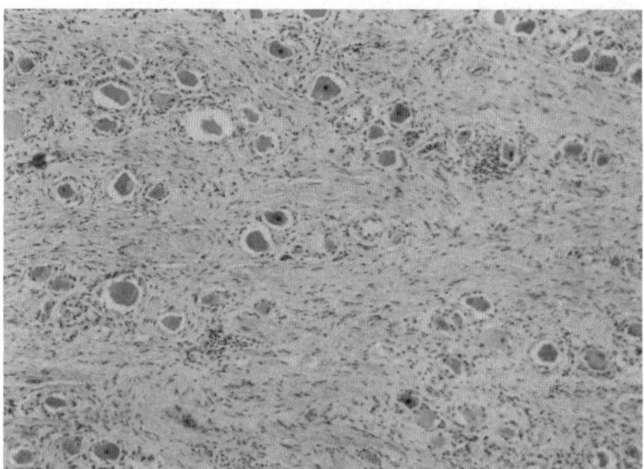

Figure 7–6 Dorsal root ganglion lymphocytic infiltration in a German patient with neuroborreliosis. Lymphocytes and plasma cells are focally positioned around some of the autonomic ganglion cells reminiscent of autoimmune effect. (Hematoxylin-eosin stain; ×100.)

feri can be demonstrated with modest ease by silver staining. The spirochetes are almost without exception visible extracellularly.[15,29]

Vasculopathy

Vascular sclerosis and hyperplasia of tunica media cells have been demonstrated in the joint, heart, soft tissues, and chronic skin infections, and focally in peripheral nerves.[12,15,21] At times, the lumina are completely obliterated by hyperplasia of the endothelial and smooth muscle cells, producing a picture of endarteritis.[25] We have seen one example of ascending aortic aneurysm in a young male patient complete with cystic medial necrosis and plasma cell aggregates in the adventitial vessels of the thoracic aorta. However, we were unable to demonstrate spirochetes (unpublished data) and cannot list this as a definite *Borrelia* effect at this writing.

CENTRAL AND PERIPHERAL NERVOUS SYSTEM

Meningoencephalitis

Rarely, CNS disturbance in the form of stupor and encephalopathic states[23,24,33] have been accompanied by perivascular cerebral edema on cerebral cortical biopsy, with mononuclear cells in the form of microglial cells and definite lymphocytes in perivascular distributions. This picture, however, is seen in only some cases, with others demonstrating only an increase in the number of oligodendrocytes. Some cases have shown a delicate spongioform encephalopathic picture on biopsy, either as an isolated finding without a change in the cellularity of the cerebral cortex or also associated with an increase in oligodendrocytes. Leptomeningeal lymphocytosis has been demonstrated in one case,

that of a young woman with clinical evidence of cerebral vasculitis. The biopsy, however, was superficial and showed a strip of lymphocytic infiltration in the leptomeningeal layers, but no vasculitis. No astrocytic cell necrosis was present in any of the eight brain biopsy samples we have studied to date, but two patients had definite neuronophagia. The limited pathology to date has not been impressive: an increase in phagocytic microglial cells, perivascular lymphocytes, and plasma cells in leptomeninges and mild spongioform changes.

Radiculitis

Ganglia, particularly dorsal root, have been examined histopathologically in two circumstances. Both cases demonstrated aggregates of lymphocytes and plasma cells within the ganglia directly involving the large ganglion cells in a satellite configuration (Fig. 7–6). One case showed striking ganglion cell loss with replacement by nests of lymphocytes.[21] The pattern is suggestive of an autoimmune effect.[38] Spirochetes were not demonstrated during a careful and exhaustive search. Such changes may account for radiculopathy as well as cranial neuropathy including Bell's palsy.

Peripheral neuropathy

In cases of peripheral neuropathy, sural nerve biopsies have shown reproducible and similar patterns both in North American and European cases.[12,15,21,30,31] Several biopsies show perivascular lymphocytic plasmacellular deposits in the perineurium, accompanied by varying degrees of pericapillary lymphocytic infiltration within the interior of the nerves (Fig. 7–7).[12,15,21,30] Mild to moderate

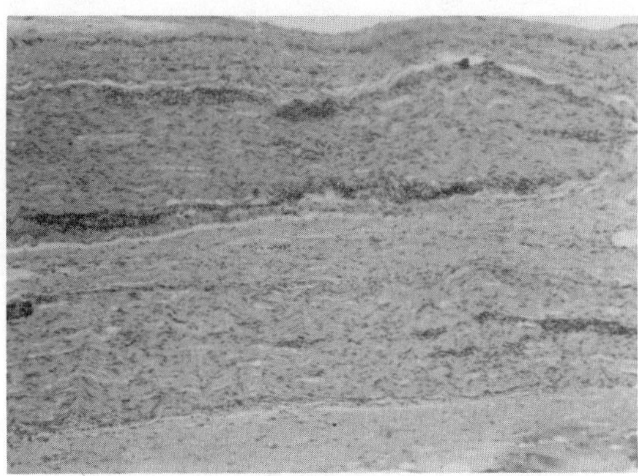

Figure 7–7 Sural nerve biopsy from a case of peripheral neuropathy. The lymphoid infiltrates in involved peripheral nerves are in perineural vascular locations and related to the small vessels within the nerve segments as well. (Hematoxylin-eosin stain; × 100.)

axonal degeneration is seen and some focal loss of myelin can be demonstrated with Luxol Blue stains. These changes are in keeping with wallerian degeneration. We have been unable to demonstrate *B. burgdorferi* directly within nerve fibers, but this does not definitively exclude the possibility that they are present. An alternative mechanism to explain the pathologic changes would be an autoimmune effect on Schwann's cells.[38] Carpal tunnel syndrome has been described in Lyme disease, reflecting another pathologic manifestation. Several midwestern cases of cutaneous disease in Lyme borreliosis have shown lymphocytes, plasma cells, and other mononuclear cells in a closely associated perineural dermal distribution, not unlike that seen in leprosy (Fig. 7–3). This pattern also suggests an autoimmune component with nerve targeted by the immune system, but the observation needs further study.

RETICULOENDOTHELIAL SYSTEM: HEPATITIS

A mild form of hepatitis has been seen on several occasions on biopsy, in patients who had modest elevations in liver enzymes.[22,34] Liver cells showed mild cytoplasmic swelling, with numerous binucleate forms and hepatocellular mitoses. Kupffer's cells were notably hyperplastic, and lymphocytes and plasma cells were found in the hepatic sinusoids as well as in the triad areas.[22] Spleen and lymph nodes demonstrate the presence of plasma cells and numerous immunoblasts (Fig. 7–8).[15,21,26] Precursor plasma cells are also evident in the lymph nodes and in the spleen. It is fairly easy to demonstrate the spirochete within the spleen in particular (Fig. 7–9).[14] Necrotic areas can be dem-

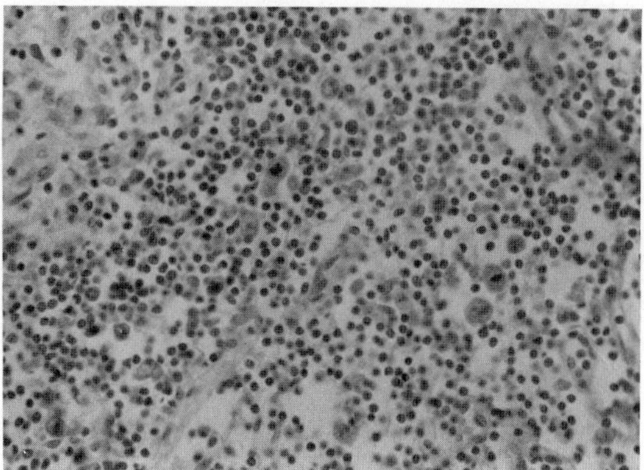

Figure 7–8 Lymph node biopsy in a case with active infection of about 7 weeks. This lymphadenitis shows the atypical lymphoblastoid cells with increased mitoses often seen in the lymph nodes and spleen of early, disseminated stage. Some of the atypical cells have immunoblastic features. Such cells are also present in the spleen at this stage. (Hematoxylin-eosin stain; × 400.)

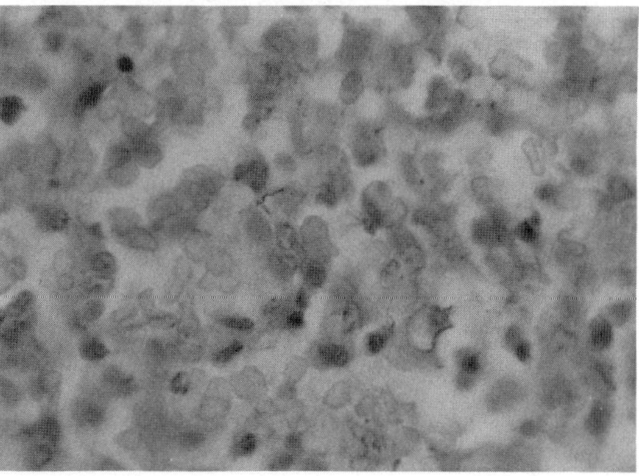

Figure 7–9 Single *B. burgdorferi* spirochete in the spleen of a newborn infant whose mother had gestational Lyme borreliosis during the first trimester. Note the extracellular location of the spirochete and the lack of atypical lymphoid cells in Fig. 7-8. Neonatal borreliosis is not associated with the degree of inflammatory cell responses seen in adult cases. (Modified Dieterle stain; × 1000.)

onstrated in the spleens of some cases, particularly in association with splenic pain and tenderness (Fig. 7–10).[35] We have had the opportunity to study two human spleens: one removed because of acute rupture, and one from a patient who succumbed to systemic infection.

MUSCULOSKELETAL SYSTEM: ARTHRITIS AND SYNOVITIS

Synovial biopsies can be very helpful in managing arthritis when the differential diagnosis is unclear.[25]

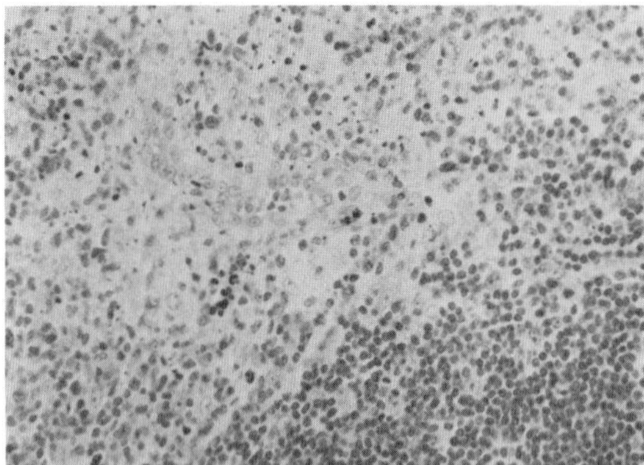

Figure 7-10 Necrosis in the spleen of a male patient with clinical presentation of acute splenic rupture secondary to Lyme splenitis. The upper left of the photomicrograph shows the well-developed necrobiotic zone with nuclear debris. (Giemsa stain; ×400.)

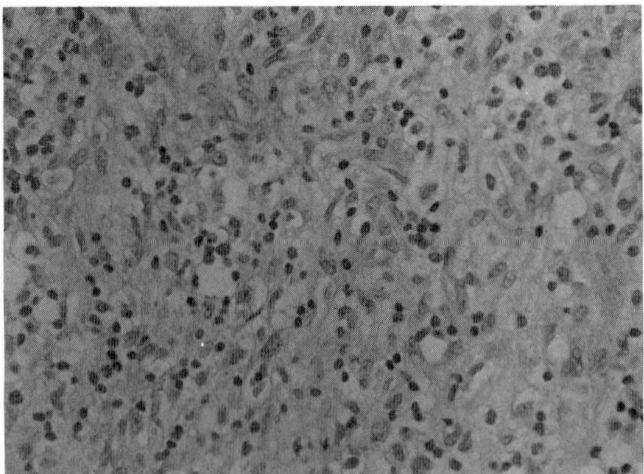

Figure 7-11 Lyme synovitis and arthritis. This synovial sample obtained at arthroscopy shows nonaggregated lymphocytes, numerous macrophages, and immunohistochemically proven synovial cells. (Hematoxylin-eosin stain; ×400.)

The synovial membrane is hypertrophic with numerous folds producing villuslike structures overlaid by hyperplastic synovial cells. Immunophenotyping shows the synovial cells to be distributed throughout the synovium in addition to the synovial villuslike surfaces. Varying degrees of synovial edema are present, but multiple aggregates of lymphocytes and plasma cells admixed with mast cells are uniformly present, provided the sample is adequate (Fig. 7-11). Rarely, giant cells can be seen, and rarer still is the presence of occasional granulomas. Fibrin deposits can be found on the surfaces of the synovial membrane, just as in Reiter's disease and in rheumatoid arthritis, but fibrin de-

Figure 7-12 Lyme synovitis. Subjacent to the upper surface lining of synovial cells is a diffuse stromal deposition of fibrin and fibrinogen material in this active case of Lyme arthritis. (Histochemical stain for fibrin; ×100.)

posits may also be seen within the stroma of the synovial membrane, at times obscuring the normal pattern of the villus stroma (Fig. 7-12). Extensive deposits within the villus stroma are highly suggestive of Lyme synovitis. In our experience, fibrin deposition in the villus stroma is less striking in Reider's disease and rheumatoid arthritis.[25] We have seen definite spirochetes within the stroma and collagen of the synovial membrane, but their presence is very difficult to discern. The majority of synovial biopsies do not readily demonstrate the presence of spirochetes. This may be a function of the volume of the synovial tissue sampled. Vascular sclerosis is generally seen in most synovial samples, and occasionally a true endarteritis is seen in a synovial vessel.[15,21,25] The presence of vasculopathy within the synovium and extensive fibrin deposits in the stroma are very suggestive of Lyme arthritis, even in the absence of clinical history.

SUMMARY

Tissue biopsies are very helpful in the following circumstances: cerebral cortex, myocardium and endocardium, synovium, soft tissue lesions including fascia and adipose tissue, deep dermis, and peripheral nerve.[42] It is generally not difficult to rule in borreliosis by demonstrating the spirochetes, especially in skin samples, but they should also be sought in cerebral cortex, myocardium, and soft tissue lesions. Tissue biopsies will be more important when wider experience has been gained in using immunohistochemistry to identify the spirochete, or portions of it, directly within tissues by DNA hybridization techniques.

The value of histopathology in the management and general understanding of the pathogenesis of these infections has been underestimated and underutilized. As greater experience is obtained in multiple laboratories, it is hoped that the procedure will be more widely used. For example, histopathologic technology may evolve to the point where patients who have an autoimmune process without spirochetes will be discerned from those with active spirochetes. In such cases, serologic tests will not be helpful. There should be no hesitation to perform a cardiobiopsy, particularly endocardial biopsies by transvenous catheter, in those institutions where the procedure is used for other diagnostic maneuvers of the myocardium. The same can be said for synovial and soft tissue lesions generally.

REFERENCES

1. Aberer E, Duray PH: Morphology of *Borrelia burgdorferi:* structural patterns of cultured borrelia in relation to staining methods, *J Clin Microbiol* 29:764, 1991.
2. Aberer E, Neumann R, Lubec G: Acrodermatitis chronica atrophicans in association with lichen sclerosus et atrophicans: tubulo-interstitial nephritis and urinary excretion of spirochete-like organisms. *Acta Derm Venereol (Stockh)* 67(1):62, 1987.
3. Ackermann R, Rehse-Kupper B, Gollmer E: Progressive borrelia encephalomyelitis, *Zentralbl Bakteriol Mikrobiol Hyg [A]* 263:201, 1986.
4. Ackermann R, Rehse-Kupper R, Gollmer E, Schmidt R: Chronic neurologic manifestations of erythema migrans borreliosis, *Ann NY Acad Sci* 539:16, 1988.
5. Asbrink E, Brehmer-Andersson E, Hovmark A: Acrodermatitis chronica atrophicans—a spirochetosis. Clinical and histopathological picture based on 32 patients, *Am J Dermatopathol* 8:209, 1986.
6. Asbrink E, Hovmark A: Comments on the course and classification of Lyme borreliosis, *Scand J Infect Dis* 77:41, 1991.
7. Asbrink E, Hovmark A, Hederstedt B: The spirochaetal etiology of acrodermatitis chronica atrophicans Herxheimer, *Acta Derm Venereol* (Stockh) 64:506, 1984.
8. Atlas E, Novack SN, Steere AC, Duray PH: Lyme myositis, *Ann Intern Med* 109:245, 1988.
9. Bafverstedt B: Uber lymphadenosis benigna cutis, *Acta Derm Venereol (Stockh)* Suppl II:1, 1943.
10. Benach JL, Villar Fernandez B, Szczeponski A, Garcia Manco JC: Lyme borreliosis: non-specific interactions of the organism with the host, *Scand J Infec Dis* 77:130, 1991.
11. Berger BW, Clemmense OJ, Ackermann AB: Lyme disease is a spirochetosis, *Am J Dermatopathol* 5:111, 1983.
12. Camponovo F, Meier C: Neuropathy of vasculitic origin in a case of Garin-Boujadoux-Bannwarth syndrome with positive borrelia antibody response, *J Neurol* 233:69, 1986.
13. Caro WA, Helwig EB: Cutaneous lymphoid hyperplasia, *Cancer* 24:487, 1969.
14. Cimmino MA, Azzolini A, Tobia F, Pesce CM: Spirochetes in the spleen of a patient with chronic Lyme disease, *Am J Clin Pathol* 91:95, 1988.
15. Duray PH: The surgical pathology of human Lyme disease: an enlarging picture, *Am J Surg Pathol* II(5):47, 1987.
16. Duray PH, Asbrink E, Weber K: The cutaneous manifestations of human Lyme disease: a widening spectrum, *Adv Dermatol* 4:255, 1989.
17. Duray PH, Burgdorf WHC, Goltz RW: Persistent cutaneous lymphoid hyperplasia of the face with conjunctival involvement, *Arch Ophthalmol* 103:555, 1985.
18. Duray PH, Johnson AC: The histopathology of experimentally infected hamsters with the Lyme disease spirochete, *Borrelia burgdorferi* (42251). *Proc Soc Exp Biol Med* 181:263, 1986.
19. Duray PH, Kusnitz A, Ryan J: Demonstration of the Lyme disease spirochete *Borrelia burgdorferi* by a modification of the Dieterle stain, *Lab Med* 16:685, 1985.
20. Duray PH, Steere AC: The spectrum of organ and systems pathology in human Lyme disease, *Zentralbl Bakteriol Mikrobiol Hyg [A]* 263:169, 1986.
21. Duray PH, Steere AC: Clinical pathologic correlations of Lyme disease by stage, *Ann NY Acad Sci* 539:65, 1988.
22. Goellner MH, Agger WA, Duray PH: Hepatitis due to recurrent Lyme disease, *Ann Intern Med* 108:707, 1988.
23. Halperin JJ: North American Lyme neuroborreliosis, *Scand J Infect Dis* 77:74, 1991.
24. Halperin JJ, Luft BJ, Anand AK: Lyme neuroborreliosis: central nervous system manifestations, *Neurology* 39:753, 1989.
25. Johnston YE et al: Lyme arthritis; spirochaetes found in synovial microangiopathic lesions, *Am J Pathol* 118:26, 1985.
26. Kirsch M et al: Fatal adult respiratory distress syndrome in a patient with Lyme disease, *JAMA* 259:2737, 1988.
27. Koning J de, Bosma RB, Hoogkamp-Korstanje JAA: Demonstration of spirochaetes in patients with Lyme disease with a modified silver stain, *J Med Microbiol* 23:261, 1987.
28. Koning J de, Hoogkamp-Korstanje JAA: Demonstration of spirochetes in biopsies, *Zentralbl Bakteriol Mikrobiol Hyg[A]* 263:179, 1986.
29. Koning J de, Hoogkamp-Korstanje JAA, Linde MR van der, Crijns HJGM: Demonstration of spirochetes in cardiac biopsies of patients with Lyme disease, *J Infect Dis* 106:150, 1989.
30. Kristoferitsch W: Neurological manifestations of Lyme borreliosis: clinical definition and differential diagnosis, *Scand J Infect Dis* 77:64, 1991.
31. Kristoferitsch W et al: Neuropathy associated with acrodermatitis chronic atrophicans, *Ann NY Acad Sci* 539:35, 1988.
32. Marcus LC et al: Fatal pancarditis in a patient with coexistent Lyme disease and babesiosis, *Ann Intern Med* 103:374, 1985.
33. Pfister HW, Einhaupl KM, Preac-Mursic V, Wilske B: The spirochetal etiology of lymphocytic meningoradiculitis of Bannwarth (Bannwarth's syndrome), *J Neurol* 231:141, 1984.
34. Prinz A, Weiss P, Stanek G: Generalized exanthema, acute hepatitis with porphyria and eosinophilia. Another clinical feature of Lyme disease? *Zentralbl Bakteriol Mikrobiol Hyg [A]* 263:389, 1987.
35. Rank EL et al: Human necrotizing splenitis caused by *Borrelia burgdorferi, Am J Clin Pathol* 91:493, 1989.
36. Reimers CD et al: Myositis caused by *Borrelia burgdorferi:* report of four cases, *J Neurol Sci* 91:215, 1989.
37. Reznick JW et al: Lyme carditis, *Am J Med* 81:923, 1986.
38. Sigal LH, Tatum AH: Lyme disease patients' serum contains IgM antibodies to *Borrelia burgdorferi* that cross-react with neural antigens, *Neurology* 38:1439, 1988.
39. Stanck G, Klein J, Bittner R, Glozar D: *Borrelia burgdorferi* as an etiologic agent in chronic heart failure? *Scand J Infect Dis* 77:85, 1991.

40. Steere AC, Duray PH, Butcher EC: Spirochetes and lymphoid cell surface markers in Lyme synovitis: comparison with rheumatoid synovium and tonsillar lymphoid tissue, *Arthritis Rheum* 31:487, 1988.
41. Steere AC et al: The early clinical manifestations of Lyme disease, *Ann Intern Med* 99:76, 1983.
42. Stiernstedt G et al: Diagnostic tests in Lyme borreliosis, *Scand J Infect Dis* 77:136, 1991.
43. Weber K, Schierz G, Wilske B, Preac-Mursic V: European erythema migrans disease and related disorders, *Yale J Biol Med* 57:463, 1984.
44. Weber K, Schierz G, Wilske B, Preac-Mursic V: Das lymphozytom—eine Borreliose? *Z Hautkr* 60:1585, 1985.
45. Weber K et al: *Borrelia burgdorferi* in a newborn despite oral penicillin for Lyme borreliose during pregnancy, *J Pediatr Infect Dis* 7:286, 1988.

SECTION TWO

Clinical Aspects

8 Overview of Spirochetal Infections

Jorge L. Benach and James L. Coleman

Spirochetal infections include diseases caused by several species within three genera: *Borrelia, Leptospira,* and *Treponema.* Although technically considered to be gram-negative organisms, these bacteria are seldom included in this major morphologic grouping and have traditionally been considered a special group. Spirochetes are flexible cells with a helical configuration and with motility conferred by endoflagella. The pathogenic species produce diseases that have both differences and similarities. The organisms themselves share the helical rod configuration and range from those with very tight coils of the helix *(Leptospira)* to coils regularly spaced 1 μm apart *(Treponema)* to coils irregularly spaced 2 to 4 μm apart *(Borrelia). Leptospira* are cultured rather easily, and this permits the isolation of the organism to be used as a means of laboratory diagnosis. *Borrelia* can be cultured in Kelly's medium[55] but are fastidious organisms that divide slowly in culture. *Treponema pallidum,* the etiologic agent of syphilis, has never been cultured in vitro. This impressive range in the ability of the various pathogenic species of the family Spirochaetaceae to survive and grow in artificial media indicates significant physiologic and metabolic differences among the species. Thus, generalizations about the organisms may be difficult to make. This also extends to generalizations regarding the various spirochetal diseases. With this caveat in mind, this chapter focuses on summaries of the major spirochetal diseases rather than presenting a detailed list of differences and similarities among them. The differences among the four major spirochetal diseases will become apparent, but the similarities, in very general terms, are quite important and should be highlighted because they have an impact on diagnosis and treatment.

1. *Spirochetal diseases are characterized by periods of clinical activity separated by periods of remission.* There is a wide range of presentations to this disease pattern. For example, leptospirosis is a biphasic illness with an initial early septicemic phase, a brief period in which the symptoms and signs of the early phase subside or disappear only to be followed by the second systemic phase. Relapsing fever, as the name implies, represents a compressed version of the relapse-remission pattern with febrile episodes separated by afebrile periods. The nature of this pattern in relapsing fever has been elucidated and is due to antigenic variability of the organism. Syphilis, at the other extreme, represents this relapse-remission pattern best in its well-known clinical stages and latent periods. Lastly, Lyme disease fits this pattern well with its distinct stages and relapses of the same manifestations or appearance of new ones.

2. *Spirochetal diseases are protean and chronic.* Syphilis and now Lyme disease have been called the "Great Imitators." There are good reasons for this. Spirochetes invade many organs and produce organ-associated disease that is often so nonspecific that it can be confused with other entities. For example, although relapsing fever is most associated with episodes of spirochetemia and thus conveys the impression of a blood infection, it is actually a systemic disease with many different manifestations. Leptospirosis is a classically protean disease with significant injury to the heart, liver, kidneys, eyes, and other organs. Lastly, the protean manifestations of syphilis and Lyme disease are well-known and need not to be reviewed here. Spirochetal diseases are of long duration. The 20 to 30 year period between primary and tertiary syphilis is the classical statement regarding the chronic condition. In this regard, we already know that certain manifestations of Lyme disease can take up to a decade to develop. With time, it may become apparent that Lyme disease has a natural course of illness which approaches that of syphilis. Another aspect that can be discussed under this heading is the apparent continuation of the disease process after the organisms are no longer detectable. The "sequestration" or disappearance from the blood of the *Borrelia* in the afebrile periods between relapses in relapsing fever may be due to the action of specific antibodies, but it can also represent the simplest example of "hiding." Why is it so difficult to culture or even visualize spirochetes in the synovium and synovial fluid of patients with Lyme arthritis of long duration? What is tertiary syphilis

in the absence of *Treponema pallidum?*

3. *With the exception of* Treponema pallidum, *all other spirochetal pathogens are zoonotic or vectorborne diseases.* This is an important epidemiologic feature of these diseases. Human leptospirosis is acquired through contact with infected animals and is most important as an occupational disease of persons engaged in some form of animal maintenance. The infections caused by *Borrelia* spp. are vectorborne or vectorborne zoonoses. Because of the intimate habits of the vector *Pediculus humanus corporis,* with man its host, louseborne relapsing fever tends to occur in epidemics where crowding and lack of hygiene may be factors. Although a vectorborne disease is by definition a zoonosis, *Borrelia recurrentis* does not appear to have other animal reservoirs. In contrast, *Borrelia burgdorferi* and the multiple species of ticks that cause relapsing fever have many animal reservoirs. This feature may explain the rural and suburban distribution of these diseases as well as their focality because access to the reservoir and to the vector are obviously critical for transmission. The focality of these last two diseases is strikingly self evident. The early epidemiologic studies of Steere and co-workers in Connecticut indicated that the incidence of Lyme disease on the two opposing shores of a river were dramatically different.[80] Today, Lyme disease has a very high incidence east of New York City (Long Island) as well as north (Westchester County), but the city itself, which lacks suitable reservoirs and vectors, has virtually no native Lyme disease.[10,93]

In the United States, there are thousands of cases of spirochetal diseases. Heading the list for the first 9 months of 1991 is syphilis with 30,658 cases (both primary and secondary), followed by Lyme disease with 6,783 cases, as reported in *Morbidity and Mortality Weekly Reports,* Oct. 4, 1991. The impact of these diseases is far greater than their numbers would suggest because of the long duration of the illnesses, the cost of parenteral antibiotic therapy, and the high morbidity of the diseases. In the United States, relapsing fever and leptospirosis are low-frequency disease. This is not so worldwide; relapsing fever can be found in large numbers in Africa. All together, these diseases are as important as they are fascinating to study. Additional reading on these topics can be found in a monograph[51] and in excellent reviews.[2,15]

BORRELIA

It is without doubt that human disease caused by spirochetes of the genus *Borrelia* was present in ancient times and was probably described by Hippocrates and by physicians in ancient Egypt.[31,63] Epidemics of borreliosis, in the form of relapsing fever, have occurred throughout recorded history,

right up until modern times,[13] and it was only with the advent of more effective control measures and improvements in treatment through the use of antibiotics that the incidence of this disease was finally brought under comparative control.

Relapsing fever in humans occurs in two forms. Both are vectorborne. The epidemic form, caused by *Borrelia recurrentis,* is transmitted from person to person by the body louse, *Pediculus humanus.* There is no animal reservoir. The endemic form is transmitted by various species of the soft tick *Ornithodoros* and is caused by a number of different species of *Borrelia* in North and South America, including *B. hermsii, B. turicatae, B. parkeri, B. mazzottii,* and *B. venezuelensis. Borrelia* species responsible for endemic relapsing fever in the Old World are *B. duttonii, B. crocidurae, B. persica, B. hispanica, B. latyschewii,* and *B. caucasica.*[11,31]

In addition to causing human disease, *Borrelia* spp. are of significant veterinary importance. *B. theileri* (bovine borreliosis)[31] and *B. coriaceae* (epizootic bovine abortion)[57] cause disease in domestic cattle. *B. anserina* is the cause of avian borreliosis.[31] *B. burgdorferi,*[16] the causative agent of Lyme disease, is transmitted by the ixodid hard ticks *Ixodes dammini* and *I. pacificus* in North America, *I. ricinus* in Europe, and *I. persulcatus* in Asia.

Borrelia spp. vary in length from 8 μm for *B. coriaceae*[57] to more than 20 μm for *B. burgdorferi,*[16,57] with widths ranging from 0.2 to 0.3 μm[16,47] for *B. burgdorferi* to 0.45 to 0.5 μm for *B. recurrentis* and *B. persica.*[44,54] Structurally, *Borrelia* spp. share many of the characteristics of other spirochetes including a fluid, lipid-rich outer envelope[6,22,52] enclosing a periplasmic space containing anywhere from 15 to 30 endoflagellae for relapsing fever borreliae[45-47] and 7 to 11 endoflagellae for *B. burgdorferi.*[16,47] The endoflagellae are not located at the cell surface as is the case for other bacterial flagellae but reside in the periplasmic space between the outer envelope and the protoplasmic cylinder.[7] These endoflagellae contain many structural similarities to the flagellae of other bacteria and also exhibit significant NH_2-terminal amino acid identity with the endoflagellae of other spirochetes.[23] The innermost component of the spirochete, the protoplasmic cylinder, which contains the cytoplasm and genomic elements as well as the peptidoglycan, is responsible for giving the spirochete its characteristic coiled appearance.

Human relapsing fever

In general, the clinical course of human relapsing fever consists of an incubation period, followed by the first attack and by a number of relapses. The incubation period for louseborne relapsing fever is generally regarded to be from 2 to 15 days, although the more common scenario would be 5 to 8 days.[31] The incubation period for the tickborne variety is generally regarded to be anywhere from 2 to 12 days.[31] Transmission from louse to human is accomplished by the infected person crushing the louse and inadvertently introducing the *Borrelia*-containing hemolymph into the bite wound. Transmission can also occur by transferring contaminated material to the conjunctiva with the fingers.[19] Transmission of the tickborne relapsing fever is accomplished as a direct result of tick feeding through introduction of saliva[34,90] or excretion.[20,90] The duration of the incubation period may depend on the spirochete burden of the arthropod vector and, thus, on the number of spirochetes that enter the body.[31] After entering the bloodstream, the borreliae rapidly multiply at the rate of approximately once every 6 hours.[28,86] In laboratory animals, the spirochetemia can be as high as 10^7 borreliae/ml of blood.[18,86] The patient may experience headache, chills, weakness, malaise, vertigo, vague aches and pains, and nausea.[31] The onset of these symptoms may be quite sudden and is usually accompanied by a high fever with some daily fluctuations. If treatment is not provided, this period of high fever normally lasts 2 to 3 days and is followed by a period in which the patient will feel well. The patient invariably experiences a number of relapses punctuated by periods of wellness. This clinical scenario of relapse followed by apparent recovery is usually sufficient for making a diagnosis in a patient.[31] Although relapsing fever does exhibit significant organ-tropisms in humans and animals,[9,18,38] with the brain being most favored, relapsing fever is primarily an infection of the bloodstream.

The relapse phenomenon characteristic of relapsing fever was an obvious point of interest for the pioneers in the study of immunology and was recognized as a potential model for the study of the immune system. Useful contributions were made as early as 1918 when Janeso[50] reported that *Borrelia* isolates made from infected mice in the relapse stage of the infection differed serologically from those of the first attack stage. The fact that the relapse isolates were different antigenically from the first attack isolates presumably allowed them to proliferate in the presence of host protective factors derived against the attack isolate. This antigenic change was subsequently shown to be reversible when the isolates were passed back into nonimmune animals. Later studies[12,65] on both louseborne and tickborne *Borreliae* showed that this antigenic variation was more complex than originally thought in that a number of distinct serotypes could be distinguished in relapse isolates. A question that still remained was whether anti-

genically distinct populations of *Borreliae* arose during the course of the infection or were present along with the first attack population in the original isolate. This was impossible to answer using nonhomogeneous populations of spirochetes. It was resolved when Schuhardt and Wilkerson,[77] using *B. turicatae* cloned from a single cell, showed that relapses still occurred. More recently, Stoenner et al.,[86] using cloned *B. hermsii* infection of mice as a laboratory model, isolated 25 separate and distinct serotypes. In recent years, studies on the biology of borreliae, most notably *B. hermsii*, have led investigators to conclude that antigenic variation in borreliae is a reversible, genetically induced antigenic change that gives the spirochete an obvious advantage in eluding the host immune response. Immunofluorescence studies[21] indicated that the variable antigens were located on the cell surface. Another study indicated that they were proteinaceous in character.[33] SDS-polyacrylamide gel electrophoresis (PAGE) and Western blot analysis of homogeneous populations of several serotypes of *B. hermsii* has revealed that antigenic variation is associated with a change in a single surface exposed protein of variable molecular weight designated the variable major protein (VMP).[5,6] Each serotype of *B. hermsii* had its own characteristic VMP, which differed from VMPs of other serotypes in molecular weight, peptide map profile, and reactivity to serotype-specific polyclonal and monoclonal antibodies.[3-5] The genes encoding for several of these VMPs have been cloned and subsequently expressed in *Escherichia coli*.[64,73] Plasterk et al[73] showed that in *B. hermsii* with regard to VMP_7 and VMP_{21}, expressed VMP genes are located on an expression plasmid adjacent to an expression sequence. Unexpressed VMP genes are located on a storage plasmid. Antigenic variation involves the removal of the expressed VMP gene and movement of the unexpressed VMP gene to a site adjacent on the expression plasmid with the concomitant transcription and translation of that particular VMP. In summary, the cyclic process of antigenic variation is due to the appearance of new antigens followed by the production of specific antibodies. Eventually, the organisms revert to the expression of antigens to which antibodies already exist, and this may signal the end of the period of febrile relapses.

The pathophysiology of relapsing fever is associated with spirochetemia in which infections with *B. recurrentis* can reach 10^5 organisms/ml[33,79] of blood. During the remission periods, surviving borreliae appear to be confined to organs, because they cannot be found in the circulation. This trafficking between circulation and organs is accompanied by the febrile-afebrile periods of this disease.

In general, the clinical course of relapsing fever is similar in infections with *B. recurrentis* and with the species associated with ticks.[13,33,79] The literature seems to convey the impression, however, that louseborne relapsing fever may last longer and be somewhat more severe. For example, the louseborne infection has longer periods of fever, but a smaller number of relapses than tickborne infection. In fact, louseborne relapsing fever often only has one relapse.

The onset of relapsing fever can be abrupt with high fever, headache, and other constitutional manifestations. Tachycardia and other cardiovascular abnormalities can be present in some patients. Myocarditis and conduction abnormalities of the heart have been reported. A rash, which can be maculopapular and/or petechial and restricted to the trunk, can be noted at the time of fever resolution of the first episode. Hemorrhage, as noted in the skin petechiae, nosebleed, and hematuria, is a common finding of acute relapsing fever.

Neurologic manifestations are common and important in relapsing fever and have been noted in 30% of the patients. These can include cranial neuritis, meningitis, encephalitis, and hemiplegia.

Increases in protein and a pleocytosis (mild to moderate) of the cerebrospinal fluid (CSF) are common in neurologic relapsing fever, but particularly in patients with central nervous system (CNS) manifestations. Borrelial organisms can be found in the CSF. The diagnosis of relapsing fever is made by direct visualization of the spirochetes in the blood during the periods of fever. Thin blood smears can be stained with Giemsa or acridine orange.[78] Because the organisms appear to be organ bound during the afebrile period, examination of the blood at these times may not be productive. Because the tickborne form of this disease is associated with production of antibodies to variable antigens, it is to be expected that serology for relapsing fever would be most productive after a full complement of specific antibodies have been formed.[32] In the United States, serology for relapsing fever is done in large reference laboratories. It should be remembered that sera from patients with relapsing fever cross-react with antigens from *B. burgdorferi*.[61] In these cases, the ease of spirochetal demonstration in the blood, the occurrence of relapsing febrile periods, and other geographic and epidemiologic features should be sufficient to establish a diagnosis. Tetracycline, chloramphenicol, penicillin, and erythromycin have been used to treat relapsing fever.[43,72] As in Lyme disease, treatment failures have been reported.[43,72,79] The Jarisch-Herxheimer reaction is typically associated with this infection with paroxysms, leukopenia, increase in fever, and a drop in blood pressure. Three studies have implicated a spirochetal endotoxin as the inducer of the Jarisch-Herxheimer reaction.[14,17,35]

Lyme disease

Lyme disease bears a resemblance to other spirochetal diseases such as syphilis and relapsing fever in that it is typically characterized by periods of acute illness followed by periods of apparent remission. It is similar to syphilis in that, if left untreated, the disease tends to progress in stages with extended periods where the patient may feel totally asymptomatic. The symptoms associated with early Lyme disease usually occur between 3 and 14 days after being bitten by a tick that is infected with *B. burgdorferi*. During this period of infection, approximately 60% of patients will experience erythema migrans[81,83] (EM), which is characterized as an expanding erythematous annular skin lesion with central clearing that usually appears at the site of the tick bite. Approximately one half of this group of patients will also develop satellite lesions in other areas of the body. Concurrent with EM, the patient may complain of low-grade fever, headache, stiff neck, lack of energy, arthralgias and myalgias, and generalized or regional lymphadenopathy.[83]

Second-stage Lyme disease normally occurs during a period of several weeks to several months after the appearance of EM and is characterized by the involvement of the cardiovascular and central nervous systems. The skin and joints may also be affected.[1,71,75,81] The cardiac disorder is primarily manifested by one or more forms of cardiac arrhythmia, with incomplete or complete heart block,[24] and is usually self-limiting.[62,67] Neurologic signs include bilateral Bell's palsy, meningitis, Bannwarth's syndrome, and encephalitis and radiculitis,[68,75,81] which may occur suddenly shortly after EM or may progress gradually over a period of months.* During this stage, the spirochete may be isolated from the CSF of patients with meningitis,[74,84] although instances are rare. *B. burgdorferi* has an affinity for glial cells of the CNS.[36] This may explain why isolations from CSF are so rare. The arthritis of second-stage Lyme disease is usually migratory and polyarticular.

Third-stage Lyme disease occurs months or years after the initial infection and is often described as the chronic phase of the disease. It is characterized by the involvement of the joints, with the knee, wrist, and shoulder most commonly involved.[41,49,81,82] Peripheral nervous system[8,69] and skin[1,48] are also involved. In third-stage Lyme disease, CNS abnormalities may be the direct result of invasion of brain tissue by *B. burgdorferi* as

---

*References 40, 42, 66, 75, 76, 85.

demonstrated by the fact that the organism has been seen in brain tissue sections.[59,60,92] *B. burgdorferi* has also been isolated from brains of infected Syrian hamsters.[53] The cutaneous disorders found in third-stage Lyme disease are lymphocytoma, which is an erythematous inflammation usually found on the ear lobe or surrounding the nipple, and acrodermatitis chronica atrophicans (ACA), a gradually progressing dermatitis usually of the feet, hands, elbows, and knees.

LEPTOSPIRA

Leptospirosis is a complex zoonosis caused by one organism, *Leptospira interrogans*, which, in turn, has numerous serotypes, known in the current literature as *"serovars."*[89] The most common serovars associated with human infection are noted in Table 8–1. Human infection tends to be an occupational occurrence and is determined by the type of contact to be had in the epizootiologic chain of this disease. Because leptospirosis is a widespread zoonosis, persons who work as veterinarians, livestock workers, ranchers, and farmers working with domestic animals are at high risk for this disease. Transmission occurs after leptospires penetrate mucous membranes or wounds. Leptospires are transmitted by way of the urine of infected animals, and contaminated water and soil. Leptospirosis can be a chronic kidney and urinary tract infection in reservoir animals[29,30] and thus can remain a source of organisms for long periods of time.

Leptospirosis has an incubation period of 6 to 13 days. The first manifestations involve fever, malaise, headache, and nausea and may last for about 1 week. Leptospires are present in the blood and CSF during this period, which is self-limited, followed by a short period of remission. The second stages of this disease can result in an immune anicteric leptospirosis, or an icteric leptospirosis also known as Weil's disease. Feigen and co-workers,[29] Edwards and Domm,[27] and Heath et al[39] have described this disease in detail; this account is extracted from their observations.

Anicteric leptospirosis is characterized by fever, headache, malaise, and weakness. The immune

stage follows the remission of the first or "septicemic" stage and presents with headache of unusual severity. Meningitis is the single most common sign of this stage but can also involve ocular abnormalities, generalized lymphadenopathy and splenomegaly, tachycardia, respiratory involvement, nausea and vomiting, and abdominal pain.

The meningitis of this immune stage of anicteric leptospirosis is usually aseptic. Leptospires can be found in the CSF during the early or septicemic stage, but, during the second phase, the CSF does not contain the organisms, which have been replaced by antibody. There is pleocytosis in the CSF, and elevated protein and pressure. In the more severe cases, myocarditis, renal failure, and hemorrhage complete the clinical presentation.

Icteric leptospirosis or Weil's syndrome has a clinical presentation that is essentially different from that described earlier. This stage of leptospirosis involves renal and hepatic disease and is considered to be significantly more severe. Hepatomegaly occurs in about one fourth of the patients; direct bilirubin is elevated, and there is a marked increase in serum creatinine phosphokinase. Alkaline phosphatase and liver transaminases are only moderately elevated. As it may be expected from these manifestations, jaundice is a primary finding. The renal involvement is associated with severe jaundice and is thought to result from the underlying vasculitis present in this disease. Urine tests are almost always abnormal with proteinuria and hematuria. Renal failure can occur.[56] Myocardial abnormalities such as congestive heart failure and hemorrhagic myocarditis have been reported in Weil's syndrome.

Microhemorrhage with capillary injury is the main organ finding in this disease and probably is the basis for the clinical manifestations. Thrombocytopenia without disseminated intravascular coagulation is very common in second phase leptospirosis.[25,26]

Leptospires are the most easily cultivated of all the spirochetes; thus, diagnosis is definitive if the organisms can be isolated from body fluids in the septicemic or early disease stages. With advancing disease, leptospires become more difficult to isolate, except for some organs such as the kidney, so diagnosis relies more on serology. A number of serologic assays are available including enzyme-linked immunosorbent assay (ELISA) and slide agglutinations based on the appearance of agglutinins.[70,91] Although the leptospiral serology is sensitive and specific, it is best to attempt to isolate the organism. Serology may not be able to identify the precise infecting serovar, whereas the organisms can be serotyped if an isolate is available.

Although leptospirosis is seldom a fatal disease,

Table 8-1 Serovars of *Leptospira interrogans* associated with human disease

Leptospira interrogans serovar australis
autumnalis
canicola
grippotyphosa
helodomidis
icterohaemor-
rhagiae
pomona

several complications, notably renal failure, hemorrhage, and hypotension, require supportive attention beyond the usually curative regimens of penicillin or tetracycline.

Leptospirosis is a major disease of dogs, and a vaccine exists for these animals. Dogs can be a major source of transmission to humans, even those who are immunized.[30]

SYPHILIS AND OTHER SIMILARITIES

A full or even partial consideration of syphilis in this overview of spirochetal diseases is beyond the scope of this chapter; therefore, the brief treatment afforded here is hardly a manifestation of its true importance. Only those areas that have specific relevance to potential similarities to Lyme disease are considered.

Endarteritis obliterans is a pathologic hallmark of syphilis. The pathology of this lesion is well-known. A similar pathologic phenomenon has been described in Lyme disease—specifically in the synovium of Lyme arthritis patients.[24] In fact, focal vasculitic lesions are becoming increasingly reported in Lyme disease.[24] Earlier, we discussed the vasculitic pathology of leptospirosis and indicated that much of the organ pathology and, hence, the disease can be the result of vessel wall damage. Experimental evidence has shown that *T. pallidum* and *B. burgdorferi* can attach and move across endothelial cell monolayers.[87,88] The collective evidence for vasculitic injury in several spirochetal diseases may not be a coincidence, and this tissue could be a primary target for spirochetes as a site outside the circulation. That inflammation of the blood vessels occurs in several spirochetal diseases may be an indication that the organisms may reside and even activate endothelium at least for a period of time leading to the production of injury.

Another area of similarity between syphilis and Lyme disease is the rapid spread of their respective agents to the CNS.[37,58] A nervous system tropism has been suggested for relapsing fever *Borrelia*. Indeed, neurologic abnormalities are common and important in all four diseases considered here. The evidence for a nervous system tropism, however, needs to be balanced against the fact that many other organ systems are affected in spirochetal diseases. Spirochetes, however, can be considered naturally neuropathogenic. That is, they invade the nervous system early and affect all patients regardless of age and with far greater frequency than other bacteria that produce neurologic abnormalities.

ACKNOWLEDGMENT

This article was supported in part by grants AI27044 and AR40445 from the National Institutes of Health and by a grant from the Mathers Charitable Foundation.

REFERENCES

1. Asbrink E, Hovmark A: Cutaneous manifestations in *Ixodes*-borne *Borrelia* spirochetosis, *Int J Dermatol* 26:215, 1987.
2. Barbour AG, Hayes SF: Biology of *Borrelia* species, *Microbiol Rev* 50:381, 1986.
3. Barbour AG, Barrera O, Judd R: Structural analysis of the variable major proteins of *Borrelia hermsii, J Exp Med* 158:2127, 1983.
4. Barbour AG, Stoenner HG: Antigenic variation of *Borrelia hermsii, UCLA Symp Mol Cell Biol New Ser* 20:123, 1984.
5. Barbour AG, Tessier SL, Stoenner HG: Variable major proteins of *Borrelia hermsii, J Exp Med* 156:1312, 1982.
6. Barbour AG, Tessier SL, Todd WJ: Lyme disease spirochetes and *Ixodes* tick spirochetes share a common surface antigenic determinant as defined by a monoclonal antibody, *Infect Immun* 41:795, 1983.
7. Barbour AG et al: *Borrelia* genus-specific monoclonal antibody binds to a flagellar epitope, *Infect Immun* 52:549, 1986.
8. Baumhackl U et al: Neurological manifestations of *Borrelia burgdorferi* infections: the enlarging clinical spectrum, *Zentralbl Bakteriol Mikrobial Hyg [A]* 263:334, 1986.
9. Beck MD: California field and laboratory studies on relapsing fever, *J Infect Dis* 60:64, 1937.
10. Benach JL, Coleman JL: Clinical and geographic characteristics of Lyme disease in New York, *Zentralbl Bakteriol Mikrobiol Hyg* 263:477, 1986.
11. Bone G: L'infection des *Ornithodorus moubata* par le spirochete di Dutton, *C R Soc Biol* 129:903, 1938.
12. Brussin AM, Rogowa GJ: Zur frage der pathogenese der rezidie beim experimentellen ruckfallfieber, *Zbl Bakt I Abt Orig* 20:39, 1927.
13. Bryceson ADM et al: Louse-borne relapsing fever. A clinical and laboratory study of 62 cases in Ethiopia and a reconsideration of the literature, *Q J Med* 39:129, 1970.
14. Bryceson ADM et al: Studies on the mechanism of the Jarisch Herxheimer reaction in louse-borne relapsing fever: evidence for the presence of circulating *Borrelia* endotoxin, *Clin Sci* 43:343, 1972.
15. Burgdorfer W: The enlarging spectrum of tick borne spirochetosis, *Rev Infect Dis* 8:932, 1986.
16. Burgdorfer W et al: Lyme disease—a tick borne spirochetosis? *Science* 216:1317, 1982.
17. Butlar T, Jones PK, Wallace CK: *Borrelia recurrentis* infection: clinical trials of antibiotics and management of the Jarisch Herxheimer-like reaction, *J Infect Dis* 137:573, 1978.
18. Chorine V, Crougue O: Virulence du sang du cobaye infecte avec le *Spirochaeta hispanica, Ann Inst Pasteur* (Paris) 68:518, 1942.
19. Chung H-L: The cerebrospinal fluid of patients suffering from the Chinese strain of relapsing fever, *Trans R Soc Trop Med Hyg* 31:625, 1938.
20. Chung H-L, Wei Y-L: Studies on the transmission of relapsing fever in north China II. Observations on the mechanism of transmission of relapsing fever in man, *Am J Trop Med* 18:661, 1938.
21. Coffee EM, Eveland WC: Experimental relapsing fever initiated by *Borrelia hermsii*. II. Sequential appearance of major serotypes in the rat, *J Infect Dis* 117:29, 1967.
22. Coleman JL, Benach JL: Isolation of the outer envelope from *Borrelia burgdorferi, Zentralbl Bakteriol Mikrobiol Hyg [A]* 263:123, 1986.
23. Coleman JL, Benach JL: Identification and characterization of an endoflagellar antigen of *Borrelia burgdorferi, J Clin Invest* 84:322, 1988.
24. Duray PH, Steere AC: Clinical pathologic correlations of Lyme disease by stage, *Ann NY Acad Sci* 539:65, 1988.
25. Edwards CN, Nicholson DG, Everard COR: Thrombocy-

topenia in leptospirosis, *Am J Trop Med Hyg* 31:827, 1982.

26. Edwards CN, et al: Thrombocytopenia in leptospirosis: The absence of evidence for disseminated intravascular coagulation, *Am J Trop Med Hyg* 35:352, 1986.

27. Edwards GA, Domm BM: Human leptospirosis, *Medicine* 39:117, 1960.

28. Eidmann E, Lippett H, Poespodihardjo S: Quantitative untersuchungen uber die vermehsung von *Borrellia erratici* in der weissen maus, *Z Tropen Med Parasitol* 10:339, 1948.

29. Feigen RD, Anderson DC: Human leptospirosis, *CRC Critical Rev Clin Lab Sci* 5:413, 1975.

30. Feigen RD et al: Human leptospirosis from immunized dogs, *Ann Intern Med* 79:777, 1973.

31. Felsenfeld O: *Strains, vectors, human and animal borreliosis*, St Louis, 1971, Warren H. Green.

32. Felsenfeld O: *Immunity relapsing fever*. In Johnson RC, editor: *The biology of parasites spirochetes*, New York, 1976, Academic Press.

33. Felsenfeld O et al: Studies in borreliae. II. Some immunologic, biochemical, and physical properties of the antigenic components of *Borrelia turicatae*, *J Immunol* 94:805, 1965.

34. Gaber MS et al: *Borrelia crocidurae* localization and transmission in *Ornithodorus erracticus* and *O. savignyi*, *Parasitology* 88:403, 1984.

35. Galloway RE et al: Activation of protein mediators of inflammation and evidence for endotoxemia in *Borrelia recurrentis* infection, *Am J Med* 63:933, 1977.

36. Garcia-Monco JC, Fernandez Villar B, Benach JL: Adherence of Lyme disease spirochetes to glial cells and cells of glial origin, *J Infect Dis* 160:497, 1989.

37. Garcia-Monco JC et al: *Borrelia burgdorferi* in the central nervous system: experimental and clinical evidence for early invasion, *J Infect Dis* 161:1187, 1990.

38. Hassan IM: Experimental observations on *Treponema recurrentis*, *J Egypt Public Health Assoc*, p 237, 1941.

39. Heath CW Jr, Alexander AD, Galton MM: Leptospirosis in the United States. Analysis of 483 cases in man, 1949-1961, *N Engl J Med* 273:857, 1965.

40. Henriksson A et al: Immunoglobulin abnormalities in cerebrospinal fluid and blood over the course of lymphocytic meningo-radiculitis (Bannwarth's syndrome), *Ann Neurol* 20:337, 1986.

41. Herzer P et al: Lyme arthritis: clinical features, serological and radiographic findings of cases in Germany, *Klin Wochenschr* 64:206, 1986.

42. Hindfett B et al: Clinical and cerebrospinal fluid findings in lymphocytic meningo-radiculitis (Bannwarth's syndrome), *Acta Neurol Scand* 66:444, 1982.

43. Horton JM, Blaser MJ: The spectrum of relapsing fever in the Rocky Mountains, *Arch Intern Med* 145:871, 1985.

44. Hovind-Hougen K: Electron microscopy of *Borrelia merionesi* and *Borrelia recurrentis*, *Acta Pathol Microbiol Scand Sect B* 82:799, 1974.

45. Hovind-Hougen K: Determination by means of electron microscopy of morphologic criteria of value for some spirochetes in particular treponemes, *Acta Pathol Microbiol Scand Suppl B* 225:1, 1976.

46. Hovind-Hougen K: Treponema *and* Borrelia *morphology*. In Johnson RC, editor: *The biology of parasitic spirochetes*, New York, 1976, Academic Press.

47. Hovind-Hougen K: Ultrastructure of spirochetes isolated from *Ixodes ricinus* and *Ixodes dammini*, *Yale J Biol Med* 57:543, 1984.

48. Hovmark A, Asbrink E, Olsson I: The spirochetal etiology of lymphadenosis benigna cutis sollitaria, *Acta Derm Venereol* 66:479, 1986.

49. Jacobs, JC, Stevens M, Duray PH: Lyme disease simulating septic arthritis, *JAMA* 256:1138, 1986.

50. Janeso N: Experimentelle untersuchung bezuglich der pathogenese der rezidive des ruckfallfiebers, *Zbl Bakt Orig* 81:457, 1918.

51. Johnson RC, editor: *The biology of parasitic spirochetes*, New York, 1976, Academic Press.

52. Johnson RC: The spirochetes, *Ann Rev Microbiol* 31:89, 1977.

53. Johnson RC, Marek N, Kodner C: Infection of Syrian hamsters with Lyme disease spirochetes, *J Clin Microbiol* 20:1099, 1984.

54. Karmi Y: *Borrelia persica* and *B. baltazardi* sp. nov.: experimental pathogenicity for some animals and comparisons of the ultrastructure, *Ann Microbiol (Paris)* 130:157, 1979.

55. Kelly R: Cultivation of *Borrelia hermsii*, *Science* 173:443, 1971.

56. Kennedy ND et al: Leptospirosis and acute renal failure—clinical experience and a review of the literature, *Post Grad Med J* 55:176, 1979.

57. Lane RS et al: Isolation of a spirochete from the soft tick *Ornithodorus coriaceus:* a possible agent of epizootic bovine abortion, *Science* 230:85, 1985.

58. Lukehart SA et al: Invasion of the central nervous system by *Treponema pallidum:* implications for diagnosis and treatment, *Ann Intern Med* 109:855, 1988.

59. MacDonald AB: *Borrelia* in the brains of patients dying with dementia, *JAMA* 256:2195, 1986.

60. MacDonald AB, Mirando JM: Concurrent neocortical borreliosis and Alzheimer's disease, *Hum Pathol* 18:759, 1987.

61. Magnarelli LA, Anderson JF, Johnson RC: Crossreactivity in serological tests for Lyme disease and other spirochetal infections, *J Infect Dis* 156:183, 1987.

62. Marcus LC et al: Fatal pancarditis in a patient with coexistent Lyme disease and babesiosis: demonstration of spirochetes in the myocardium, *Ann Intern Med* 103:374, 1985.

63. Martini E: Zur alteren geschichte der recurrens im europaischen raum, *Ergeb Hyg Bakteriol Immunitaetsforsch Exp Thec* 29:213, 1955.

64. Meier JT, Simon MI, Barbour AG: Antigenic variation is associated with DNA rearrangements in a relapsing fever *Borrelia*, *Cell* 41:403, 1985.

65. Meleney HE: Relapse phenomena of *Spironema recurrentis*, *J Exp Med* 48:65, 1928.

66. Murray N et al: Specificity of CSF antibodies against components of *Borrelia burgdorferi* in patients with meningopolyneuritis Garin-Bujadoux-Bannworth, *J Neurol* 233:224, 1986.

67. Olson LJ, Okafon EC, Clements IP: Cardiac involvement in Lyme disease: manifestations and management, *Mayo Clin Proc* 61:745, 1986.

68. Pachner AR, Steere AC: The triad of neurologic abnormalities of Lyme disease: meningitis, cranial neuritis, and radiculoneuritis, *Neurology* 35:47, 1985.

69. Pachner AR, Steere AC: CNS manifestations of third stage Lyme disease, *Zentralbl Bakteriol Mikrobiol Hyg [A]* 263:301, 1986.

70. Pappas MG et al: Rapid serodiagnosis of leptospirosis using the IgM specific dot ELISA: comparison with the microscopic agglutination tests, *Am J Trop Med Hyg* 34:346, 1985.

71. Park HK, Jones BE, Barbour AG: Erythema chronicum migrans: diagnosis by monoclonal antibodies, *J Am Acad Dermatol* 15:406, 1986.

72. Perine PL, Teklu B: Antibiotic treatment of louse borne relapsing fever in Ethiopia: a report of 377 cases, *Am J Trop Med Hyg* 32:1096, 1983.

73. Plasterk RHA, Simon MI, Barbour AG: Transposition of structural genes to an expression sequence on a linear plasmid causes antigenic variation in the bacterium *Borrelia hermsii, Nature* 318:257, 1985.

74. Preac-Mursic V et al: Repeated isolation of spirochetes from the cerebrospinal fluid of a patient with meningoradiculitis Bannwarth, *Eur J Clin Microbiol* 3:564, 1984.

75. Reik L et al: Neurologic abnormalities of Lyme disease, *Medicine (Baltimore)* 58:281, 1979.

76. Ryberg B et al: Antineural antibodies in Guillain-Barre syndrome and lymphocytic meningoradiculitis (Bannwarth's syndrome), *Arch Neurol* 41:1277, 1984.

77. Schuhardt VT, Wilkerson M: Relapse phenomena in rats infected with single spirochetes (*Borrelia recurrentis* var. turicatae), *J Bacteriol* 62:215, 1951.

78. Sciotto CG et al: Detection of *Borrelia* in acridine orange blood smears by fluorescence microscopy, *Arch Pathol Lab Med* 107:384, 1983.

79. Southern PM Jr, Sanford JP: Relapsing fever, a clinical and microbiological review. *Medicine* 48:129, 1969.

80. Steere AC, Malawista SE: Cases of Lyme disease in the United States: locations correlated with the distribution of *Ixodes dammini, Ann Intern Med* 91:730, 1979.

81. Steere AC et al: Erythema chronicum migrans and Lyme arthritis: the enlarging clinical spectrum, *Ann Intern Med* 86:685, 1977.

82. Steere AC et al: Chronic Lyme arthritis: clinical and immunogenetic differentation from rheumatoid arthritis, *Ann Intern Med* 90:896, 1979.

83. Steere AC et al: The early clinical manifestations of Lyme disease, *Ann Intern Med* 99:76, 1983.

84. Steere AC et al: The spirochetal etiology of Lyme disease, *N Engl J Med* 308:733, 1983.

85. Stiernstedt GT et al: Diagnosis of spirochetal meningitis by enzyme-linked immunosorbent assay and indirect immunofluorescence assay in serum and cerebrospinal fluid, *J Clin Microbiol* 21:819, 1985.

86. Stoenner HG, Dodd T, Larsen C: Antigenic variation of *Borrelia hermsii, J Exp Med* 156:1297, 1982.

87. Szczepanski A et al: The interaction between *Borrelia burgdorferi* with endothelium in vitro, *J Clin Invest* 85:1637, 1990.

88. Thomas DD et al: *Treponema pallidum* invades intercellular junctions of endothelial cell monolayers. *Proc Natl Acad Sci USA* 85:3608, 1988.

89. Turner LH: *Classification of spirochetes in general and of the genus* Leptospira *in particular.* In Johnson RC, editor: *The biology of parasitic spirochetes,* New York, 1976, Academic Press.

90. Varma MGR: Comparative studies on the transmission of two strains of *Spirochaeta duttoni* by *Ornithodorus moubata* and of *S. turicatae* by *Q. turicata, Ann Trop Med Parasitol* 50:1, 1956.

91. Watt G et al: The rapid diagnosis of leptospirosis: a prospective comparison of the dot enzyme linked immunosorbent assay and the genus specific microscopic agglutination test at different stages of illness, *J Infect Dis* 157:840, 1988.

92. Weber K et al: *Borrelia burgdorferi* in a newborn despite oral penicillin for Lyme borreliosis during pregnancy, *Pediatr Infect Dis* 7:286, 1988.

93. White DJ et al: The geographic spread and temporal increase of the Lyme disease epidermic. *JAMA* 266:1230, 1991.

9 Dermatologic Aspects

Bernard W. Berger

Erythema migrans,[10,11,16,30] acrodermatitis chronica atrophicans,[7] and borrelial lymphocytoma[23] have been established as cutaneous markers of Lyme disease. The expanding knowledge of this illness has led to the introduction of additional cutaneous entities thought to be directly associated with a *Borrelia burgdorferi* infection. This association is not without controversy, particularly with sclerotic lesions, and until definitive studies are forthcoming, an open mind is in order.

ERYTHEMA MIGRANS
Clinical appearance

Erythema migrans (EM) is the most common and distinctive cutaneous manifestation of Lyme disease.[13,14,29] The clinical diagnosis of Lyme disease can be established by correctly identifying this lesion. This is particularly important because serologic tests are frequently not reactive during the first few weeks of the illness, a time when EM is most likely to be present.[17,25,29]

EM is a dynamic lesion whose clinical appearance changes dramatically over a period of days. It occurs in 60% to 80% of the patients with Lyme disease.[29] The more thorough the cutaneous examination, the greater the likelihood of discovering the lesion.

EM appears 8 to 9 days (range: 2 to 28 days) after the bite of an infected Ixodid tick. It begins as a red macule, which becomes papular before expanding into an annular erythematous plaque. The erythema is generally uniform in intensity initially, but, as the lesion expands, some areas within the plaque may pale or fade completely, resulting in two general forms: an expanding red plaque with varying intensities of redness within the plaque (see Color Plate Fig. 1); or a central red plaque surrounded by normal appearing skin, which, in turn, is surrounded by an expanding red band resembling a target or a ring within a ring configuration.[11]

There is considerable variation in the appearance of EM, particularly its central portion, which usually persists as an erythematous plaque but may appear edematous, vesicular (see Color Plate Fig. 2), or crusted. In some lesions, there is complete clearing of the central erythema. However, the centrifugally enlarging periphery tends to remain a distinct erythematous band until the lesion resolves. Although circular lesions predominate, triangular (see Color Plate Fig. 3) or elongated oval lesions may occur. As its name indicates, most EM lesions are reddish in color, but some lesions, particularly those appearing on the lower extremities, may present with a blue-red hue.[11,14]

A review of 200 consecutive patients with solitary EM lesions showed they appeared most commonly on the trunk (38%) and lower extremities (38%). The upper extremities were next in frequency (11%), followed by the pelvic region (7%), and the head and neck (6%). Although children under 5 years of age accounted for only 6% of these 200 patients, they represented 40% (5 of 12) of the patients presenting with EM of the head and neck.[15]

EM lesions are frequently warmer than the surrounding clinically normal skin. They are usually asymptomatic but have been described as being pruritic or painful.

The size and rate of expansion of EM are also variable. Most lesions demonstrate gradual centrifugal enlargement, whereas others expand rapidly, forming a large plaque in a relatively short time (see Color Plate Fig. 4). For example, patients seen 8 to 14 days after the appearance of EM had lesions ranging in size from 4 by 6 cm to 20 by 42 cm (median: 12 by 17 cm).[14]

Although EM appears as a solitary lesion in most instances, multiple lesions also occur (see Color Plate Fig. 5). Multiple lesions represent dissemination of *B. burgdorferi* from the original EM to other skin sites by way of the blood or lymphatics. The frequency of occurrence of these secondary EM lesions ranged from 6% to 48%[10,14,30] and probably depended on when in the course of the illness the patient was evaluated. Patients evaluated 6 to 7 days after the appearance of EM had multiple lesions 17% of the time.[14] They tend to be smaller than the primary EM lesion, are more likely to have clear centers, occur on any skin surface except the palms and soles, and are asymptomatic. Secondary EM lesions do not appear on mucous membranes.

Extracutaneous signs and symptoms

When EM appears alone or in combination with minor constitutional symptoms, Lyme disease is considered to be localized. If EM is accompanied by extracutaneous signs and symptoms of major intensity, or if EM appears in multiplicity, Lyme disease is considered to be disseminated. The significance of this distinction is in the patient's response to treatment, in that patients with localized disease usually experience a favorable response to initial antibiotic treatment, whereas patients with disseminated illness may require retreatment.[12]

In a study of 237 patients with EM in which the initial evaluation took place within the first 4 weeks of their illness, 128 (54%) of the patients had disseminated Lyme disease. The most frequently experienced extracutaneous signs and symptoms were fever (55%), fatigue (48%), musculoskeletal discomfort (47%), headache (38%), and chills (23%). Also described were eye complaints (9%), cardiac rate and rhythm abnormalities (9%), irritability (9%), gastrointestinal complaints (9%), Bell's palsy (6%), sore throat (2%), numbness or tingling sensation of an extremity (1%), shortness of breath (1%), and memory lapses (1%). These signs and symptoms could precede the appearance of EM, occur concurrently with EM, or follow the appearance of EM lesions.[14]

Complete heart block and meningitis caused by *B. burgdorferi* have been diagnosed in patients presenting with EM.

Thin plaques of granuloma annulare and fixed drug eruptions may be difficult to differentiate from EM. Cellulitis, contact dermatitis, cutaneous arthropod reactions, and dermatophytosis appearing as reddish, annular lesions should also be considered in the differential diagnosis. The usual absence of EM lesions on the palms, soles, and mucous membranes helps to differentiate a patient with multiple EM lesions from one with erythema multiforme.

Microbiology

Cultivation of the etiologic agent of Lyme disease, *B. burgdorferi,* from EM lesions provides a definite laboratory diagnosis of the illness as well as firmly establishing the association between the organism and EM. Until recently, attempts to isolate this spirochete from EM lesions of patients in the United States have met with limited success ranging from 5% to 43%.[18,31] However, *B. burgdorferi* was isolated from EM lesions of 18 of 21 (86%) patients with untreated Lyme disease.[19] Organisms were cultivated from typical and atypical EM lesions, secondary EM lesions, EM lesions smaller

than 5 cm in diameter, and from clinically normal perilesional skin. It appears that cultivation of *B. burgdorferi* from EM lesions can be a high-yield procedure.

Histopathology

The variable clinical picture of EM is reflected in its histopathology. Three general patterns are seen.[16] The most common is a superficial and deep perivascular and interstitial infiltrate, composed mostly of lymphocytes but containing plasma cells. The second pattern consists of a superficial and deep perivascular and interstitial lymphocytic infiltrate with eosinophils but devoid of plasma cells. The third pattern has the same lymphocytic infiltrate picture but is devoid of both plasma cells and eosinophils.

With Warthin-Starry or Dieterle silver staining, spirochetes can be identified in EM lesions. The spirochetes are found mostly in specimens obtained from the borders of EM lesions and in biopsy specimens containing plasma cells (see Color Plate Fig. 6).[16]

The absence of the described histopathologic patterns or of spirochetes on silver staining does not rule out EM. *B. burgdorferi* has been cultivated from EM lesions showing only a perivascular lymphocytic infiltrate or an arthropod reaction pattern on hematoxylin and eosin staining, and from EM lesions negative for spirochetes on silver staining.[18]

Serologic testing

Serologic tests are concerned with recognizing a specific immune response to *B. burgdorferi,* but, because of a delayed antibody response in Lyme disease, serologic tests are frequently not reactive during the first few weeks of the illness.[20,25,29] Therefore, a positive serologic test can be supportive of the diagnosis, but a negative result certainly does not rule out Lyme disease.[17]

BORRELIAL LYMPHOCYTOMA AND ACRODERMATITIS CHRONICA ATROPHICANS

B. burgdorferi has been cultivated from borrelial lymphocytoma (BL) lesions,[23] also known as lymphocytoma benigna cutis, as well as from acrodermatitis chronica atrophicans (ACA) lesions,[8] which convincingly supports the association of these entities to the spirochete. Whereas EM is the most common cutaneous manifestation of Lyme disease on both sides of the Atlantic, BL and ACA are predominantly European manifestations.

Borrelial lymphocytoma

BL is a bluish-red tumorlike skin lesion that has a predilection for the ear lobes of children and the nipple/areolar region of adults. BL is an early cutaneous manifestation of Lyme disease that may be preceded by or may appear with EM. BL may be accompanied by signs and symptoms of meningoradiculitis or acute arthritis.[9]

Acrodermatitis chronica atrophicans

ACA is the characteristic cutaneous lesion of late Lyme disease. It occurs predominantly in women between 40 and 70 years of age and begins as a bluish-red edematous lesion, usually on an extremity, most commonly on the lower leg or foot. There are variations in the amount of erythema and edema present. Fibrous bands may develop, particularly in the ulnar and tibial regions, and fibrous nodules may form near joints. Associated regional lymphadenopathy is often present. Years later, the skin of the involved area becomes atrophic and develops a wrinkled appearance.[9]

Extracutaneous complications of the skeletal and neurologic system can occur. Subluxations of the small joints of the hands and feet and sensory peripheral neuropathies of the ACA-involved extremities are the most common of these organ system complications.[9]

The clinical diagnosis of ACA can be supported by serologic and histopathologic findings. ACA patients usually have an elevated antibody response to *B. burgdorferi* on enzyme-linked immunosorbent assay (ELISA).[9] The histopathologic picture of ACA is that of proliferation and dilation of cutaneous vessels in combination with a patchy or interstitial infiltrate composed primarily of lymphocytes with an admixture of plasma cells. As the lesion progresses to an atrophic stage, there is a decrease in the inflammatory cell infiltrate along with pronounced atrophy of the epidermis and dermis.[7]

ADDITIONAL CUTANEOUS DISORDERS
Morphea and lichen sclerosus et atrophicus

The borrelial origin of morphea (localized scleroderma) and lichen sclerosus et atrophicus has been proposed on the basis of serologic and immunohistochemical studies and the isolation of *B. burgdorferi* from patients with morphea.[4-6,32] However, using serologic and microbiologic methods, other studies have concluded that there is no evidence of a common etiology for Lyme disease and localized scleroderma.[21,22,24]

This continuing controversy can be explained in part by the observation that sclerotic lesions (morphea or lichen sclerosus et atrophicus) can develop in 10% of patients with ACA, and that these lesions may be clinically and histologically indistinguishable from non-ACA morphea and lichen sclerosus et atrophicus.[9]

The association of *B. burgdorferi* to other sclerotic skin conditions includes anetoderma,[27] atro-

phoderma,[32] eosinophilic fasciitis,[28] and progressive facial hemiatrophy.[3] These conditions are probably multifactorial in origin and, as exemplified by progressive facial hemiatrophy, can occur without an associated *B. burgdorferi* infection.[1,26]

Cutaneous reaction patterns or coincidental findings

Granuloma annulare, erythema nodosum, urticaria, and Schönlein-Henoch–like purpura have been identified on patients with serologic and extracutaneous symptomatology of Lyme disease.[14] *B. burgdorferi* infections have also been associated with cutaneous B cell lymphoma[21] and benign lymphocytic infiltration of the skin.[2]

CONCLUSION

With improved microbiologic procedures at hand and with the advent of a reliable, standardized, polymerase chain reaction assay, we will be able to determine with certainty the skin diseases associated with a *B. burgdorferi* infection.

REFERENCES

1. Abele DC, Bedingfield RB: Progressive facial hemiatrophy (Parry-Romberg syndrome) and antibodies to *Borrelia*: reply, *J Am Acad Dermatol* 25:579, 1991.
2. Abele DC, Anders KH, Chandler FW: Benign lymphocytic infiltration (Jessner-Kanof): Another manifestation of borreliosis? *J Am Acad Dermatol* 21:795, 1989.
3. Abele DC et al: Progressive facial hemiatrophy (Parry-Romberg syndrome) and borreliosis, *J Am Acad Dermatol* 22:531, 1990.
4. Aberer E, Stanek G: Histological evidence for spirochetal origin of morphea and lichen sclerosus et atrophicus, *Am J Dermatopathol* 9:374, 1987.
5. Aberer E et al: Evidence for spirochetal origin of circumscribed scleroderma (morphea), *Acta Derm Venereol* 67:225, 1987.
6. Aberer E et al: Neuroborreliosis in morphea and lichen sclerosus et atrophicus, *J Am Acad Dermatol* 19:820, 1988.
7. Asbrink E, Brehmer-Andersson E, Hovmark A: Acrodermatitis chronica atrophicans—a spirochetosis. Clinical and histopathological picture based on 32 patients, *Am J Dermatopathol* 8:209, 1986.
8. Asbrink E, Hovmark A: Successful cultivation of spirochetes from skin lesions of patients with erythema chronica migrans and acrodermatitis chronica atrophicans, *Acta Pathol Microbiol Immunol* 66:161, 1985.
9. Asbrink E, Hovmark A: Early and late cutaneous manifestations in *Ixodes*-borne borreliosis, *Ann NY Acad Sci* 539:4, 1988.
10. Asbrink E, Olsson I: Clinical manifestations of erythema chronicum migrans Afzelius in 161 patients, *Acta Derm Venereol* 65:43, 1985.
11. Berger BW: Erythema chronicum migrans of Lyme disease, *Arch Dermatol* 120:1017, 1984.
12. Berger BW: Treatment of erythema chronicum migrans of Lyme disease, *Ann NY Acad Sci* 539:346, 1988.
13. Berger BW: Cutaneous manifestations of Lyme borreliosis, *Rheum Dis Clin North Am* 15:627, 1989.
14. Berger BW: Dermatologic manifestations of Lyme disease, *Rev Infect Dis* 11(suppl 6):S1475, 1989.
15. Berger BW: Diagnosis and treatment of Lyme disease, *Clin Courier-National Institutes of Health* 9:2, 1991.

16. Berger BW, Clemmensen OJ, Ackerman AB: Lyme disease is a spirochetosis: a review of the disease and evidence of its cause, *Am J Dermatopathol* 5:111, 1983.
17. Berger BW, MacDonald AB, Benach JL: Use of an autologous antigen in the serologic testing of patients with erythema migrans of Lyme disease, *J Am Acad Dermatol* 18:1243, 1988.
18. Berger BW et al: Isolation and characterization of the Lyme disease spirochete from the skin of patients with erythema chronicum migrans, *J Am Acad Dermatol* 15:459, 1986.
19. Berger BW et al: Cultivation of *Borrelia burgdorferi* from erythema migrans lesions and perilesional skin, *J Clin Microbiol* 30:359, 1992.
20. Craft JE, Grodzicki RL, Steere AC: Antibody response in Lyme disease: evaluation of diagnostic tests, *J Infect Dis* 149:789, 1984.
21. Garbe C et al: *Borrelia burgdorferi*-associated cutaneous B cell lymphoma: clinical and immunohistologic characterization of four cases, *J Am Acad Dermatol* 24:584, 1991.
22. Hoesly JM, Mertz LE, Winkelmann RK: Localized scleroderma (morphea) and antibody to *Borrelia burgdorferi*, *J Am Acad Dermatol* 17:455, 1987.
23. Hovmark A, Asbrink E, Olsson I: The spirochetal etiology of lymphadenosis benigna cutis solitaria, *Acta Derm Venereol* 66:479, 1986.
24. Lupoli S et al: Lyme disease and localized scleroderma— no evidence for a common aetiology, *Br J Rheumatol* 30:154, 1991.
25. Rahn DW, Malawista SE: Lyme disease: recommendations for diagnosis and treatment, *Ann Intern Med* 114:472, 1991.
26. Ribot TE et al: Progressive facial hemiatrophy (Parry-Romberg syndrome) and antibodies to *Borrelia burgdorferi*, *J Am Acad Dermatol* 25:578, 1991.
27. Rufli T et al: Zum erweiteren Spektrum zeckenubertragener Spirochatosen, *Hautartz* 37:597, 1986.
28. Stanek G et al: Schulman syndrome, a scleroderma subtype caused by *Borrelia burgdorferi*, *Lancet* 1:1490, 1987.
29. Steere AC: Lyme disease, *N Engl J Med* 321:586, 1989.
30. Steere AC et al: The early clinical manifestations of Lyme disease, *Ann Intern Med* 99:76, 1983.
31. Steere AC et al: The spirochetal etiology of Lyme disease, *N Engl J Med* 308:733, 1983.
32. Weber K, Preac-Mursic V, Reimers C: Spirochetes isolated from two patients with morphea, *Infection* 16:25, 1988.

10 Rheumatic Manifestations

Alan T. Kaell, Ronald S. Bennett, and Max I. Hamburger

Lyme disease was first recognized in the United States as an epidemic of inflammatory arthropathy.[147,148] Since the 1982 discovery of *Borrelia burgdorferi* as the causative agent[17,154] and the advent of serologic tests, many rheumatic symptoms have been attributed to Lyme disease.[9,143] Such rheumatic manifestations include myalgia, arthralgia, arthritis, fibrositis, myositis, and bone and joint involvement secondary to acrodermatitis chronicum atrophicans (ACA).[109,143] This chapter reviews these rheumatic manifestations and their differential diagnostic considerations.

HISTORICAL PERSPECTIVE OF RHEUMATIC MANIFESTATIONS

Lyme disease was originally reported in the United States in 1977 as a distinct inflammatory arthropathy.[148] In a 1975 epidemic near Lyme, Connecticut, 39 children and 12 adults presented with rheumatic symptoms. Fifty-nine percent (23 of 39) of the children were said to have met the American Rheumatism Association (ARA) criteria for the diagnosis of juvenile rheumatoid arthritis (JRA). However, atypical features for JRA were noted, including familial and geographic clustering, seasonal onset, brief duration of joint effusions, and the lack of positive antinuclear antibodies (ANA) or iritis. An antecedent rash, identified as erythema migrans (EM), prompted the recognition of Lyme arthritis (LA) as a distinct inflammatory arthropathy.

Arthritis was associated with EM in a case report from Germany in 1974.[163] The "rheumatism" described in patients with Bannwarth's syndrome as early as 1941 may have been the first reported cases of rheumatic manifestations of *B. burgdorferi* infection.[8]

The earliest case of probable LA in the United States, purported to occur in 1962, was identified in a 1986 epidemiologic study of Great Island, Massachusetts.[157] A 35-year-old woman with high serum titer antibodies to *B. burgdorferi* reported a history of transient knee arthritis recurring between 1962 and 1964. She did not recall a history of EM. No long-term sequelae were noted, although the

patient described episodes of hand stiffness and fatigue over the next 15 years.

Clinicoepidemiologic definition of Lyme arthritis

In an effort to establish uniformity in counting cases of Lyme disease, the Centers for Disease Control (CDC) adopted clinical and serologic criteria for the disease.[111] This uniform case definition is used for the purpose of epidemiologic surveillance. Such criteria are intentionally specific but lack sensitivity. Table 10-1 describes the 1989 CDC criteria for Lyme arthritis.

Symptomatic people infected with *B. burgdorferi* may fail to meet these CDC criteria and yet warrant treatment for LA.[111] Up to 50% of patients presenting with LA may not recall the pathognomonic EM rash, flulike illness, or deer tick bite.[143] The availability of Lyme serology since 1982 has enabled clinicians to "confirm" such cases of LA. However, both false-positive and false-negative test results complicate accurate diagnosis.[9,109] The challenge to physicians is to diagnose and treat rheumatic symptoms in people who fail to meet the CDC criteria.[9,111] A clinician's diagnostic reasoning process may be improved by studying the clinical characteristics of a disease. The natural history of *B. burgdorferi* infection and its rheumatic manifestations are reviewed below. These manifestations are divided into early and late features, but the distinction is often arbitrary.

EARLY RHEUMATIC MANIFESTATIONS

Within days or weeks after *B. burgdorferi* infection, the organism may disseminate to the joints, bone, or muscle.[143] Musculoskeletal symptoms occurring during this time include arthralgias, myalgias, stiff neck, backache, and hand stiffness. Abnormal physical findings include pain on neck flexion, malar rash, muscle tenderness, and periorbital edema (Table 10-2).[153,155]

Before the discovery of the bacterial etiology of Lyme disease in 1982, patients in the United States with EM were not routinely treated with antibiotics. These patients, therefore, afford the opportu-

Table 10–1 Lyme disease national surveillance case definition for Lyme arthritis

A case of Lyme arthritis is defined as follows:
A person with a late musculoskeletal manifestation of Lyme disease and
1. A history of erythema migrans (as defined by the CDC); or
2. Laboratory confirmation of *B. burgdorferi* infection.

Late musculoskeletal manifestations of *B. burgdorferi* infection (when an alternate explanation is not found):
Recurrent, brief attacks (lasting weeks or months) of objective joint swelling in one or a few joints sometimes followed by chronic arthritis in one or a few joints.

Manifestations that are not considered to be criteria for diagnosis include chronic progressive arthritis that is not preceded by brief attacks and chronic symmetric polyarthritis. Additionally, arthralgias, myalgias, or fibromyalgia syndromes alone are not accepted as criteria for musculoskeletal involvement.

This epidemiologic case definition is intended for surveillance purposes only.

Modified from Rahn D, Malawista S: Lyme disease: recommendations for diagnosis and treatment, *Ann Intern Med* 114:473, 1991.

Table 10–2 Early musculoskeletal symptoms of Lyme disease*

	Number of patients (*n* = 314)	(%)
Symptoms		
Malaise, fatigue, lethargy	251	(80)
Stiff neck	151	(48)
Arthralgias	150	(48)
Myalgias	135	(43)
Backache	81	(26)
Hand stiffness	16	(5)
Signs		
Pain on neck flexion	52	(17)
Malar rash	41	(13)
Muscle tenderness	12	(4)
Periorbital edema	10	(3)

Modified from Steere AC et al: The early clinical manifestations of Lyme disease, *Ann Intern Med* 99:78, 1983.
*Erythema migrans was required for inclusion in this study.

nity to study the natural history of *B. burgdorferi* infection. In a landmark report of untreated EM, 55 patients from Connecticut were followed prospectively for 3 to 8 years.[146] Twenty percent (11 of 55) of these patients had no further manifestations of Lyme disease. Eighty percent (44 of 55) developed rheumatic symptoms and signs.

Arthralgias

Fifty-four percent (29 of 55) of patients with untreated EM develop episodes of musculoskeletal pain without objective findings.[146] Pain can occur in specific joints, periarticular areas, tendons, bursa, enthesis, muscle, and cervical or lumbar spine regions. The area involved does not appear to correlate with the location of the EM rash. Each episode is characterized by pain on motion and at rest, without objective findings of joint effusion, warmth, erythema, or synovial swelling. Unlike fibrositis, the pain typically affects only one or two regions at a time. Episodes resolve within a few hours to several days but may recur within several months. This syndrome has been referred to as "localized, intermittent musculoskeletal pain" (LIMP).[71] It can involve up to 10 different regions over time.

One third of patients with LIMP resolve within a mean of 3.1 years (range: 1 month to 6 years) after the EM rash. Two thirds ultimately develop objective rheumatic features. Overall, 50% of patients with LIMP develop episodic synovitis and 18% develop chronic synovitis (greater than 1 year of continuous inflammation in a specific joint).

Although inflammatory arthritis can occur as early as 2 weeks after EM, its pathogenesis may differ from the other early symptoms and is, therefore, discussed as a late rheumatic manifestation of *B. burgdorferi* infection.

LATE RHEUMATIC MANIFESTATIONS
Inflammatory arthritis

Although inflammatory LA can occur without an antecedent EM rash,[143,148] most reports on the natural history of Lyme disease include only patients with EM. Sixty percent (34 of 55) of patients with untreated EM develop inflammatory arthritis evidenced by synovial effusion or pain on motion.[146] The mean interval from onset of disease to frank arthritis is 6 months (range: 4 days to 2 years). Fifty-six percent (19 of 34) have antecedent LIMP symptoms.[71] The most common arthritis pattern is intermittent, asymmetric synovitis of one or more large joints. A monoarticular or oligoarticular (less than four joints) pattern is seen in 70% to 80% of patients. The frequency of joints involved, in descending order, is knee, shoulder, ankle, elbow, temporomandibular joint, wrist, hip, fingers, toes, sternoclavicular joint. A similar pattern of joint involvement has been described in other regions of the United States.*

The knee is the most commonly involved joint in LA. Typically, patients develop a relatively painless, large effusion and Baker's cyst.[146] A ruptured cyst causing pseudophlebitis may be the presenting feature. On occasion, a patient can present with a painful, red-hot, swollen joint, which mimics septic arthritis.[38,60]

The TMJ may be the initial joint involved in up to 25% of cases of LA.[70,146] In contrast, TMJ pain is usually seen as a late feature in other inflammatory arthropathies.[45]

Polyarticular inflammation is seen in only 21% of patients with transient synovitis.[146] Although a pseudorheumatoid pattern has been attributed to *B. burgdorferi* infection,[32] less than 10% of patients have symmetric joint involvement that mimics rheumatoid arthritis (RA).[146,149]

The initial reports of LA suggested that Lyme disease could mimic JRA.[148] However, in a recent report of 46 children with LA, none fulfilled strict criteria for JRA (that is, persistence of synovitis for 6 weeks from onset).[159]

In most patients, individual attacks of synovitis remit spontaneously after a few days to a few weeks (range: 3 days to 11.5 months). One third have an isolated attack of synovitis. Two thirds have recurrent attacks of synovitis of variable frequency and duration. In general, the frequency and duration of attacks diminish over time, with 10% to 20% of patients entering long-term remission each year.[147,159] Children and adults with LA have a similar course.†

Up to 17% (6 of 34) of patients with an attack of synovitis develop chronic, persistent synovitis lasting 1 year or longer.[146]

Chronic arthritis

Overall, 11% (6 of 55) of patients with untreated EM develop chronic arthritis lasting 1 year or longer.[146,159] The onset of this persistent synovitis averages 12 months (range: 4 months to 48 months) after the untreated EM rash. Typically, only one or two joints are involved. In 85% (5 of 6), there is antecedent LIMP and transient arthritis of the specific joints.[71,146] In two thirds (4 of 6) of chronic LA patients, one or both knees are affected. Other joints involved include the shoulder and hip. Untreated, the arthritis may persist for at least 4 years or spontaneously resolve in 1.5 to 3 years. Patients with the class II human leukocyte antigen (HLA) phenotype DR4 and/or DR2 appear to be at risk

of developing chronic LA.[145,149] If antibodies to outer surface proteins develop in these DR4 or DR2 patients, they are less likely to respond to antibiotic therapy.[65]

UNUSUAL RHEUMATIC MANIFESTATIONS
Acrodermatitis chronica atrophicans

ACA is a late cutaneous manifestation of *B. burgdorferi* infection (see Chapter 9). It is recognized more often in Europe but is well documented in the United States.[67,157] ACA appears as a bluish-red lesion, which may become atrophic or sclerotic. Periostitis, bone erosion, and small joint subluxations may occur beneath such lesions.[4,5,55] Peripheral neuropathy is often noted in the involved region. Focal nodular myositis has also been described in some ACA patients.[114] To date, *B. burgdorferi* infection has not been associated with neuropathic, or Charcot, osteoarthropathy in the United States.

Myositis

Myalgias are common in both early and late Lyme disease.[143,146,153] *Borrelia burgdorferi* has not been successfully cultured from muscle tissue, although it has been seen between muscle fibers by silver stain technique in patients with focal muscle complaints.[7,114] An interstitial lymphoplasmacytic infiltrate of non-necrotic muscle has been associated with focal muscle pain and tenderness.[7,114,122] In addition, a noninflammatory necrotizing myopathy has been described.[126] Both chronic inflammatory and necrotic muscle changes have occurred as a focal nodular myositis in patients with ACA.[114,122] Proximal muscle weakness and elevated creatine kinase in conjunction with meningopolyneuritis has been reported.[114,122] Symmetric upper and lower extremity weakness typical of polymyositis has not been attributed to *B. burgdorferi* infection.

OTHER COUNTRIES

LA occurs throughout Europe,* Russia,[31] China,[2] Japan,[68] and Australia.[158] The incidence and prevalence of LA in these countries vary considerably. In some reports, LA appears to be less prevalent in Europe than in the United States.[56,141] Geographic variation may be attributed to several factors, including (1) the practice of treating EM with antibiotics in Europe since 1950,[54] (2) differences in physician recognition of rheumatic manifestations due to *B. burgdorferi* infection,[28,44] (3) a diverse response of the host to *B. burgdorferi* infection,[143,145] and (4) regional variations in the *B. burgdorferi* strain.[3,10,168] Although strain variation

---

*References 1, 6, 12, 14, 38, 77, 82, 98, 159, 167.
†References 6, 12, 38, 58, 98, 159, 167.

*References 13, 44, 54, 56, 75, 101, 141, 162.

of *B. burgdorferi* has been shown to be a crucial factor in the development of LA in experimental animal models,[3] its role in humans is not established. In general, the clinical features of LA appear similar throughout the world. However, in contrast to the United States, LA presenting as persistent, chronic synovitis without antecedent episodic synovitis has often been described in Europe.[20,54]

PATHOGENESIS

The pathogenesis of the diverse rheumatic manifestations of Bb infection is unknown.[134,142] *Borrelia burgdorferi* has been shown to disseminate hematogenously to the joints early during the course of infection.[102] Although *B. burgdorferi* can be visualized in synovium,[72,137,144] it rarely can be cultured from synovial fluid.[112,121] This may reflect technical difficulties in *B. burgdorferi* culture technique. However, it appears that most joints affected by LA are sterile and not "septic" in the usual sense of the word.

The mechanism by which *B. burgdorferi* triggers acute or chronic synovitis is unknown. The human host immune response appears to be important in the rheumatic manifestations of *B. burgdorferi*.[134,142] Class II major histocompatibility complex (MHC) genes HLA DR 4 and HLA DR 2 appear to be associated with chronic LA and failure to respond to antibiotics.[65,142,145] Cellular or humoral immune responses to *B. burgdorferi* heat-shock proteins may play a role in the immunopathogenesis of LA.[19,49,61,131,169,173] The molecular basis of how infectious agents may cause rheumatic disease has been reviewed.[91,100,123,129,169] Another explanation for the diversity of rheumatic manifestations ascribed solely to *B. burgdorferi* is that *Ixodes* ticks may transmit viruses or other bacteria, alone or simultaneously, with *B. burgdorferi*.[128]

LABORATORY TESTS AND RADIOGRAPHS
Blood tests

Routine laboratory testing is often not helpful in the differential diagnosis of LA.[50,111,133] Some patients with LA may not have any laboratory abnormalities. Laboratory findings in early Lyme disease are summarized in Table 10–3. Anemia and leukocytosis were not found in the original 51 patients with LA.[148] Twenty of these 51 patients had active joint disease at the time of evaluation and erythrocyte sedimentation rate (ESR) averaged 15 mm/hr (range 4 to 55). Of the 31 asymptomatic patients, ESR averaged 8 mm/hr (range 4 to 22). Nine of the 20 symptomatic patients had C3 less than 70 mg%, compared to none of the 31 asymptomatic patients.

Patients with LA can have elevated serum IgM levels, elevated ESR (range 6 to 177 mm/hr), and mixed cryoglobulins.[76,149,150] The IgM component of the cryoprecipitate does not appear to be an antiglobulin. The presence of mixed cryoglobulins may predict the development of arthritis early in the course of Lyme disease. However, late arthritis can occur in patients without detectable mixed cryoglubulins.[150]

Rheumatoid factor (RF) and ANA are typically absent from the sera of LA patients.[148] Transient low titer ANA[38,41,88] and anticardiolipin antibodies have been reported. Low titer RF has occurred in up to 25% of cases.[1,76]

Synovial fluid (SF)

Routine SF analysis (cell count, glucose, total protein, Gram's stain, culture, crystal) is usually nondiagnostic in LA. Such analysis, however, is essential to rule out other causes of monoarthritis[132] (for example, crystals, tuberculosis fungi, other bacterial infections). Culture of SF for *B. burgdorferi* has a low yield and is not routinely available. *Borrelia burgdorferi* has rarely been identified or cultured from joint fluid.[112,121,137]

The synovial fluid is often inflammatory with white blood cell (WBC) count averaging 25,000 cells per ml (range 500 to 110,000 cells).[143] Polymorphonuclear (PMN) leukocytes predominate, averaging 80% of the white blood cells in synovial effusions. However, eosinophilia (79% of 18,100 WBC/ml) has rarely been reported.[69] Synovial fluid glucose is typically normal and total protein is modestly elevated (range 4.3 to 9 g).

Many other SF findings of interest have been

Table 10–3 Laboratory findings in early Lyme disease

	Number of patients *n* = 314 (%)	Median (range)
Hematocrit < 37%	37 (12)	35 (31-36)
Leukocytes > 10,000 cells/mm	24 (8)	12 (11-18)
ESR > 20 mm/hr	166 (53)	35 (21-68)
IgM > 250 mg/dl	104 (33)	310 (252-930)

Modified from Steere AC et al: The early clinical manifestations of Lyme disease, *Ann Intern Med* 99:78, 1983.

reported but have unknown clinical significance.[24,25,97,136] Cryoglobulins and Clq-reactive material are present in SF.[51] These correlate with total SF granulocyte count, but are not of clinical importance. SF complement levels are normal, and RF and ANA are usually absent. Interleukin-1 (IL-1), which activates collagenase, is found in the SF.[46] Elevated levels of collagenase and prostaglandin E_2 from synovial explants of a patient with erosive LA have been demonstrated.[152] A host-derived novel chemoattractant isolated from the SF has been recently described in LA patients.[39] Further studies are needed to confirm these findings.

Synovial pathology

Synovial biopsy is often not diagnostically helpful. The histopathology is similar to that described in RA and Reiter's syndrome.[36,37] Biopsy can demonstrate villous hypertrophy, fibrin deposition, and infiltrates of activated lymphocytes, plasma cells, macrophages, and mast cells in subsynovial tissue. It is unusual to identify spirochetes in the synovium by Dieterle silver stain or immunoperoxidase techniques.[37,61,72,144] Spirochetes may be seen in a perivascular location associated with a form of endarteritis obliterans characterized by luminal obliteration due to intimal ("onion skin") and adventitial cell proliferation.[36,62]

The polymerase chain reaction (PCR) technique for identification of *B. burgdorferi* DNA in synovial tissue or fluid may help distinguish LA from other inflammatory arthritides.[42,106,115] If this technique proves to be sensitive and specific for diagnosing LA, the role of synovial biopsy may be expanded.[106]

Radiographs

Radiographs of symptomatic joints are not particularly useful in the diagnosis of either early or late LA.[81,81a] Radiologic findings observed in LA (for example, osteoarthritis, chondrocalcinosis, or enthesitis) may be coincidental to *B. burgdorferi* infection. Early in LA, radiographs can demonstrate intraarticular effusion, prepatellar bursal fluid, or infrapatellar fat pad edema.[81] In LIMP syndrome patients, radiographs of symptomatic joints are usually normal.[71] In chronic arthritis, a nonspecific "mixed-bag" of radiographic findings may be seen, including (1) enthesis changes (for example, calcifications of quadriceps tendon and ossification in the patellar ligament), (2) calcification of menisci and patella, (3) subchondral cysts in the shoulder, hip, and tibia, (4) joint space narrowing, and (5) osseous changes.[54,81,148] When osseous changes are present, features suggestive of inflammatory arthritis (periarticular osteopenia and symmetric joint space narrowing) are seen in 40%; features suggestive of osteoarthritis (osthophytosis and subchondral sclerosis) are seen in 30%; and features sugges-

tive of both are seen in 30%.

Erosive disease is seen on radiographs of symptomatic joints in less than 5% of patients with untreated EM.[54,81,148,152] In patients with chronic knee synovitis, erosive changes typically occur at the cartilage-bone margin of the femur or tibia. These marginal erosions are similar to those seen in many other types of chronic inflammatory arthritides. Erosions at the posterosuperior aspect of the calcaneus have been reported in an HLA B27 patient with Achilles tenosynovitis.[81]

LYME SEROLOGY

Serologic assays for antibodies to *B. burgdorferi* lack both standardization and 100% specificity.[9,23,118] Problems in interlaboratory variation are well documented.[52,53,87,130] Nevertheless, Lyme enzyme linked immunosorbent assay (ELISA) is the best screening test available for confirming *B. burgdorferi* exposure in patients in whom LA is suspected.[35,111] Nearly all patients with LA have antibodies to *B. burgdorferi* detectable in their sera. Most commercial assays use whole sonicated *B. burgdorferi* and thus detect antibodies to multiple spirochetal antigens. False-positive results attributable to antibodies cross-reactive to *B. burgdorferi* can be seen in the serum of patients with (1) other spirochetal infections,[22,118] (2) disorders associated with polyclonal B cell activation[50] (for example, infectious mononucleosis and sarcoidosis), (3) nonspirochetal subacute bacterial endocarditis (SBE),[63,64] and (4) commensal, nonpathogenic oral treponemes.[90]

Western blot analysis can help document true exposure to Bb.[34,43] Although there are no uniformly established criteria for defining a true positive Western blot analysis,[23] results can be used to confirm exposure to *B. burgdorferi* in patients with suspected LA. However, documenting a true humoral response to *B. burgdorferi* does not necessarily imply that the patient's rheumatic condition is attributable to active *B. burgdorferi* infection.[63] For instance, patients with well-defined inflammatory arthritides (for example, RA) who reside in Lyme endemic areas may be truly seropositive based on a prior asymptomatic infection with *B. burgdorferi*.[18,48,80,109,139]

SERONEGATIVE LYME ARTHRITIS

Nearly all patients with LA have antibodies to *B. burgdorferi* detectable in their sera. However, patients with objective rheumatic features and a history of tick exposure or EM rash may fail to mount a detectable humoral response to *B. burgdorferi*.[30,33] The incidence of seronegative LA appears to be low (less than 5%). Several possible explanations for seronegative LA include[33] (1) blunting or abrogation of the humoral immune response by early antibiotic therapy,[30,133] (2) antibodies to *B.*

burgdorferi may be sequestered in putative immune complexes[127] (others have not been able to corroborate this finding[33]), and (3) the serum humoral immune response to Bb may be delayed as long as 18 months after EM and LA.[78]

In seronegative LA patients, a T-cell mediated immune (CMI) response to *B. burgdorferi* may be demonstrated and used to confirm exposure to *B. burgdorferi*.[30,33,99,104] In 12 seronegative patients with active LA who had received early antibiotic treatment for EM, elevated *B. burgdorferi*-induced T-cell lymphoproliferative responses were evident and patients responded to subsequent antibiotic therapy.[30]

Although some investigators have found T-cell responses to Bb to be nonspecific (occurring in 67% of healthy controls),[174] others have demonstrated a 95% specificity.[33] In the latter study, none of nine healthy subjects were positive, whereas four of nine asymptomatic *Borrelia* laboratory workers were positive. Only 4 of 77 control subjects had T-cell proliferative responses to *B. burgdorferi*. These four control subjects had undifferentiated neurologic or rheumatologic syndromes but did not respond to antibiotic therapy. Several factors may explain positive CMI responses in people without active *B. burgdorferi* infections. First, a nonspecific response to cross-reactive spirochetal polypeptides, including the 41- and 58-kD proteins, may occur.[172] Second, a specific response to fragments of borrelial proteins may occur in laboratory workers with airborne or contact exposure to *B. burgdorferi* protein fragments during sonication.[33]

Both chronicity and severity of LA have been associated with a greater T-cell proliferative response.[33] However, the sensitivity of the T-cell proliferative assay is low in both active and inactive LA. T-cell responses to Bb are seen in only 45% (12 of 27) of active LA patients and 25% of inactive LA patients. These findings are consistent with the notion that the cellular immune (CMI) response may be localized to the joint.[134,136] In one case, a patient with apparent LA failed to mount either a humoral or CMI response to *B. burgdorferi*.[33]

DIFFERENTIAL DIAGNOSIS

Patients with rheumatic manifestations in whom the diagnosis of Lyme disease is "confirmed" solely on serologic grounds require careful evaluation to exclude other differential diagnostic entities before institution of empiric antibiotic therapy.[85,109-111,143]

The differential diagnostic considerations of the various rheumatic manifestations of Lyme disease are detailed below.

Arthralgia/myalgia

Fibrositis. The fibrositis syndrome typically is associated with at least 18 specified symmetric tender muscle trigger points.[170] Some patients with objective signs of Lyme disease may develop a typical fibrositis syndrome.[135] More often, patients with Lyme disease develop a localized, intermittent musculoskeletal pain or LIMP syndrome confined to one or two joint regions.[71,146] In patients with positive Lyme serology and fibrositis without objective clinical features of *B. burgdorferi* infection, the diagnosis of Lyme disease should be made with caution.[135,143] If a patient with LIMP or fibrositis has cognitive complaints, it is important to rule out subtle Lyme encephalopathy.[84]

Polymyalgia rheumatica (PMR). In older patients with arthralgia/myalgia, PMR should be considered.[57] Symmetric stiffness of the shoulder and pelvic girdle regions is the hallmark of PMR. In contrast to most cases of Lyme disease, the ESR is often dramatically elevated in PMR. A careful search for associated symptoms or signs of temporal arteritis (for example, amaurosis fugax, headache, jaw claudication) should be conducted in patients with elevated ESR or symptoms compatible with PMR.

Psychogenic rheumatism. When objective features of Lyme disease are lacking, patients of all ages should be suspected of having psychogenic rheumatism[116] or somatization disorder. It is important to consider subtle Lyme encephalopathy in these patients.[84]

Trichinosis. Symptoms and signs suggestive of trichinosis have been reported in cases of early Lyme disease. These include diarrhea (2%), myalgia (43%), periorbital edema (3%), muscle tenderness (4%), and abdominal pain (8%).[153] If these signs or symptoms are present, a history of raw meat ingestion should be sought.

Monoarticular arthritis

Temporomandibular joint. In LA, the TMJ is the fourth most commonly involved joint.[146] Symptoms typically occur early in the course of Lyme disease.[70,146] In other rheumatic conditions, TMJ involvement usually occurs as a late feature of the disease (for example, JRA).[45] However, the TMJ joint may be affected early in the course of gonococcal arthritis.[92] In addition, the temporal headache and jaw claudication secondary to temporal arteritis may be potentially confused with Lyme TMJ involvement.[57]

Crystalline arthropathies. First, metatarsophalangeal (MTP) joint inflammation or podogra has been described in LA and may mimic gout.[146] Ulnar nodules can occur in LA and may be confused with gouty tophi. Low-dose aspirin taken for the pain of LA can lead to serum uric acid elevation. SF analysis with polarizing microscopy confirms the presence of uric acid or calcium pyrophosphate deposition (CPPD) crystals.

Infectious arthritis. LA has been reported clinically to mimic pyogenic or septic arthritis.[38,60] As in acute bacterial arthritis, the SF WBC count in monoarticular LA may be greater than 100,000 cells, with a predominance of PMN leukocytes. SF cultures for bacteria known to cause septic arthritis should be obtained in cases of suspected pyogenic arthritis.

Migratory arthritis

Acute rheumatic fever (ARF). The arthritis of ARF is typically additive in adults and migratory in children.[11,95] None of the original 39 children with LA had elevated anti-streptolysin-O (ASO) titers or met Jones' criteria for ARF.[148] The *Erythema marginatum* rash of ARF may be confused with the secondary EM rash of Lyme disease. The former tends to change borders within minutes to hours whereas EM changes over days. An antecedent sore throat can be seen in both LA and ARF.[153] Similarly, carditis and heart block can be seen in both diseases.[143] Unlike the prompt response of ARF arthritis to aspirin, salicylates are not effective in LA.[148]

Neisseria **gonococcal (GC) and meningitides infections.** Migratory arthritis can occur in both of these neisserial infections.[15,92,107] Tenosynovitis is more typical of GC infection. Joint aspiration is often sterile, yet pharyngeal, anal, or cervical cultures may reveal the neisserial organism. A distinctive "gun powder" rash seen in disseminated GC infection or *N. meningitides* infection may clarify the diagnosis. In a patient with suspected sexually transmitted disease, syphilis serology should be obtained. Syphilis may be associated with false-positive Lyme serology, even if VDRL is negative. The arthritic involvement caused by spirochetal organisms has been recently reviewed.[22,113]

Subacute bacterial endocarditis (SBE). Arthralgias and arthritis can occur in SBE caused by nonspirochetal organisms.[63] Antibodies cross-reactive to *B. burgdorferi* can be demonstrated in up to 40% of SBE patients.[64] The presence of these antibodies can lead to misdiagnosis.[63]

Vasculitis. Henoch-Schönlein purpura[117] and polyarteritis nodosa[161] can be associated with arthritis, rash, neuropathy, and testicular and abdominal pain. Both testicular and abdominal pain have been reported in Lyme disease.[153]

Monoarticular or oligoarticular synovitis persisting longer than 6 weeks

Seronegative spondyloarthropathy. Reiter's syndrome, ankylosing spondylitis, or reactive arthritis may be confused with LA. Organisms capable of triggering reactive arthritis are either gut associated (for example, *Yersinia, Salmonella, Klebsiella*) or sexually acquired (for example, *Chlamydia*). Patients susceptible to reactive arthritis often have the genetic marker HLA B27. Although patients with LA may carry the HLA B27 marker, the incidence of B27 in patients with chronic LA does not differ from the normal population.[159]

Adding to the differential diagnostic confusion is the possibility of a "reactive arthropathy" to *B. burgdorferi* infection.[165] In German study, 18% of patients with reactive arthritis or Reiter's syndrome had antibodies and proliferative T-cell responses to *B. burgdorferi* (3% of normal and fibrositis control groups had antibodies to *B. burgdorferi*). Antibiotic treatment did not abrogate the reactive synovitis. Although it is unclear whether these patients had active *B. burgdorferi* infection, antibiotics may be necessary to diminish the risk of long-term sequelae from *B. burgdorferi* infection.

Psoriatic (PS) arthritis. A subtype of PS arthropathy is asymmetric and oligoarticular. Careful search for nail pitting, occult patches of psoriasis in the scalp, buttock cleft, and umbilicus should help clarify the diagnosis. Sausage digits, typical of psoriatic arthritis, have also been noted in LA.[146]

Seronegative rheumatoid arthritis (SNRA). This type of arthritis may present in an asymmetric oligoarticular pattern. The diagnosis of SNRA requires the persistence of synovitis for at least 6 weeks. Patients with SNRA living in Lyme endemic areas may have antibodies to *B. burgdorferi* in their sera.[32] Of 102 patients with SNRA in Wisconsin, 27 were positive on Lyme serology and 75 were negative.[32] Of the 27 positive Lyme disease patients with SNRA, 18 (67%) "resolved" with antibiotic treatment not otherwise specified (N.O.S.) at a mean follow-up of 7.4 months. Of 75 negative Lyme patients, 22 (29%) spontaneously resolved at mean follow-up of 16 months. Antibiotic treatment appears effective among some SNRA patients with antibodies to *B. burgdorferi* who lack other features of Lyme disease.[32,162a] In a similar clinical setting, others have found antibiotics may be effective, although relapses are common 6 months after completion of therapy.[18]

Pauciarticular JRA. The diagnosis of JRA requires persistent synovitis for at least 6 consecutive weeks at onset and exclusion of other rheumatic disorders.[16] Although 59% of the original 39 children with LA were said to fulfill JRA criteria,[148] a recent prospective study of 46 children with LA found that none fulfilled strict JRA criteria.[159] In the United States, chronic LA is often preceded by recurrent bouts of synovitis lasting less than 6 weeks. In Europe, however, up to 50% of patients with chronic arthritis have synovitis that is unremitting from the onset.[54] In general, LA is not associated with a positive ANA, although transient low titer ANAs have been described.[1,41,60] Pauciarticular JA is associated with a positive ANA, especially in females. A slit lamp ocular examination is necessary to diagnose occult uveitis in JRA. Although *B. burgdorferi* has been associated with ocular involvement,[143] *B. burgdorferi* infection has only rarely been associated with late onset ocular involvement in children with LA.[159] Symptomatic or asymptomatic keratitis has been described, occurring 6 years after EM onset.

Systemic lupus erythematosus. Malar rash can be noted in patients with early Lyme disease.[153] Although the ANA is usually negative,[148] transient ANAs have been noted in some cases of LA.[38,41,60] In addition, up to 45% of patients with early Lyme arthritis may have low C3 serum complement levels.[148]

Sarcoidosis. Because Lyme disease has been associated with erythema nodosum or septal panniculitis, sarcoidosis is in the differential diagnosis.[73] Sarcoidosis may present as periarthritis of the knees and ankles with or without erythema nodosum.[66] A chest x-ray film that reveals bilateral hilar adenopathy confirms Lofgren's syndrome. Other clinical features shared by LA and sarcoidosis (for example, Bell's palsy and lymphocytic pleocytosis) may add to diagnostic confusion. In addition, both disorders may have chronic osseous and joint involvement.[119,140] Because sarcoidosis is associated with polyclonal B cell activation, false-positive Lyme serology may occur.[50]

Hemophiliac arthropathy. In a young child with monoarticular or oligoarticular arthritis, hemarthrosis should be considered.[40] A detailed personal and family history as well as a coagulopathy screen with prothrombin time (PT), partial thromboplastin time (PTT), and platelet count should be obtained. To date, LA has not been associated with hemarthrosis.

Traumatic arthritis. In the absence of an underlying coagulopathy, spontaneous hemarthrosis is unusual. The author has seen several children present with Lyme synovitis whose initial swelling had been attributed to post-traumatic synovitis.[60] Conversely, if a patient presents with traumatic meniscal or ligament tear associated with a synovial effusion, a true positive Lyme serology (for example, from previous asymptomatic *B. burgdorferi* infection) would be unrelated to the problem.

Viral arthritis. Many viruses have been associated with epidemic arthritis in children and adults.[59] These include rubella,[171] varicella, rubeola, hepatitis B,[105] mumps,[138] echovirus type 6, adenovirus type 7, and group A arboviruses. Parvovirus B19, the cause of erythema infectiosum, has been associated with epidemic arthritis in adults[47,94,103,166] and confused with LA.[94] In addition, recurrent knee arthritis after rubella vaccination of women can occur, although the onset and duration of this synovitis are variable.[160] Similar reactions may occur after hepatitis B vaccination. Although the group A arbovirus can cause epidemic arthritis, it does not recur and differs in joint pattern from LA.[59,148] Chikungunya and O'nyongnyong are denguelike illnesses that affect large joints. In contrast to epidemic LA, Ross River virus in Australia affects small joints of the hand.

TREATMENT

The optimal therapy for early or late rheumatic manifestations of Lyme disease has yet to be determined.[86,88,108,111,143]

Early rheumatic symptoms

Although several oral antibiotic regimens shorten the duration of EM and diminish the frequency of Lyme arthritis, minor rheumatic symptoms recur in 50% of patients.[26,93,151,155] The development of these symptoms does not correlate with the choice of antibiotic or the duration of therapy. It is not clear that these symptoms indicate antibiotic failure. The severity of the initial illness may indicate early disseminated disease and herald recurrent arthralgia, musculoskeletal pain, and fatigue. Short-term non-narcotic analgesics and nonsteroidal antiinflammatory (NSAID) drugs may be used to diminish these symptoms.[108,110,124] In most patients, such symptoms usually resolve. Others develop a syndrome suggestive of fibrositis[135] (see below).

Failure of oral antibiotic treatment for EM to prevent subsequent Lyme arthritis has been well documented.[28] The arthritis, however, may be milder in patients who have received early antibiotic therapy compared to arthritis occurring in untreated EM patients. Whether more prolonged oral antibiotic therapy or intravenous treatment for early disseminated *B. burgdorferi* infection will ameliorate or prevent frank arthritis is not known.

Acute arthritis

Acute synovitis may spontaneously remit within days to weeks, although recurrences are common.[146,159] Oral or intravenous antibiotic therapy is recommended to hasten resolution of arthritis and diminish the frequency of recurrence[88,143] (Table 10–4).

If the clinical picture suggests pyogenic infection, the joint should be drained by needle aspiration and immobilized to control pain. Temporary protected weight-bearing may be necessary in cases of lower extremity joint involvement.[110]

Although NSAIDs control pain and inflammation, their efficacy in patients with intermittent LA

Table 10–4 Antibiotic regimens for Lyme arthritis

Amoxicillin and probenecid	500 mg each PO qid × 30 days
Doxycycline	100 mg PO bid × 30 days
Penicillin	20 million U IV qd in divided doses × 14 days
Ceftriaxone	2 g IV qd × 14-21 days

These guidelines are to be modified by new findings and should always be applied with close attention to the clinical course of individual patients.

Modified from Rahn DW, Malawista SE: Lyme disease: recommendations for diagnosis and treatment, *Ann Intern Med* 114:475, 1991.

is difficult to assess. In addition, NSAID use makes it difficult to assess the response to antibiotics.

Persistent arthritis

Response to antibiotic treatment of established Lyme arthritis may be slow or not at all. In general, the duration of therapy is based on clinical response.[88,111] In a double-blind placebo-controlled trial in patients with LA, only 7 of 20 (35%) patients responded to IM penicillin G benzathine given weekly for three doses, whereas none of 20 patients responded to placebo.[156] High-dose (20 million U) IV penicillin given for 14 days cured 11 of 20 (55%) patients. Similarly, 5 of 10 (50%) responded to IV penicillin in another study.[29] More prolonged IV treatment (14 to 21 days) with high-dose IV penicillin does not appear to be effective in chronic LA.

The efficacy of ceftriaxone therapy varies among different studies. Initial reports found that 12 of 13 patients (90%) responded to ceftriaxone.[29] There was no difference between 2 g and 4 g of ceftriaxone. In a randomized trial of doxycycline versus amoxicillin/probenecid for treatment of Lyme arthritis, nonresponders were treated with IV penicillin or ceftriaxone.[83] Response rates were similar in all groups.

After successful antibiotic treatment, patients with LA often remain seropositive, although antibody levels to *B. burgdorferi* tend to diminish within a year.[159] No data are available on the use or role of serial antibody determination to assess persistent infection or disease. The presence of these antibodies may be protective against reinfection with *B. burgdorferi*. No case of reinfection (that is, new case of EM) has been documented in treated LA patients with an expanded humoral response.[143] This is in contrast to patients with EM treated early in the disease in whom antibodies to *B. burgdorferi* are not detected. Reinfection has been documented to occur in these patients.[164]

In patients in whom antibiotic therapy for LA is unsuccessful, the mechanism of persistent or recurrent arthritis is unclear.[91,134,142] The presence of viable organisms may not be required to maintain an untoward immune response. Failure of antibiotic therapy has been correlated with HLA-DR4.[65,142,145] Although immunogenetics may predict which patients with LA are unlikely to respond to antibiotic treatment (see above), the absence of 100% specificity limits the predictive value of this test and mandates antibiotic treatment for all patients with LA. Thus, there is no current role for routine HLA-DR typing of patients with LA.

Patients unresponsive to antibiotic therapy

Refractory synovitis. The role of intraarticular corticosteroids remains controversial. Their use has been associated with a diminished response to antibiotic therapy.[29,83,86] However, in antibiotic-resistant cases, intraarticular corticosteroids may be of use.[21,96,125] NSAID agents may help with symptomatic control in patients with LA pain but does not abate the synovitis. In refractory knee synovitis, synovectomy is beneficial in up to 80% of patients.[21,96,126] The role for slow-acting antirheumatic drugs such as hydroxychloroquine or azulfidine is unknown.[125]

Fibrositis. Patients with Lyme disease and fibrositis or fibrositis and antibodies to *B. burgdorferi* without other features of Lyme disease do not appear to respond to intravenous or oral antibiotics.[135] The fibrositis syndrome may respond clinically to regimens geared toward fibrositis (for example, low-dose tricyclic antidepressant medication or cyclobenzaprine). To date, however, no randomized, prospective trials of antibiotic treatment for such patients have been performed. This does not imply that antibiotic treatment of such individuals is unnecessary. Such treatment may prevent more serious rheumatic or neurologic sequelae if active *B. burgdorferi* infection is present.

Diverse inflammatory arthritides. Patients with well- or ill-defined chronic (greater than 6 months' duration) inflammatory arthropathies may have positive Lyme serology without other features of Lyme disease.[12,18,120,139,162a] Such patients should not be diagnosed as having LA.[143] The antibodies detected by ELISA may be false-positive or truly positive yet unrelated to the underlying rheumatic problem. However, some patients may respond to antibiotic therapy. In a double-blind, placebo-controlled trial of intravenous ceftriaxone, 27 of 58 patients with diverse arthritides responded to treatment.[18] Sixteen of 27 relapsed 6 to 18 months after the initial response. Although responders may have had LA, it is more likely that ceftriaxone suppressed the occult source of chronic antigenic stimulation caused by some other bacteria.[18,79] Alternatively, ceftriaxone may have unrecognized antirheumatic properties.

Other antibiotic regimens have not proven effective in treating patients with well-defined chronic inflammatory arthropathies and antibodies to *B. burgdorferi* without other features of Lyme disease.[12]

REFERENCES

1. Agger W et al: Lyme disease: clinical features, classification, and epidemiology in the upper mid-west, *Medicine* 70(2):83, 1991.
2. Ai X et al: Clinical manifestations and epidemiological characteristics of Lyme disease in Hailin County, Heilongjiang Province, China, *Ann NY Acad Sci* 539:302, 1988.
3. Anderson JF, Barthold SW, Magnarelli LA: Infectious but nonpathogenic isolate of *Borrelia burgdorferi, J Clin Microbiol* 28:2693, 1990.
4. Asbrink E, Brehmer-Andersson E, Hovmark A: Acrodermatitis chronica atrophicans—a spirochetosis: clinical and histopathological picture based on 32 patients, *Am J Dermatopathol* 8:209, 1986.
5. Asbrink E, Hovmark A: Early and late cutaneous manifestations of *Ixodes*-borne borreliosis, *Ann NY Acad Sci* 539:4, 1988.
6. Athreya BH: Childhood Lyme arthritis: experience in an endemic area, *J Pediatr* 109(5):753, 1986.
7. Atlas E et al: Lyme myositis: muscle invasion by *Borrelia burgdorferi, Ann Intern Med* 109:245, 1988.
8. Bannwarth A: Chronische lymphocytare meningitis entzundliche polyneuritis und "rheumatismus," *Arch Psychiatr Nervenkr* 113:284, 1941.
9. Barbour AG: The diagnosis of Lyme disease: rewards and perils, *Ann Intern Med* 110:501, 1989.
10. Barbour AG, Heiland RA, Howe TR: Heterogeneity of major proteins in Lyme disease borreliae: a molecular analysis of North American and European isolates, *J Infect Dis* 152:478, 1985.
11. Barnert AL, Terry EE, Persellin RH: Acute rheumatic fever in adults, *JAMA* 232:925, 1975.
12. Belani K, Regelmann WE: Lyme disease in children, *Rheum Dis Clin North Am* 15:679, 1989.
13. Bianchi G et al: Articular involvement in European patients with Lyme disease. A report of 32 Italian patients, *Br J Rheumatol* 29:178, 1990.
14. Bowen GS: Clinical manifestations and descriptive epidemiology of Lyme disease in New Jersey 1978-82, *JAMA* 251:2236, 1984.
15. Brandt KD, Cathcart ES, Cohen AS: Gonococcal arthritis, *Arthritis Rheum* 17:503, 1974.
16. Brewer EJ et al: Current proposed revision of JRA criteria, *Arthritis Rheum* 20:195, 1977.
17. Burgdorfer W et al: Lyme disease: tick-borne spirochetosis? *Science* 216:1317, 1982.
18. Caperton EM et al: Ceftriaxone therapy of chronic inflammatory arthritis. A double-blind placebo controlled trial, *Arch Intern Med* 150:1677, 1990.
19. Carriero MM, Laux DC, Nelson DR: Characterization of the heat shock protein antigens of *Borrelia burgdorferi, Infect Immun* 58:2186, 1990.
20. Chakravarty KK, Webley M, Summers GD: A case of chronic Lyme arthritis in England, *Ann Rheum Dis* 50:134, 1991.
21. Cohen S, Jones R: An evaluation of the efficacy of arthroscopic synovectomy of the knee in rheumatoid arthritis: 12-24 month results, *J Rheumatol* 14:452, 1987.
22. Cooke WD, Dattwyler RJ: Spirochetal arthritis, including Lyme disease, *Curr Opin Rheumatol* 2:622, 1990.
23. Corpuz M et al: Problems in the use of serologic tests for the diagnosis of Lyme disease, *Arch Intern Med* 151:1837, 1991.
24. Cruz MH et al: Intrasynovial production of oligoclonal specific antibodies in Lyme arthritis, *N Engl J Med* 322:1889, 1990.
25. Cruz M et al: Lyme arthritis: oligoclonal anti-*Borrelia burgdorferi* IgG antibodies occur in joint fluid and serum, *Scand J Immunol* 33:61, 1991.
26. Dattwyler RJ: Amoxycillin plus probenecid versus doxycycline for treatment of erythema migrans borreliosis, *Lancet* 336:1404, 1990.
27. Dattwyler RJ, Halperin JJ: Failure of tetracycline therapy in early Lyme disease, *Arthritis Rheum* 30:448, 1987.
28. Dattwyler RJ et al: Lyme disease in Europe and North America, Lancet 1:681, 1987.
29. Dattwyler RJ et al: Treatment of late Lyme borreliosis—randomised comparison of ceftriaxone and penicillin, *Lancet* 1:1191, 1988.
30. Dattwyler RJ et al: Seronegative Lyme disease: dissociation of specific T- and B-lymphocyte responses to *B. burgdoferi, N Engl J Med* 319:1441, 1989.
31. Dekonenko EJ et al: Lyme borreliosis in the Soviet Union: a cooperative US-USSR report, *J Infect Dis* 158:748, 1988.
32. Dlesk A et al: Lyme disease presenting as seronegative rheumatoid arthritis, *Ann NY Acad Sci* 539:454, 1988.
33. Dressler F, Yoshinari NH, Steere AC: The T-cell proliferative assay in the diagnosis of Lyme disease, *Ann Intern Med* 115:533, 1991.
34. Dressler F et al: Western blotting in the serodiagnosis of Lyme disease (abstract #B94), *Arthritis Rheum* 34(Suppl):S113, 1991.
35. Duffy J et al: Diagnosing Lyme disease: the contribution of serologic testing, *Mayo Clin Proc* 63:1116, 1988.
36. Duray PH: The surgical pathology of human Lyme disease. An enlarging picture, *Am J Surg Pathol* 11(Suppl):47, 1987.
37. Duray PH, Steere AC: Clinical pathologic correlations of Lyme disease by stage, *Ann NY Acad Sci* 539:65, 1988.
38. Eichenfeld AH et al: Childhood Lyme arthritis: experience in an endemic area, *J Pediatr* 109:753, 1986.
39. Georgilis K et al: Neutrophilic chemotactic factors in synovial fluids of patients with Lyme disease, *Arthritis Rheum* 34:770, 1991.
40. Gilbert MS: Musculoskeletal manifestations of hemophilia, *Mt Sinai J Med* 44:339, 1977.
41. Goebel KM, Krause A, Neurath F: Acquired transient autoimmune reactions in Lyme arthritis: correlation between rheumatoid factor and disease activity, *Scand J Rheum* 75(Suppl):314, 1988.
42. Goodman JL et al: Molecular detection of persistent *Borrelia burgdorferi* in the urine of patients with active Lyme disease, *Infect Immun* 59:269, 1991.
43. Grodzicki RL, Steere AC: Comparison of immunoblotting and indirect enzyme-linked immunosorbent assay using different antigen preparations for diagnosing early Lyme disease, *J Infect Dis* 157:790, 1988.
44. Guerrero A et al: Joint manifestations of Lyme disease in Spain, *Br J Rheumatol* 30:71, 1991.
45. Guralnick W, Kaban LB, Merrill RG: Medical progress: temporomandibular joint afflictions, *N Engl J Med* 299:123, 1978.
46. Habicht GS et al: Lyme disease spirochetes induce human and murine interleukin 1 production, *J Immunol* 134:3147, 1985.

47. Haile CA: Parvovirus and epidemic arthritis, *Md Med J* 39:939, 1990.

48. Hanrahan JP et al: Incidence and cumulative frequency of endemic Lyme disease in a community, *J Infect Dis* 150:489, 1984.

49. Hansen K et al: Immunochemical characterization of and isolation of the gene for a *Borrelia burgdorferi* immunodominant 60-kilodalton antigen common to a wide range of bacteria, *Infect Immun* 56:2047, 1988.

50. Hardin J: Lyme disease, *Clin Aspects Autoimmunity* 4:23, 1990.

51. Hardin JA, Steere AC, Malawista SE: Immune complexes and the evolution of Lyme arthritis: dissemination and localization of abnormal C1q binding activity, *N Engl J Med* 301:1358, 1979.

52. Hedberg CW, Osterholm MT: Serologic test for antibody to *Borrelia burgdorferi*, *Arch Intern Med* 150:732, 1990.

53. Hedberg CW et al: An interlaboratory study of antibody to *Borrelia burgdorferi*, *J Infect Dis* 155:1325, 1987.

54. Herzer P et al: Lyme arthritis: clinical features, serological and radiographic findings of cases in Germany, *Klin Wochenschr* 64:206, 1986.

55. Hovmark A, Asbrink E, Olsson I: Joint and bone involvement in Swedish patients with *Ixodes ricinus*-borne *Borrelia* infection, *Zentralbl Bakteriol Mikrobiol Hyg [A]* 263:275, 1986.

56. Huaux JP et al: Pattern of Lyme arthritis in Europe: report of 14 cases, *Ann Rheum Dis* 47:164, 1988.

57. Hunder GG, Michet CJ: Giant cell arteritis and polymyalgia rheumatica, *Clin Rheum Dis* 11:471, 1985.

58. Huppertz HI: Childhood Lyme borreliosis in Europe, *Eur J Pediatr* 149(12):814, 1990.

59. Hyer FH, Gottlieb NL: Rheumatic disorders associated with viral infections, *Semin Arthritis Rheum* 8:17, 1978.

60. Jacobs JC, Stevens M, Duray PH: Lyme disease simulating septic arthritis, *JAMA* 256:1138, 1986.

61. Jarjour WN et al: Auto antibodies to human stress proteins. A survey of various rheumatic and other inflammatory diseases, *Arthritis Rheum* 34:1133, 1991.

62. Johnston YE et al: Lyme arthritis: spirochetes found in synovial microangiopathic lesions, *Am J Pathol* 118:26, 1985.

63. Kaell AT et al: Positive Lyme serology in subacute bacterial endocarditis: a study of four patients, *JAMA* 264:2916, 1990.

64. Kaell AT et al: Thirty cases of non-spirochetal subacute bacterial endocarditis (SBE): the occurrence of antibodies reactive to *B. burgdorferi* (Bb), (Abstract # B91), *Arthritis Rheum* 34:S113, 1991.

65. Kalish RA, Leony JM, Steere AC: Delay in the immune response to outer-surface proteins (OSP) A and B of *B. burgdorferi:* correlation with arthritis and treatment failure in susceptible patients with Lyme disease (abstract #66), *Arthritis Rheum* 34(Suppl):S43, 1991.

66. Kaufman LD: Lofgren's syndrome (acute sarcoidosis) sine erythema nodosum mimicking acute rheumatoid arthritis, *NY State J Med* 90:463, 1990.

67. Kaufman LD et al: Late cutaneous Lyme disease: acrodermatitis chronica atrophicans, *Am J Med* 86:828, 1989.

68. Kawabata M et al: Lyme disease in Japan and its possible incriminating tick vector, *Ixodes persulcatus, J Infect Dis* 156:854, 1987.

69. Kay J et al: Synovial fluid eosinophilia in Lyme disease, *Arthritis Rheum* 31(11):1384, 1988.

70. Kelsey JH: Lyme disease: an important consideration in the differential diagnosis of TMD, *J Mich Dent Assoc* 72(4-5):209, 1990.

71. Kolstoe J, Messner RP: Lyme disease: musculoskeletal manifestations, *Rheum Dis Clin North Am* 15:649, 1989.

72. Koning J, Bosma RB, Hoogkam JA: Demonstration of spirochetes in patients with Lyme disease with a modified silver stain, *J Med Microbiol* 23:261, 1987.

73. Kramer N et al: Septal panniculitis as a manifestation of Lyme disease, *Am J Med* 81:149, 1986.

74. Krause A et al: Lyme borreliosis. Autologous serum required for optimum stimulation, *Arthritis Rheum* 34(4):393, 1991.

75. Kryger P et al: Lyme borreliosis among Danish patients with arthritis, *Scand J Rheumatol* 19(1):77, ISSN 0300-9742, 1990.

76. Kujala GA, Steere AC, Davis JS IV: IgM rheumatoid factor in Lyme disease: correlation with disease activity, total serum IgM and IgM antibody to *Borrelia burgdorferi*, *J Rheumatol* 14:772, 1987.

77. Lane RS, Lavoie PE: Lyme borreliosis in California: acarological, clinical, and epidemiological studies, *Ann NY Acad Sci* 539:192, 1988.

78. Lastavica CC et al: Rapid emergence of a focal epidemic of Lyme disease in coastal Massachusetts, *N Engl J Med* 320:133, 1989.

79. Laumio A et al: Double-blind placebo-controlled study of three month treatment with lymecycline on reactive arthritis, *Arthritis Rheum* 34:6, 1991.

80. Lavoie PE, Burgdorfer W: Serological reactivity to *Borrelia burgdorferi* in rheumatoid arthritis patients, *Ann NY Acad Sci* 539:461, 1988.

81. Lawson JP, Steere AC: Lyme arthritis: radiologic findings, *Radiology* 154(1):37, 1985.

81a. Lawson JP, Rahn DW: Lyme disease and radiologic findings in Lyme arthritis, *AJR,* 158:1065, 1992.

82. Levine JF et al: Indigenous cases of Lyme disease diagnosed in North Carolina, *South Med J* 84(1):27, ISSN 0038-4348, 1991.

83. Liu NY et al: Randomized trial of doxycycline vs. amoxicillin/probenecid for the treatment of Lyme arthritis: treatment of non-responders with IV penicillin or ceftriaxone, *Arthritis Rheum* 32:S46 1989 (abstract).

84. Logigian EL, Kaplan RF, Steere AC: Chronic neurologic manifestations of Lyme disease, *N Engl J Med* 323:1438, 1990.

85. Longworth DL: The clinical challenge of Lyme disease, *Cleve Clin J Med* 57:453, 1990.

86. Luft BJ, Dattwyler RJ: Treatment of Lyme borreliosis, *Rheum Clin North Am* 15:747, 1989.

87. Luger SW, Krauss E: Serologic tests for Lyme disease: interlaboratory variability, *Arch Intern Med* 150:761, 1990.

88. Lyme Lines: Lyme Disease Research News from NIH: 1-9, July 1991.

89. Mackworth-Young CG et al: Anticardiolipin antibodies in Lyme disease, *Arthritis Rheum* 31:1052, 1988.

90. Magnarelli LA et al: Cross reactivity of non-specific treponemal antibody in serologic tests for Lyme disease, *J Clin Microbiol* 28:1276, 1990.

91. Malawista SE, Steere AC: Lyme disease: infectious in origin, rheumatic in expression, *Adv Intern Med* 31:147, 1986.

92. Masi AT, Eisenstein BI: Disseminated gonococcal infection (DGI) and gonococcal arthritis (GCA), *Semin Arthritis Rheum* 10:173, 1981.

93. Massarotti E et al: A multicenter, randomized trial of doxycycline, amoxicillin/benemid, and azithromycin for the treatment of early Lyme disease, *Arthritis Rheum* 33:S37, 1990.

94. Mayo DR, Vance DW Jr: Parvovirus B19 as the cause of a syndrome resembling Lyme arthritis in adults, *N Engl J Med* 324(6):419, 1991.

95. MacDonald EC, Weisman NH: Articular manifestations of rheumatic fever in adults, *Ann Intern Med* 89:917, 1978.

96. McLaughlin TP et al: Chronic arthritis of the knee in Lyme disease: a review of the literature and report of two cases treated by synovectomy, *J Bone Joint Surg* 68A:1057, 1986.

97. Mensi N et al: Characterization of *Borrelia burgdorferi* proteins reactive with antibodies in synovial fluid of a patient with Lyme arthritis, *Infect Immun* 58(7):2404, SSN 0019-9567, July 1990.

98. Miller LC: Musculoskeletal manifestations of infectious disease in children, *Curr Opin Rheumatol* 2(5):817, 1990.

99. Moffat CM et al: Cellular immune findings in Lyme disease: correlation with serum IgM and disease activity, *Am J Med* 77:625, 1984.

100. Moreland LW, Koopman WS: Infection as a cause of arthritis, *Curr Opin Rheumatol* 3:639, 1991.

101. Muhlemann MF, Wright DJM: Emerging pattern of Lyme disease in the United Kingdom and Irish Republic, *Lancet* I:260, 1987.

102. Nadelman RB et al: Isolation of *Borrelia burgdorferi* from the blood of seven patients with Lyme disease, *Am J Med* 88:21, 1990.

103. Naides SJ et al: Rheumatologic manifestations of human parvovirus B19 infection in adults, *Arthritis Rheum* 33:1297, 1990.

104. Neumann A et al: Frequency of *Borrelia burgdorferi*-reactive T lymphocytes in Lyme arthritis, *Rheumatol Int* 9:237, 1989.

105. Pease C, Keat A: Arthritis as the main or only symptom of hepatitis B infection, *Post Grad Med J* 61:545, 1985.

106. Persing DH et al: Multi-target detection of *B. burgdorferi* associated DNA sequences in synovial fluids of patients with arthritis. *Arthritis Rheum* 33:536, 1990 (abstract).

107. Pinals RS: Meningococcemia presenting as acute polyarthritis, *J Rheumatol* 4:420, 1977.

108. Rahn DW: Treatment of Lyme disease, *Post Grad Med* 87:159, 1990.

109. Rahn DW: Lyme disease: clinical manifestations, diagnosis, and treatment, *Semin Arthritis Rheum* 20(4):201, 1991.

110. Rahn DW, Malawista SE: Clinical judgment in Lyme disease, *Hosp Pract*, p 39, Mar 30, 1990.

111. Rahn DW, Malawista SE: Lyme disease: recommendations for diagnosis and treatment, *Ann Intern Med* 114(6):472, 1991.

112. Rawlings JA, Foernier PV, Teltow GJ: Isolation of *Borrelia* spirochetes from patients in Texas, *J Clin Microbiol* 25:1148, 1987.

113. Reginato AJ et al: Synovitis in secondary syphilis: clinical, light and electron microscopic studies, *Arthritis Rheum* 22:170, 1979.

114. Reimers CD et al: Myositis caused by *Borrelia burgdorferi:* report of four cases, *J Neurol Sci* 91:215, 1989.

115. Rosa PA, Schwan TG: A specific and sensitive assay for the Lyme disease spirochete *Borrelia burgdorferi* using the polymerase chain reaction, *J Infect Dis* 160:1018, 1989.

116. Rotes-Querol J: *The syndromes of psychogenic rheumatism in soft tissue rheumatism.* In Dickson ASJ, editor: *Clinical rheumatism disease,* London, 1979, WB Saunders.

117. Roth DA, Wilz DR, Theil GB: Schönlein-Henoch syndrome in adults, *Q J Med* 55:145, 1985.

118. Russell H et al: Enzyme-linked immunosorbent assay and indirect immunofluorescence assay for Lyme disease, *J Infect Dis* 149:465, 1984.

119. Sartoris DJ et al: Musculoskeletal manifestations of sarcoidosis, *Semin Roentgenol* 20:376, 1985.

120. Saulsbury FT, Katzmann JA: Prevalence of antibody to *Borrelia burgdorferi* in children with juvenile rheumatoid arthritis, *J Rheumatol* 17(9):1193, 1990.

121. Schmidli J et al: Cultivation of *Borrelia burgdorferi* from joint fluid three months after treatment of facial palsy due to Lyme borreliosis, *J Infect Dis* 158:905, 1988.

122. Schmutzhard E, Willeit J, Gerstenbrand F: Meningopolyneuritis Bannwarth with focal nodular myositis: a new aspect in Lyme borreliosis, *Klin Wochenschr* 64:1204, 1986.

123. Schoen RT: Pathogenesis, diagnosis, manifestations and treatment of Lyme disease, *Curr Opin Rheumatol* 3:610, 1991.

124. Schoen R, Rahn D: Lyme disease update: tips on recognition and treatment, *J Musculoskel Med* 8(5):75, 1991.

125. Schoen RT et al: Treatment of refractory chronic Lyme arthritis with arthroscopic synovectomy, *Arthritis Rheum* 34:1056, 1991.

126. Schoenen J et al: Myositis during *Borrelia burgdorferi* infection (Lyme disease), *J Neurol Neurosurg Psychiatry* 52:1002, 1989.

127. Schutzer SE et al: Sequestration of antibody to *Borrelia burgdorferi* in immune complexes in seronegative Lyme disease, *Lancet* 335:312, 1990.

128. Schwan TG, Simpson WJ: Diagnosing Lyme disease, *Ann Intern Med* 115:577, 1991.

129. Schwartz BD: Infectious agents, immunity and rheumatic diseases, *Arthritis Rheum* 33:457, 1990.

130. Schwartz BS et al: Antibody testing in Lyme disease: a comparison of results in four laboratories, *JAMA* 262:3431, 1989.

131. Shanafelt MC et al: T cell and antibody reactivity with the *Borrelia burgdorferi* 60 kDa heat shock protein in Lyme arthritis, *J Immunol* 146(11):3985, 1991.

132. Shmerling RH et al: Synovial fluid tests: what should be ordered? *JAMA* 264:1009, 1990.

133. Shrestha M, Grodzicki RL, Steere AC: Diagnosing early Lyme disease, *Am J Med* 78:235, 1985.

134. Sigal LH: Lyme disease 1988: immunologic manifestations and possible immunopathogenetic mechanisms, *Semin Arthritis Rheum* 18:151, 1989.

135. Sigal L: Summary of the first 100 patients seen at a Lyme disease referral center, *Am J Med* 88:577, 1990.

136. Sigal LH et al: Proliferative responses of mononuclear cells in Lyme disease: reactivity to *Borrelia burgdorferi* antigens is greater in joint fluid than in blood, *Arthritis Rheum* 29:761, 1986.

137. Snydman DR et al: *Borrelia burgdorferi* in joint fluid in chronic Lyme arthritis, *Ann Intern Med* 104:798, 1986.

138. Solem JH: Mumps arthritis without parotitis, *Scand J Infect Dis* 3:173, 1971.

139. Sood SK et al: Positive Lyme disease (LD) serology in juvenile rheumatoid arthritis (JRA) in a LD endemic area: analysis by immunoblot (IB), *Arthritis Rheum* 34:537, 1991 (abstract #29).

140. Spilberg I, Siltzbach LE, Mc Ewen C: The arthritis of sarcoidosis, *Arthritis Rheum* 12:126, 1969.

141. Stanek G et al: European Lyme borreliosis, *Ann NY Acad Sci* 539:274, 1988.

142. Steere AC: The pathogenesis of Lyme disease: implications for rheumatic disease, *Ann NY Acad Sci* 539:87, 1988.

143. Steere AC: Lyme disease, *N Engl J Med* 321:586, 1989.

144. Steere AC, Duray PH, Butcher EC: Spirochetal antigens and lymphoid cell surface markers in Lyme synovitis: comparison with rheumatoid synovium and tonsillar lymphoid tissue, *Arthritis Rheum* 31:487, 1988.

145. Steere AC, Dwyer E, Winchester RJ: Association of chronic Lyme arthritis with HLA-DR4 and HLA-DR2 alleles, *N Engl J Med* 323:219, 1990.

146. Steere AC, Schoen RT, Taylor E: The clinical evolution of Lyme arthritis, *Ann Intern Med* 107:725, 1987.

147. Steere AC et al: Erythema chronicum migrans and Lyme arthritis: the enlarging clinical spectrum, *Ann Intern Med* 86:685, 1977.

148. Steere AC et al: Lyme arthritis: an epidemic of oligoarticular arthritis in children and adults in three Connecticut communities, *Arthritis Rheum* 20(1):7, 1977.

149. Steere AC et al: Chronic Lyme arthritis: clinical and immunogenetic differentiation from rheumatoid arthritis, *Ann Intern Med* 90:896, 1979.

150. Steere AC et al: Lyme arthritis: correlation of serum and cryoglobulin IgM with activity, and serum IgG with remission, *Arthritis Rheum* 22:471, 1979.

151. Steere AC et al: Antibiotic therapy in Lyme disease, *Ann Intern Med* 93:1, 1980.

152. Steere AC et al: Elevated levels of collagenase and prostaglandin E_2 from synovium associated with erosion of cartilage and bone in a patient with chronic Lyme arthritis, *Arthritis Rheum* 23:591, 1980.

153. Steere AC et al: The early clinical manifestations of Lyme disease, *Ann Intern Med* 99:76, 1983.

154. Steere AC et al: The spirochetal etiology of Lyme disease, *N Engl J Med* 308:733, 1983.

155. Steere AC et al: Treatment of the early manifestations of Lyme disease, *Ann Intern Med* 99:22, 1983.

156. Steere AC et al: Successful parenteral penicillin therapy of established Lyme arthritis, *N Engl J Med* 312:869, 1985.

157. Steere AC et al: Longitudinal assessment of the clinical and epidemiological features of Lyme disease in a defined population, *J Infect Dis* 154:295, 1986.

158. Stewart A et al: Lyme arthritis in the Hunter Valley, *Med J Aust* 1:139, 1982.

159. Szer IS, Taylor E, Steere AC: The long-term course of Lyme arthritis in children, *N Engl J Med* 325:159, 1991.

160. Thompson GR et al: Intermittent arthritis following rubella vaccination, *Am J Dis Child* 125:526, 1973.

161. Travers RK et al: Polyarteritis nodosa: a clinical and angiographic analysis of 17 cases, *Semin Arthritis Rheum* 8:181, 1979.

162. Valesova M, Trnavsky K: Joint manifestations of Lyme borreliosis in Czechoslovakian patients, *Z Rheumatol* 49(4):192, 1990.

162a. Watanakunakorn C, Tolivar J: Lyme arthritis with subarticular cyst formation in metacarpal and metatarsal bones, *South Med J* 85:187-88, 1992.

163. Weber K: Erythema chronicum migrans meningitis—eine bakterielle infections—kraukheit? *Munch Med Wochenschr* 46:1993, 1974.

164. Weber K et al: Reinfection with erythema migrans disease, *Infection* 14:32, 1986.

165. Weyand CM, Goronzy JJ: Immune responses to *Borrelia burgdorferi* in patients with reactive arthritis, *Arthritis Rheum* 32:1057, 1989.

166. White DG et al: Human parvovirus arthropathy, *Lancet* i:419, 1985.

167. Williams CL et al: Lyme disease in childhood: clinical and epidemiologic features of ninety cases, *Pediatr Infect Dis J* 9(1):10, 1990.

168. Wilske B et al: Antigenic variability of *Borrelia burgdorferi*, *Ann NY Acad Sci* 539:126, 1988.

169. Winfield JB: Stress proteins, arthritis and autoimmunity, *Arthritis Rheum* 32:1497, 1989.

170. Wolfe F et al: The American College of Rheumatology 1990 criteria for the classification of fibromyalgia: report of the Multi Center Criteria Committee, *Arthritis Rheum* 33:160, 1990.

171. Yanez JE et al: Rubella arthritis, *Ann Intern Med* 64:772, 1966.

172. Yoshinari NH, Reinhardt BN, Steere AC: T-cell responses to polypeptide fractions of *Borrelia burgdorferi* in patients with Lyme arthritis, *Arthritis Rheum* 34:707, 1991.

173. Yssel H et al: *Borrelia burgdorferi* activates a T helper type 1-like T-cell subset in Lyme arthritis, *J Esp Med* 174:593, 1991.

174. Zoshke DC, Skemp AA, Defosse DL: Lymphoproliferative responses to *Borrelia burgdorferi* in Lyme disease, *Ann Intern Med* 114:285, 1991.

11 Cardiac Manifestations

Stephen C. Vlay

Lyme disease, caused by the spirochete *Borrelia burgdorferi* and transmitted by the deer tick, may result in a variety of clinical manifestations. Originally associated with arthritis in children in Lyme, Connecticut, it soon became apparent that dermatologic, cardiac, and neurologic disorders could follow.[10,21-23] Often, when arthritis is not a prime manifestation of the disease, and a patient is evaluated for a problem such as atrioventricular (A-V) block, recognition of an earlier skin rash such as erythema migrans (EM) points to the diagnosis of Lyme disease.

The most important message for the physician is to be aware of the disorder and to include Lyme disease in the differential diagnosis, particularly when the patient has been exposed to an endemic area.

Lyme disease is a global disorder and has been reported in North America, Europe (Germany, Austria, Switzerland, France, Sweden, Czechoslovakia), Russia, China, Japan, and possibly Brazil in South America. In North America, the vast majority of reported cases have been found in Connecticut, New York, Massachusetts, Rhode Island, Wisconsin, and Minnesota.[2] Certain areas are particular focal points such as Lyme, Connecticut; and Long Island and Westchester in New York state. Other endemic areas include Virginia, Maryland, North Carolina, Missouri, California, and Oregon. As endemic areas increase in scope, the disorder and its variations become more apparent.[15]

In North America, the spirochete is carried by the tick *Ixodes dammini* in the northeast and midwest and the tick *Ixodes pacificus* in the western states. In Europe a different tick is involved, *Ixodes ricinus;* in Asia the tick vector is *Ixodes persulcatus.*[21] In North America, joint abnormalities seem to be one of the most common findings. In Europe, cutaneous manifestations such as lymphadenosis cutis benigna and acrodermatitis chronica atrophicans are frequent.

As physician awareness of Lyme disease increases, this infectious disorder will more often be included in the differential diagnosis and the diagnosis is likely to be made with increasing frequency. Lyme disease may not always be seropositive, particularly if the patient has received partial but ineffective treatment shortly after initial infection. The phenomenon of seronegative Lyme disease is a real one, and it is likely that the incidence of *B. burgdorferi* infection is even higher than current numbers indicate. Seronegative Lyme disease may certainly have as dire consequences as the seropositive form.

CARDIAC INVOLVEMENT

Cardiac involvement is the least documented major organ system involvement in Lyme disease. In North American patients, it has been estimated to occur in 4% to 10%[3] to as many as 8% to 20%.[13] It is less common than skin, joint, or nervous system involvement. European patients appear to have a much lower incidence of cardiac involvement, but it does occur on both continents.[24] There is a 3:1 male predominance, and cardiac involvement may occur several days to several months after the initial illness. It may rarely present as a late chronic infectious complication.

When considering myocarditis secondary to *B. burgdorferi,* it is useful to review other infectious myocarditities (Table 11-1)[31] and specifically examine those produced by other spirochetal infections. Syphilitic inflammation characteristically involves plasma cell and lymphocytic infiltration with perivascular accentuation and obliterative endarteritis. Syphilis is perhaps best known for its effect on the arterial tree with aortitis being a prime feature. The ascending aortitis results in a dilated aneurysmal ascending aorta and widened aortic root, often with aortic regurgitation. (It is this anatomy that gives credence to the adage that the murmur of syphilitic aortic regurgitation is heard to the right of the sternum, and that related to rheumatic disease is heard to the left.) In the myocardium, gummas may be seen and the conducting system may be affected by A-V block. These cardiovascular complications of untreated syphilis are infrequently seen today.

Leptospirosis can affect the heart to cause petechiae or larger foci of hemorrhage on the epi-

Table 11–1 Infections that may involve the heart

Bacterial
Brucella
Clostridium
Diphtheria
Legionella
Neisseria meningitidis
Salmonella
Streptococcus (acute rheumatic fever)
Tuberculosis
Also myocardial involvement related to infectious endocarditis

Spirochetal
Lyme disease
Leptospirosis
Relapsing fever
Syphilis

Rickettsial
Rocky Mountain spotted fever
Q fever
Scrub typhus

Viral
Adenovirus
Arbovirus A + B
Coxsackie B + A
Cytomegalovirus
Echovirus
Enterovirus
Herpes simplex
Hepatitis
Human immunodeficiency virus
Influenza
Measles (rubeola)
Mumps
Rubella
Poliomyelitis
Vaccinia
Variola
Yellow fever

Fungal
Mycoplasma
Actinomycosis
Aspergillosis
Blastomycosis
Candidiasis
Coccidioidomycosis
Cryptococcus
Histoplasmosis

Parasites
Protozoa
Malaria
Trypanosoma cruzi (Chagas' disease)
Trypanosomiasis
Toxoplasmosis

Metazoal
Cysticercosis
Echinococcus
Heterophyiasis
Schistosomiasis
Trichinosis
Visceral larva migrans

cardium. The conduction system may be involved. Atrial (atrial fibrillation, atrial flutter) and ventricular (ectopy, ventricular tachycardia) arrhythmias may be noted. Rarely, the patient may develop dilatation of the heart, left ventricular (LV) failure, and pulmonary congestion. Pericarditis may be part of the entire presentation.

Relapsing fever in Ethiopia has been reported to have cardiac involvement resulting in conduction system disease with A-V block, tachyarrhythmias, and a diffuse histiocytic interstitial infiltrate in the myocardium.

With regard to the bacterial, rickettsial, viral, mycoplasma, fungal, and parasitic infections in general, it becomes apparent that these various infectious processes may affect the heart in different ways. Not all patients with these infections have cardiac involvement. In the small percentage that do, the involved area may be the pericardium, myocardium, or conduction system. Atrial and ventricular arrhythmias may result. The severity of the illness may vary from being barely noticeable to a progressive fatal pancarditis. Fortunately, such fatal involvement is rare. It is not known why the heart is spared in some patients and damaged in others, or why the severity of cardiac involvement is so variable.

Viral myocarditities are very difficult to document. With all of the different possible viruses and strains, it may be fortuitous if one obtains the appropriate acute and convalescent titers and can demonstrate a change. Some of the other infectious myocarditities have associated noncardiac findings that point to the diagnosis. Nevertheless, many conditions may remain undiagnosed and may be labeled "idiopathic" because one does not consider the specific infection in the differential diagnosis or there is limited ability to make the diagnosis for technical reasons.

If one were to predict, on the basis of knowing how other infectious myocarditidies present, the manifestations of cardiac infection with the spirochete *B. burgdorferi,* one would be concerned about effects on the conduction system and varying forms of myocarditis and pericarditis. In fact, Lyme carditis may cause pericarditis and myocarditis, with cardiomyopathy and congestive heart failure; conduction disorders; and atrial and ventricular arrhythmias. Each condition must be considered individually. Some of the manifestations may be a result of direct infiltration of the tissue by spirochetes. It is also possible, although not proven, that circulating immune complexes may be responsible for some of the inflammatory changes.

Myocardium and pericardium

Patients with Lyme disease are occasionally noted to have nonspecific ST-T wave changes on the electrocardiogram.[22] Although these findings are truly nonspecific, they certainly could represent an inflammatory process of the pericardium and myocardium. With further evaluation, radionuclide studies provided supporting evidence with gallium-67 scintigraphy demonstrating left ventricular uptake consistent with focal inflammation of the myocardium.[11,16,17] Indium cardiac antimyosin scans have also been used[8] to demonstrate cardiac inflammation resulting from Lyme disease.

A few patients have experienced severe forms of carditis and have undergone myocardial biopsy. Rare patients have died and were autopsied. Microscopic analysis of the specimens revealed lymphoplasmocytic pericarditis as well as spirochetal forms in the myocardium.[4,6,11,27] These data provided definite evidence that Lyme disease may result in a spirochetal infection of the heart and associated inflammatory response. In its worst form, cardiomegaly and pancarditis may result.

Two recent reports[19,30] documented cases of myocarditis and its complications (cardiomegaly, congestive heart failure, and arrhythmias) in patients with spirochetes demonstrated on the myocardial biopsy. In both of these cases, there was no other identifiable cause to explain the myocardial dysfunction (no coronary artery disease, no evidence for other cardiomyopathic process or toxin). It seems reasonable to attribute the process to infection with *B. burgdorferi*.

In the first case,[19] no further deterioration occurred after antibiotic therapy. In the second,[30] left ventricular dysfunction actually improved. These developments have important implications for the clinician. First, one must be more hesitant to make a diagnosis of "idiopathic" cardiomyopathy. We must be more aggressive in attempting to make the diagnosis, and it may mean more myocardial biopsies. One must not forget to consider Lyme disease in the differential diagnosis, to obtain serologic tests, as well as to send blood for other relevant possibilities (such as viral titers). The fact that ventricular function improved in the second case justifies the additional cost and risk of the myocardial biopsy procedure. The difference between treatment response (stabilization versus improvement) in the two cases may relate to the duration and extent of the infection. After a certain point, it is likely that left ventricular dysfunction becomes irreversible. Although some of these comments remain speculative, the implications of these cases cannot be dismissed, particularly when considering the potential consequences for the patient with carditis. A recent report from Europe has also suggested a relationship between serologic evidence of *B. burgdorferi* infection and dilated cardiomyopathy.[20]

Table 11–2 describes the various microscopic pathologic findings in Lyme carditis. In some patients, the myocardial biopsy may be normal or may show mild fibrosis, but in others, the biopsy may demonstrate perivascular lymphocytic infiltration in addition to more extensive involvement. In the above cited case,[30] myocardial spirochetes were demonstrated despite the absence of an inflammatory cell response. Other findings may include diffuse infiltration of the interstitium by lymphocytes, plasma cells and macrophages, myocyte necrosis, endocardial and interstitial fibrosis.[4,6,11,26,27] The pathologic picture may vary from a focal area of myocarditis to an extensive pancarditis. Immunohistochemical studies may demonstrate spirochetelike organisms (Color Plate 7).[30]

Conduction system abnormalities

Atrioventricular (A-V) block was the first recognized conduction abnormality in Lyme disease.[21,23] It is also the most common cardiac abnormality, overall, associated with this infection. The location of the block is usually at or above the A-V node and may be manifest as first- (12%), second- (16%), or third-degree (49%) A-V block.[24] Occasionally, patients may be symptomatic from the bradycardia and require a temporary pacemaker.* Most cases improve within 3 to 7 days, but some cases of high-degree A-V block may not resolve for 2 to 3 weeks. Improvement is usually gradual. Block usually retreats from third to second to first degree over the above noted time frame. First-degree A-V block, however, may persist for up to 6 months. Rarely, infra-His block has been described.[12,18] Isolated cases of persistent high degree A-V block related to Lyme borreliosis have required permanent pacemakers.[26]

The sinus node may also be involved. In 1986, sinus node dysfunction was reported in the United States[28] and in France.[7,16] It may take the form of sinoatrial (SA) block or abnormalities in sinus node recovery time. The patient may have sinus bradycardia.

In both SA block and A-V block, it is conceiv-

---

*References 1, 9, 12, 18, 25, 28.

Table 11–2 Occasional microscopic findings in Lyme carditis

Pericardium
Lymphoplasmocytic pericarditis

Myocardium
Perivascular lymphocytic infiltration
Diffuse infiltration of interstitium by lymphocytes, plasma cells, and macrophages
Myocyte necrosis
Endocardial and interstitial fibrosis

Findings may be a focal area of myocarditis or be extensive as a pancarditis

Indirect immunofluorescence
May demonstrate spirochete-like organisms

Table 11–3 Lyme carditis: Making the diagnosis

Clinical suspicion	If you forget to include it in the differential, you will never make the diagnosis.
Conduction system disease	Look for A-V block or sinus node dysfunction.
Arrhythmias	Atrial arrhythmias may be associated with pericarditis. Ventricular arrhythmias may be associated with myocarditis. Ventricular arrhythmias may vary from ventricular ectopy to ventricular tachycardia.
Pericarditis Myocarditis	Signs of pericarditis ECG: Nonspecific ST-T wave changes Left ventricular dysfunction S₃ gallop Altered contractility

able that the problem may be related to an inflammatory response to the borrelial infection, rather than irreversible damage due to borrelial infiltration of the node. This possibility has been raised because the heart block may resolve, even without antibiotic therapy.[9]

The typical patient presents with fatigue and lethargy and is found to be in complete heart block with an idioventricular or high nodal escape rhythm. Occasionally, the sinus rate is also slow. If the heart rate is considered to result in hemodynamic instability, temporary pacing is initiated. Antibiotic therapy is started. Usually, the heart block starts to resolve within a few days to 1 week. First-degree A-V block may persist for months. It is important to make the diagnosis of Lyme disease because almost all patients recover from high-degree A-V block and do not require a permanent pacemaker, as compared with other etiologies of high-degree A-V block.

Atrial and ventricular arrhythmias

Because of the associated pericarditis, some patients with Lyme disease develop atrial arrhythmias. Inflammation in the atrium may predispose to irritability, atrial premature beats, and atrial fibrillation. These types of arrhythmias are usually self-limited in scope.

Ventricular ectopy is not unexpected in any patient with myocarditis. In a patient with Lyme carditis, inflammation related to myocardial borreliosis is the most likely etiology for ventricular arrhythmia. The greater the inflammatory process, the greater the extent of left ventricular dysfunction, and the more likely the patient will have complex ventricular ectopy. Ventricular tachycardia has been reported both in Europe[19] and the United States.[30] In the latter reported case, the ventricular tachycardia was difficult to control and required electrophysiologic testing. Treatment against both the underlying problem (myocardial borreliosis) and the arrhythmia (antiarrhythmic drugs) is necessary.

The typical patient with Lyme myocarditis has isolated ventricular ectopy and, in the more advanced forms, nonsustained or rarely sustained ventricular tachycardia.

MAKING THE DIAGNOSIS

Table 11–3 provides clues to making the diagnosis. Perhaps the key is to remember to include Lyme disease in the differential diagnosis when faced with a new case of heart block or myopericarditis. This advice is particularly important when dealing with a patient who has no other known cardiac disease and no cardiac risk factors and who has been in an endemic area.

If a patient with known Lyme disease is evaluated, one must exclude cardiac involvement by looking for the major clinical features: conduction system abnormalities, arrhythmias, pericarditis, and myocarditis (see Table 11–3).

The clinical diagnosis of Lyme disease is confirmed serologically as described in detail in Chap-

Table 11–4 Lyme carditis: Confirming the diagnosis

Serology	ELISA for anti-*B. burgdorferi* antibodies Initially high IgM Later IgG May also have cryoprecipitates, circulating immune complexes Rarely rheumatoid factor, antinuclear antibodies or anticardiolipin antibodies *Remember:* Some patients are seronegative.
Myocardial biopsy	Microscopic findings (as in Table 11–2) or no inflammatory infiltrate Immunofluorescence may demonstrate spirochetes Culture of organism (very difficult)

ters 6 and 14. The enzyme-linked immunosorbent assay (ELISA) is used to determine a titer (Table 11–4). Values more than three standard deviations above the mean indicate a high likelihood of infection with *B. burgdorferi*. One must always remember that some patients may have Lyme disease despite being seronegative, possibly as a result of partial and incomplete treatment (see Chapter 25).

To be absolutely certain about myocarditis, a variety of diagnostic studies of left ventricular function may be performed. These include an echocardiogram, a radionuclide ventriculogram (multiple gated acquisition scan), or a formal left ventriculogram (contrast angiogram as part of a left heart cardiac catheterization). Radionuclide scans (gallium, antimyosin) may demonstrate abnormal uptake if myocarditis is present. In an attempt to document that Lyme disease is the cause of the carditis, myocardial biopsy may be necessary.

Pathologic findings may be negative or as described in Table 11–2. Special immunohistochemical preparations may demonstrate spirochetes. Culture of the organism is also possible but difficult to accomplish.

Table 11–5 Lyme carditis: Therapy

1. *Symptomatic bradycardia* or *Symptomatic heart block*	Temporary pacing until improvement* in symptoms and rhythm

2. *Antibiotic therapy* is recommended for all patients with Lyme carditis.
3. *Corticosteroid therapy* has been considered for some patients with A-V block, and some physicians believe the A-V block may resolve several days earlier. However, there are few randomized controlled studies to recommend this measure routinely.
4. Symptomatic therapy for symptoms of congestive heart failure
5. Appropriate antiarrhythmic drug therapy for symptomatic atrial and ventricular arrhythmias

*Once a patient is asymptomatic, pacemaker can be removed. It is not necessary to wait for complete resolution of A-V block. In fact, first degree A-V block may persist for months.

Table 11–6 Lyme carditis: Antibiotic regimens*

For serious manifestations (LV dysfunction, high-degree A-V block)

1. Ceftriaxone or	2 g IV/day × 14 days
2. Penicillin G	20 million U IV in six divided doses for 14 days

For patients with less serious manifestations of Lyme disease

1. Doxycycline or	100 mg PO bid or tid × 2 to 4 weeks
2. Amoxicillin	500 mg PO qid (± probenecid) × 2 to 4 weeks

*Azithromycin, a new erythromycinlike antibiotic, has shown promise in some preliminary clinical trials. It has the advantage of oral administration and may avoid the need for prolonged IV therapies. Its role in serious infections remains to be determined.

THERAPY OF LYME CARDITIS

Antibiotic therapy is obviously the mainstay of therapy (Table 11–5). The more serious the clinical manifestations of Lyme disease, the more necessary it is to provide aggressive antibiotic regimens.[5,21] The patient with a recent tick bite, minor constitutional symptoms, and EM may respond well to doxycycline, 100 mg PO bid or tid for 2 to 4 weeks, or amoxicillin, 500 mg PO qid ± probenecid for 2 to 4 weeks (Table 11–6). With evidence of myocarditis, most physicians would recommend ceftriaxone, 2 g IV/day for 14 days. Preliminary data with a new oral erythromycin derivative (azithromycin) appear promising. Its long half-life and penetration into the cell may allow oral therapy, but its utility for serious manifestations remains undetermined at this time.

Corticosteroid therapy has been advocated for some patients with heart block. In a few nonrandomized, uncontrolled reports with limited numbers of patients, it was felt that the administration of corticosteroids may have shortened the recovery of A–V block.[14,21,22] However, there are insufficient data to recommend corticosteroid use routinely. There is also a concern that steroids may potentiate neurologic or joint involvement in Lyme disease patients.

If the patient has symptomatic bradycardia or heart block, a temporary pacemaker may be necessary until it resolves. The important fact to remember is that this etiology of heart block and bradycardia is most often self-limited and does *not* require a permanent pacemaker.

If patients have symptomatic arrhythmias, appropriate antiarrhythmic drugs may be necessary. With atrial fibrillation, digoxin may be necessary to control the ventricular response. If the patient has an active pericarditis, attempts to restore and maintain sinus rhythm should be delayed until resolution of the pericarditis. Ventricular ectopy does not require specific treatment unless symptomatic. Usually, only sustained ventricular tachycardia (VT) or long runs of nonsustained VT require treatment with type 1 antiarrhythmic drugs. Management of life-threatening ventricular arrhythmias may require electrophysiology study.

If patients progress to congestive heart failure, appropriate management may include afterload reduction (for example, ACE inhibitor), diuretics, or digoxin. Therapy must be tailored to the individual patient.

CHRONIC LYME DISEASE

It is unknown how many patients have untreated Lyme carditis and have stabilized or progressed to left ventricular (LV) dysfunction.[29] As with syphilis, the chronic manifestations may continue undetected for years. Physicians may encounter many patients being treated for another illness who fortuitously undergo a test for Lyme disease and are found to have highly elevated titers. Yet they seem asymptomatic. It is unclear what therapeutic interventions should follow, but further evaluation, particularly to exclude cardiac or neurologic disorders, may be indicated. If, for example, central nervous system involvement is found, aggressive antibiotic therapy is indicated. If only elevated titers are noted, perhaps treatment with doxycycline might be considered. The final answers are not in, but one course of antibiotic therapy may not be unreasonable for these patients.

In addition to chronic infection, it should be remembered that, once treated, patients may become reinfected with borreliosis if exposed again.

LESSONS FOR THE FUTURE

Perhaps the most important lesson is that all the manifestations of Lyme disease may not yet be apparent. For the cardiologist, it is important to keep Lyme carditis in the differential diagnosis when dealing with a patient exposed in an endemic area who presents with a constellation of signs and symptoms as described. Antibiotic therapy may be able to halt progression of left ventricular dysfunction when it occurs and, if early enough, allow some recovery of function. How often this will be possible is unknown because the number of documented cases is few.

REFERENCES

1. Bedell SE, Pator BM, Cohen SI: Symptomatic high grade heart block in Lyme disease, *Chest* 79:236, 1981.
2. Ciesielski CA et al: Lyme disease surveillance in the United States, 1983-1986, *Rev Infect Dis* 11 (Suppl 6):S1435, 1989.
3. Cox J, Kraden M: Cardiovascular manifestations of Lyme disease, *Am Heart J* 122:1449, 1991.
4. Cray NR et al: Fatal Lyme carditis and endodermal heterotopia of the atrioventricular node, *Postgrad Med J* 66:134, 1990.
5. Dattwyler RJ et al: Ceftriaxone, an effective agent for refractory Lyme disease, *J Infect Dis* 155:1322, 1987.
6. deKoning J et al: Demonstration of spirochetes in cardiac biopsies of patients with Lyme disease, *J Infect Dis* 160:150, 1989.
7. Kapusta P et al: Troubles conductifs sina-auriculaires et auriculo-ventriculaires de la maladie de Lyme, *Arch Mal Coeur* 70:1361, 1986.
8. Kimball SA, Janson PA, LaRaia PJ: Complete heart block as the sole presentation of Lyme disease, *Arch Intern Med* 149:1897, 1989.
9. L'orincz I et al: Temporary pacing in complete heart block due to Lyme disease: a case report, *PACE* 12:1433, 1989.
10. Malawista SE, Steere AC: Lyme disease: infectious in origin, rheumatic in expression, *Adv Intern Med* 31:147, 1986.
11. Marcus LC et al: Fatal pancarditis in a patient with coexistent Lyme disease and babesiosis, *Ann Intern Med* 103:374, 1985.

12. McAlister HF et al: Lyme carditis: an important cause of reversible heart block, *Ann Intern Med* 110:339, 1989.
13. Nadelman RB, Wormser GP: A clinical approach to Lyme disease, *Mt Sinai J Med* 57:144, 1990.
14. Olson LJ, Okafor EC, Clements IP: Cardiac involvement in Lyme disease: manifestations and management, *Mayo Clin Proc* 61:745, 1986.
15. Petersen LR et al: Epidemiological and clinical features of 1,149 persons with Lyme disease identified by laboratory-based surveillance in Connecticut, *Yale J Biol Med* 62:253, 1989.
16. Ponsonnaille J et al: Myocarditie aigue cours d'un syndrome de Lyme, *Arch Mal Coeur* 79:1946, 1986.
17. Reznick VW et al: Lyme carditis: electrophysiologic and histopathologic study, *Am J Med* 81:923, 1986.
18. Rubin DA et al: Acute reversible conduction system disease due to Lyme disease, *PACE* 13:1367, 1990.
19. Stanck G et al: Isolation of *Borrelia burgdorferi* from the myocardium of a patient with longstanding cardiomyopathy, *N Engl J Med* 25:249, 1990.
20. Stanek G et al: *Borrelia burgdorferi* as an etiologic agent in chronic heart failure? *Scand J Infect Dis* S77:85, 1991.
21. Steere A: Lyme disease, *N Engl J Med* 321:585, 1989.
22. Steere AC et al: Erythema chronicum migrans and Lyme arthritis: the enlarging clinical spectrum, *Ann Intern Med* 86:685, 1977.
23. Steere AC et al: Lyme carditis: cardiac abnormalities of Lyme disease, *Ann Intern med* 93:8, 1980.
24. van der Linde MR: Lyme carditis: clinical characteristics of 105 cases, *Scand J Infect Dis* S77:81, 1991.
25. van der Linde MR, Crijins HJ, Lie KI: Transient complete AV block in Lyme disease. Electrophysiologic observations, *Chest* 96:219, 1989.
26. van der Linde MR et al: Range of atrioventricular conduction disturbances in Lyme borreliosis: a report of four cases and review of other published reports, *Br Heart J* 63:162, 1990.
27. Veyssier P et al: Atteintes cardiaques au cours de la maladie de Lyme. Deux observations, *Rev Med Interne* 8:357, 1987.
28. Vlay SC: Complete heart block due to Lyme disease, *N Engl J Med* 315:1418, 1986.
29. Vlay SC: Cardiac manifestations of Lyme disease, *Practical Cardiol* 16:63, 1990.
30. Vlay SC et al: Ventricular tachycardia associated with Lyme carditis, *Am Heart J* 121:1558, 1991.
31. Wynne J, Braunwald E: *The cardiomyopathies and myocarditidies*. In Braunwald E, editor: *Heart disease: a textbook of cardiovascular medicine,* ed 3, Philadelphia, 1988, WB Saunders.

12 Ophthalmic Manifestations

John R. Wittpenn and Patrick A. Sibony

The ophthalmic manifestations of Lyme disease have received widespread interest over the past several years paralleling the increasing frequency and spread of the disease.[1,52] A variety of ophthalmic conditions have been described in patients in each stage of Lyme disease. Despite these multiple descriptions, however, the extent and character of the eye findings in Lyme disease have yet to be clearly defined because of uncertainties in establishing a causal relationship between the ocular condition and the infection by the *Borrelia burgdorferi* spirochete. In some of the reported cases, the occurrence of ocular findings may be coincidental and unrelated to the presence of Lyme disease. In other cases, strict etiologic criteria have not been applied in making a diagnosis of Lyme disease, further complicating attempts to determine any causal relationship between Lyme disease and the ocular condition. These cases often rely only on positive Lyme serology to establish the diagnosis without acknowledging the well-known limitations of serologic testing.[1,5,13] For example, many of the reported cases have been observed in endemic areas with significant rates of positive serology (5% to 15% or more) among otherwise asymptomatic individuals.[15,16,25,59] The high background rate of seropositivity limits the usefulness of a positive Lyme titer when evaluating the etiology of an ophthalmic condition that is characteristically common and idiopathic. Seropositivity does not differentiate between past exposure or active ongoing infection. Moreover, the differences in sensitivity and specificity of various serologic assays, interlaboratory variability, and the absence of antibody formation early in the disease add to the difficulties in interpreting the significance of positive Lyme serologies.[35,37,38,54,56]

Despite these limitations, there is strong evidence for ocular involvement in Lyme disease. The evidence is primarily found in case reports underscoring the fact that ocular manifestations of Lyme disease are uncommon. Nonetheless, because uveitis, papilledema, optic neuropathy, or ocular motor palsy may be the earliest presenting sign of disease, both ophthalmologist and non-ophthalmologist should be aware of the various ocular findings in Lyme disease.

OCULAR SURFACE

Steere et al[57] were the first to note that Lyme disease affects the ocular surface in a study of 314 patients with erythema migrans (EM). They noted that 11% developed conjunctivitis within several days of the onset of the skin lesion, 6% complained of photophobia, and 3% had periorbital edema. There was no further elaboration of the ocular findings. The implication of the study as well as the anecdotal experience of clinicians frequently involved in the treatment of primary-stage Lyme disease is that these external ocular manifestations are mild and short-lived and do not require treatment.

Flach and Lavoie[20] described a 35-year-old woman with a history of acrodermatitis chronica atrophicans (ACA) who presented with a bilateral chronic follicular conjunctivitis, followed by a keratitis, who later developed episcleritis, which they attribute to late-stage Lyme disease. Immunofluorescent antibodies (IFA) to *B. burgdorferi* were slightly elevated at 1:128. She ultimately responded to topical steroids and systemic antibiotics. Similarly, Zaidman[69] described a 42-year-old man with a history of migratory arthritis, lethargy, and a suggestive rash who, two years later, developed similar systemic symptoms with a stromal keratitis. Serum IgM for Lyme disease was recorded at 1:128, and the patient improved on topical prednisone and IV ceftriaxone. Six months later, the patient developed an episcleritis and symblepharon attributed to his Lyme disease. There have been no other reports of chronic follicular conjunctivitis or episcleritis associated with Lyme disease. Therefore, the etiology in these cases should be viewed with circumspection.

Exposure keratoconjunctivitis or corneal ulceration may develop as a complication of facial paralysis, a well-established manifestation of Lyme disease.[14,43,47] Because the duration of the cranial neuropathy is short and the weakness often begins

"

improving within a few weeks,[43] exposure problems can be treated conservatively with ocular lubricants or temporary tarsorrhaphy.

LYME KERATITIS

There have been several reported cases of a keratitis occurring as a late manifestation of Lyme disease.* Patients present months to years after the onset of the disease with a painless, progressive blurring of vision and photophobia. The keratitis is characterized by focal infiltrates in a nebular pattern with indistinct borders. The infiltrates are located in the subepithelial layer and throughout the corneal stroma. Occasionally, the keratitis is associated with corneal edema or fine white keratic precipitates.

Cases treated with topical steroids responded with clearing of the lesions. There were some recurrences when steroids were discontinued, but they resolved with reinstitution of the steroid and a slow tapering of the dose. In two cases, the patients were not treated with topical steroids.[32] In the first case, the keratitis developed 5 years after the diagnosis of Lyme disease. The lesions waxed and waned over 12 months and did not respond to systemic antibiotics. The vision was not affected. In the second case, the patient had definite Lyme disease 6 months before the onset of the keratitis. She did not receive any topical steroids nor was there any mention of treatment with systemic antibiotics. Over the next 3 months, the lesions became more faint and diffuse with a return of normal vision. Eighteen months later, however, the patient developed a quadrant of stromal edema and mild neovascularization, which responded to topical steroids. The vision, however, was reduced secondary to scarring.

Another report of Lyme keratitis developed in conjunction with Lyme meningitis.[34] In this case, the opacities were described as being subepithelial corneal infiltrates without overlying epithelial defects or vascularization. The authors state that both the meningitis and keratitis resolved completely after treatment with intravenous (IV) ceftriaxone. The response of the keratitis to IV antibiotics alone differs from the other reported cases, which did not respond to systemic antibiotic treatment without the additional use of topical steroids.

Fox and colleagues[21] described a patient from the British West Indies with a history of recurrent Bell's palsy, "classic" interstitial keratitis, and hearing loss (Cogan's syndrome). The patient had a borderline positive enzyme-linked immunosorbent assay (ELISA) and a negative IFA for Lyme disease. The patient was treated with IV steroids

and ceftriaxone, which transiently improved her hearing. The diagnosis of Lyme disease in this case is questionable.

These limited case reports strongly suggest that keratitis is an ocular manifestation of late-stage Lyme disease. The judicious use of topical steroids is indicated in the treatment of Lyme keratitis, especially those cases in which the lesions involve the visual axis. The pathogenesis of Lyme keratitis is not known. Most authors,[6,32,41] however, postulate either reactivation of a previous infection, recurrence of an infection secondary to inadequate treatment, or a hypersensitivity response to *B. burgdorferi* antigen. The prompt resolution of the keratitis to topical steroids and the lack of response to systemic antibiotics, in most cases, would seem to support an immunologically mediated mechanism.

INTRAOCULAR INFLAMMATION

Patients with Lyme disease can develop a variety of intraocular inflammations including iridocyclitis, vitritis, choroiditis, or panuveitis. It has been suggested that the inflammation may be secondary to an immune reaction or direct infection of the intraocular tissues by the spirochete. Experimental studies have demonstrated hematogenous spread of the spirochete into the vitreous after intraperitoneal inoculations of live spirochete into Syrian hamsters.[17,30]

There has been only one reported case in which a spirochete, presumably *B. burgdorferi*, was recovered from a human eye.[31,58] In this case, the uveitis was unusually severe and developed in the early stage of Lyme disease rather than the more common and milder presentations seen in the later stage. The case involved a 45-year-old woman from an endemic area who developed constitutional symptoms and erythema migrans (EM), which responded to IV cefazolin and oral tetracycline. Two weeks later, after a bee sting, she developed an acute iritis with posterior synechiae. The inflammation progressed to a panuveitis with hypopyon despite the use of topical, subconjunctival, and systemic prednisone. Further treatment with IV antibiotics had no effect. The patient ultimately required two vitrectomies with administration of intravitreal antibiotics. The eye eventually became phthisical. In addition to the clinical evidence of Lyme disease, serum analysis showed an IgM titer of 1:64 and IgG of 1:512 during the acute stages and later testing showed a fall in the IgG to 1:64 and an undetectable IgM titer. Examination of the vitrectomy specimen showed marked necrosis, many neutrophils and lymphocytes. Dieterle stains revealed an occasional "spirochete" that was "morphologically compatible" with *B. burgdorferi*.

---

*References 6, 8, 9, 20, 32, 34, 41, 69.

The remaining cases of uveitis described in the literature all occur in the late stages of the disease. Winward and colleagues[66] described a series of five patients who presented with vitritis and iridocyclitis. The posterior inflammatory reaction resembled a pars planitis with peripheral "snowbanking" in one case. All patients exhibited vitreous infiltrates. Unlike typical pars planitis, however, the patients also showed significant anterior inflammation with keratic precipitates, posterior synechia, and iris nodules. Two of the five patients had a history of recurrent facial palsies 2 to 9 years before the onset of uveitis. None of the five patients had EM, although one had a history of rash 9 years earlier described as granuloma annulare. Mild cerebrospinal fluid (CSF) pleocytosis was noted in two of the three patients who underwent lumbar puncture. Four of the five patients had mild elevations of either the IFA or ELISA for Lyme borreliosis; the seronegative patient had a positive Western blot for Lyme disease. Four of five patients were initially treated with topical steroids with little or no response. All patients treated with antibiotics were also on topical steroids. Of the four treated with oral antibiotics, only one patient recovered completely. The remaining three, however, improved with IV antibiotics, although recovery in some instances was transient and required repeated courses of antibiotics.

Occasionally, uveitis may be associated with optic disc edema as shown in the case reported by Boutros.[12] The disc edema in this case was presumably secondary to a vitritis because there were no signs of optic neuropathy or intracranial hypertension. This patient also failed to respond to topical steroids and oral antibiotics, but improved after IV ceftriaxone.

There have been several cases of Lyme borreliosis affecting the posterior pole. For example, in a case described by Bialasiewicz,[10] a 32-year-old woman with constitutional symptoms presented with iridocyclitis, mild vitritis, cystoid macular edema, and exudative retinal detachments. These findings in association with lymphocytic pleocytosis initially led to the diagnosis of Vogt-Koyanagi-Harada syndrome. Lyme serologies, however, were quite elevated (IgG 1:640, IgM 1:40), and the patient improved with oral doxycycline. Similarly, Wong[67] described a 70-year-old man exposed to multiple tick bites who subsequently developed a rash with fever, headaches, myalgias, and arthralgias. Lumbar puncture showed CSF pleocytosis, and Lyme serologies were positive. After completing a 1-month course of oral tetracycline and prednisone, he developed a mild vitritis with exudative retinal detachments and shallow choroidals. He slowly improved with repeated courses of topical steroids, tetracycline, and periocular steroids. Finally, Tonjes[62] described a young patient with acute multifocal placoid pigment epitheliopathy (AMPPE), CSF pleocytosis, and positive Lyme serologies that improved on IV antibiotics.

Anterior uveitis may, in some cases, be associated with Lyme keratitis.[20,41,69] This anterior uveitis produces fine, white keratic precipitates on the corneal endothelium and generally is not associated with synechial formation. In at least one case, the author states that cells could not be seen floating through the anterior chamber although there were endothelial deposits present.[41]

Although anecdotal evidence suggests that the uveitis responds to systemic antibiotic treatment,[10,12,33,62,65-67] many of these patients were treated simultaneously with topical or systemic prednisone. Moreover, uveitis may worsen with initiation of antibiotic treatment. For example, one patient with uveitis, a CSF pleocytosis, and positive Lyme serologies was placed on IV antibiotics.[42] Two days after the onset of treatment, he developed an anterior uveitis, which subsequently resolved. Kuiper and colleagues[33] described a 39-year-old woman with a history of tick bites, EM, bilateral sixth nerve palsies, and CSF pleocytosis. The clinical picture resolved without treatment, but 1 month later she developed bilateral vitreous clouding. She underwent a vitrectomy in the right eye with improvement, but the clouding persisted in the left eye. One year later, she developed migratory arthralgias and a clinical diagnosis of Lyme disease was made despite a negative serology. She was treated with IV ceftriaxone, which initially produced an increase in clouding of the vitreous on the left, but subsequent clearing with restoration of vision to 20/20 and no further recurrences of any systemic symptoms. This apparent worsening with treatment has led some authors to suggest a mechanism similar to the Herxheimer reaction seen in the treatment of syphilis.[33,36] At least one author recommends the concurrent administration of corticosteroids with the antibiotic treatment for patients with ocular or central nervous system borreliosis.[36]

OPTIC NEUROPATHY

The most common and unequivocal manifestation of Lyme disease involving the optic nerve is papilledema, defined as optic disc swelling secondary to intracranial hypertension from Lyme meningitis.[28,34,45,48] In our experience, it is most commonly observed in children with early disseminated disease who present with headache, vomiting, or listlessness, and who occasionally complain of a horizontal binocular diplopia. On examination, they are found to have normal visual acuity, enlargement of the blindspot, optic disc swelling, and, in some cases, display signs of a sixth nerve palsy. Lumbar puncture reveals an elevated opening pressure and CSF pleocytosis. These patients generally have very positive Lyme titers (in our cases, the ELISA IgG ranged from 0.40 to 0.65 with negative controls of 0.095 to 0.115). They uniformly do well with complete resolution of the papilledema and meningitis after treatment with IV ceftriaxone.

Similar cases, all seen in children, have been reported in the literature.[28,45] The term *pseudotumor cerebri* has mistakenly been used to describe these cases. However, because these patients almost always had CSF pleocytosis, it would be more correct to attribute the papilledema to meningitis. Occasionally, a spinal tap performed early in the presentation of the disease might fail to detect CSF pleocytosis or elevated protein, thereby simulating pseudotumor cerebri. As was shown in one case, however, subsequent taps show abnormal fluid.[45] Therefore, in those patients who present with optic disc swelling, intracranial hypertension, positive Lyme titers, and a normal CSF, a repeat lumbar puncture might reveal a pleocytosis, thereby confirming a diagnosis of Lyme meningitis.

Reik,[48] in a series of Lyme patients with neurologic involvement, noted five patients with transient visual obscurations (TVOs), a nonspecific symptom associated with all forms of optic disc edema and optic disc drusen. TVOs commonly occur in patients with papilledema. Only two of their five patients with TVOs were noted to have swelling of the optic disc. Three additional patients had optic disc edema without TVOs. Only one of the eight patients, however, had intracranial hypertension. Based on this report and others,[48,68] it has been surmised that patients with normal intracranial pressures and optic disc edema have optic perineuritis, an infiltrating inflammation along the optic nerve sheath that simulates papilledema.[27] Because there were few details concerning the neurovisual status of these patients (for example, acuity, visual fields, pupillary findings, disc photographs, color vision, and so forth), it is difficult to assess the significance or reasons for TVOs without disc edema or disc edema without intracranial hypertension. Furthermore, without radiographic confirmation of optic nerve sheath thickening or enhancement, we would be reluctant, on the basis of this report alone, to conclude that Lyme disease causes an optic perineuritis. It is, however, a well-established form of luetic optic neuropathy and might yet be shown to occur in Lyme disease.

An optic neuropathy can develop in the late stages of Lyme disease in association with meningoencephalitis. Lesser described two such cases.[34]

In the first case, a 59-year-old man presented with a history of endemic exposure, facial paresis, sixth nerve palsy, and Lyme titers of 1:6400! Despite multiple courses of treatment, symptoms persisted. Five years after the initial presentation, the patient developed a rapidly progressive vision loss of 20/400, an afferent pupillary defect, and bilateral pallor of the optic discs. Magnetic resonance imaging (MRI) showed multiple white matter lesions, and CSF was positive for oligoclonal bands, but myelin basic protein was normal. In the second case, a 39-year-old woman presented with a history of erythema migrans, facial palsy, radiculoneuritis, spastic hemiparesis, a positive T cell response to *B. burgdorferi* and a Lyme titer (IgG) of 1:400. Initial exam showed normal acuities, dyschromatopsia, a mild central scotoma in the left eye (OS), pallor of the optic disc OS, and bilateral sixth nerve palsies. MRI showed multiple areas of demyelination in the brainstem and cortex. Despite treatment with IV ceftriaxone, 5 months later, she went on to develop an acute optic neuropathy in the right eye. Syphilis serologies were presumably negative, although the results were not reported in either case.

Several series describing the clinical features of Lyme meningoencephalitis have included some patients with optic neuropathies.[3,24,43,63] Because the primary focus of these papers did not emphasize the ophthalmic features, few details are provided. Jacobson has observed a few similar cases,[27] and we have also seen one such patient. It would appear that optic neuropathy is an element of Lyme disease with central nervous system involvement, although the specific features have yet to be fully described.

Whether isolated optic neuritis, defined as a rapid decline in vision associated with pain, objective signs of optic neuropathy, and improvement, can be a manifestation of Lyme disease is less clear. Unfortunately, most cases of "Lyme optic neuritis" are difficult to distinguish from the demyelinating form of optic neuritis commonly seen in patients with or without multiple sclerosis or in children with antecedent viral syndromes. For example, in the series reported by Lesser,[34] there was one patient with retrobulbar optic neuritis and another patient with neuroretinitis (papillitis associated with stellate macular exudates). Both patients had mild elevation of their Lyme titers, and both improved with antibiotic treatment. Similarly, Wu[68] described a 7-year-old boy who developed an annular rash from an insect bite followed by a generalized maculopapular rash and fevers. Several weeks later, he was diagnosed with an aseptic meningitis and "papilledema." However, the presence of a normal intracranial pressure, diminished acuity, cecocentral scotomas, and macular exudates more accurately identifies this case as an optic neuritis or neuroretinitis. Immunofluorescent antibody to Lyme disease was 1:256, and the patient improved on IV penicillin. Except for the Lyme titer, this patient's course was entirely consistent with a postviral optic neuritis commonly seen in childhood. Winterkorn,[64] in a review, also briefly described a patient with neuroretinitis and positive Lyme titer in which the diagnosis remained unresolved.

We have examined nine patients (seven female, two male) ages 19 to 41 with the rapid onset of vision loss, painful eye movements, and objective signs of optic neuropathy. The findings were all consistent with a clinical diagnosis of optic neuritis. Most of these cases had borderline positive Lyme titers, and improvement occurred without specific treatment for Lyme disease. None of the patients had a history of EM or facial palsies and all patients resided in an endemic area for Lyme disease. Those cases of optic neuritis associated with other neurologic signs such as CSF abnormalities or MRI lesions of the white matter were all consistent with multiple sclerosis.

The most cogent case made for an isolated optic neuritis as a manifestation of Lyme disease has been put forth by Jacobson who had 20 consecutive patients with isolated optic neuritis undergo a battery of serologic tests for Lyme disease (IFA, ELISA for IgG, IgM, Western immunoblots).[29] Patients with positive titers underwent CSF analysis. Four of the 20 patients (20%) had positive Lyme serologies. In each case, the clinical presentation was typical for optic neuritis. Two of the four cases showed a rise in titer for IgM, the presence of specific antibody reactions to *Borrelia* antigens on immunoblot, unusually high cell counts in the CSF, an absence of oligoclonal bands, and an elevation in the Lyme antibody index, leading the author to conclude that these two cases were probably related to Lyme disease. The author cautions, however, that all of the patients came from a hyperendemic region with a reported asymptomatic seropositivity rate as high as 15% to 20%,[15,16] identical to the rate observed among his patients with optic neuritis. It is possible that seropositivity in these patients may be the result of prior asymptomatic seroconversion.

There are scattered reports of people with nonarteritic anterior ischemic optic neuropathy (AION), positive Lyme serologies, and nonspecific constitutional symptoms attributed to Lyme disease.[23,51] An ischemic presentation would be consistent with histopathologic changes reported in Lyme disease. Duray and Steere reported vascular damage including hypercellular vascular occlusion after infection with the *B. burgdorferi* spirochete.[18]

Nevertheless, the case for Lyme disease causing a nonarteritic AION remains unconvincing. For example, one report described a 65-year-old man with myalgias and a "strongly positive" Lyme titer who developed a sudden and persistent vision loss with disc edema.[23] Unfortunately, the details concerning the eye exam and Lyme serologies, as well as the absence of other features specific to Lyme disease, make it difficult to evaluate the cause of vision loss in this case. In another case, a 53-year-old patient with steroid-responsive myalgias, cutaneous hypersensitivity, fevers, paresthesias, and an elevated erythrocyte sedimentation rate (ESR) developed a possible AION associated with a mildly elevated Lyme titer (1:256).[51] Because vasculitis could not be entirely excluded, the etiology of the optic neuropathy remains unclear. Finally, another report describes a 71-year-old man with classic AION caused by biopsy-proven giant cell arteritis.[44] The authors claim to have observed a spirochete within a giant cell. Lyme titer in this patient was not considered significant at 1:64. Histopathologic diagnosis of *B. burgdorferi* can be difficult, if not misleading.

Jacobson[27] reported seeing several patients with typical non-arteritic AION and positive Lyme titers but no other clinical features suggestive of Lyme disease within an endemic area. The CSF in these patients was normal. No treatment was given for Lyme disease. Subsequent follow-up showed no systemic sequelae of Lyme disease in these patients. Our own experience with two similar cases confirms Jacobson's observations.

OCULAR MOTOR PALSY

Neurologic complications occur in at least 10% of patients with disseminated and late infection Lyme disease, and half of these cases have cranial neuropathies.[47] The development of cranial neuropathies is commonly associated with CSF pleocytosis (93%).[46] As has already been noted, facial paralysis is the single most common cranial neuropathy in Lyme disease.[43,47] Approximately 13% of the cranial neuropathies involve the ocular motor nerves (III, IV, and VI).[46] According to Reik, the sixth nerve (unilateral or bilateral) is most commonly involved (9% of cranial neuropathies)* followed by the third nerve (3%)[2,3,50,53,61] and fourth cranial nerve (1%).[66]

In most instances, sixth nerve palsies represent a false localizing sign because many of these patients will have intracranial hypertension, meningitis, and papilledema.[27,34,45] Abducens palsies can also develop as a consequence of meningitis alone without intracranial hypertension.[24,34,50] In either

---

*References 2, 11, 40, 43, 50, 53, 60, 61.

case, sixth nerve palsies are frequently associated with other cranial neuropathies, especially the seventh nerve.[2,34,43,50] Although most cases presumably affect the peripheral fibers of the sixth nerve, the occurrence of sixth nerve palsies in patients with Lyme encephalitis probably includes some patients with pontine lesions affecting the fascicular portion of the nerve. Such cases may be difficult to distinguish from multiple sclerosis.

Lyme disease presenting as an isolated sixth nerve palsy is most unusual.[27] We, however, saw an 86-year-old woman with a history of cataract surgery and hyperparathyroidism who presented with a painless, binocular horizontal diplopia. She denied headaches, neurologic, or dermatologic complaints. The examination revealed only a left sixth nerve palsy and bilateral intraocular lenses. Computed tomography (CT) scan and blood work including ESR, thyroid studies, Tensilon test, and RPR were normal. An ELISA IgG for Lyme disease was extraordinarily elevated with an optical density of 0.891 (negative control 0.099). CSF showed 18 monocytes with a CSF:serum antibody index of 1.34. The sixth nerve palsy resolved shortly after completion of IV ceftriaxone. Two months later the serum ELISA was 1.009 (cutoff 0.125), and 6 months later serum ELISA decreased to 0.290 (0.089). We are not aware of isolated third or fourth nerve palsies presenting in a similar fashion.

MISCELLANEOUS

There has been one report of an orbital myositis attributed to a presumed case of Lyme disease.[55] The case involved a 5-year-old girl who developed a suggestive rash followed by Bell's palsy with CSF pleocytosis. The rash and pleocytosis resolved without treatment. Four months later, she developed arthritis involving the knee, and shortly thereafter developed a painful ophthalmoplegia. CT scan of the orbit showed evidence of orbital myositis, which responded to steroid therapy. Serologies were not reported nor was she apparently treated with antibiotics for Lyme disease. Thus, the etiology of the orbital myositis in this case remains uncertain, although Lyme disease has been documented to cause myositis elsewhere.[4]

There have been a few isolated reports of pupillary abnormalities associated with Lyme disease.[22,34,47] Glauser[22] described a 30-year-old man with a positive history for a tick bite and EM. He subsequently developed headache, fever, myalgia, malaise, and a stiff neck. His constitutional symptoms improved on oral tetracycline, but, shortly thereafter, he developed a preganglionic Horner's syndrome on the left side, which resolved after 10 days of IV ceftriaxone. Reik[47] described eight patients with neurologic complications of Lyme disease. One of the complications mentioned is an Argyll Robertson pupil, but no further details were provided. Finally, Lesser[34] refers to a patient with Lyme meningitis and associated Lyme keratitis who after treatment developed one pupil that reacted in a "tonic fashion."

CONCLUSION

Despite the remaining uncertainties regarding the clinical manifestations of ocular Lyme disease, it is clear that there is a considerable overlap with the ophthalmic manifestations of syphilis. This seems especially true in cases of patients with optic neuropathies, keratitis, uveitis, and ocular motor nerve palsies. Because all spirochetes share common antigens, serologic tests may cross react. Depending on the method, Lyme titers may be positive in approximately 20% to 60% of patients with syphilis[39,49]; and 20% of patients with Lyme disease may have a weakly positive FTA-Abs (usually <1:10).[26] Among patients with Lyme disease, the RPR and MHA-TP are usually negative.[26] However, a positive Lyme titer with a negative VDRL does not completely rule out syphilis because nearly 30% of patients with primary, latent, or late syphilis will also have a negative VDRL and positive FTA.

Some of the published cases purporting to describe the ophthalmic manifestations of Lyme disease have omitted serologic testing for syphilis (or at least failed to mention the results),[34] and where these studies were performed the results suggest that syphilis is at least a plausible alternative, if not the actual cause.[19,65,70] One must be especially cautious when diagnosing Lyme disease in patients from nonendemic regions. For example, one report describes a 39-year-old Oklahoman woman who presented with a skin lesion on her breast, diffuse pains, myelopathy, bilateral sixth nerve palsies, and lymphocytic pleocytosis.[19] This patient developed what clinically resembled an optic neuritis with mildly elevated Lyme titer (1:128) and a negative VDRL, but the FTA and MHA-TP were positive. Similar concerns can be raised in other cases with bilateral optic atrophy,[65] ischemic optic neuropathy,[65] and uveitis.[70] Demonstration of specific antibodies to Lyme specific surface antigens (31kD, 34kD) by Western blot may be the only practical means by which to distinguish the two diseases when serologies are both positive.[7] However, although these antigen studies are highly specific, sensitivity is low, and, therefore, the test is not always helpful.

Distinguishing some of the ophthalmic manifestations of Lyme disease from multiple sclerosis can be even more difficult. If isolated optic neuritis occurs in Lyme disease, it appears to be clinically indistinguishable from the ordinary form of demyelinating optic neuritis except for the elevated Lyme titer. The absence of any other findings suggestive of Lyme disease, such as EM or facial palsies, in these cases is noteworthy. Moreover, the presence of other neurologic findings, such as CSF pleocytosis or white matter lesions on MRI, may not permit a clear distinction between Lyme disease and multiple sclerosis. Finally, optic neuritis frequently resolves spontaneously. Thus, response to antibiotics is by no means a reliable criterion for establishing the diagnosis of Lyme optic neuritis. Although the demonstration of intrathecal production of Lyme disease antibodies may help, the possibility that such associations are merely coincidental must be considered, and, in some cases, treatment will be initiated even when the diagnosis remains uncertain.

Finally, other diseases may mimic the ocular manifestations of Lyme disease, including viral and postviral syndromes, sarcoidosis, Behçets, Vogt-Koyanagi-Harada, lymphoma, vasculitis, Guillain-Barré, herpes zoster, and others. Consider, for example, a patient we saw with a 5-year history of progressive optic atrophy in one eye and positive Lyme titer. A CT scan performed 5 years earlier was said to be normal, but repeat MRI scan revealed an ipsilateral sphenoid wing meningioma compressing the optic nerve. Thus, until we have a better understanding of the full ophthalmic spectrum of Lyme disease, patients presenting with ocular conditions possibly related to Lyme disease need to be carefully and fully evaluated to rule out all other possible etiologies.

REFERENCES

1. Aaberg TM: The expanding ophthalmologic spectrum of Lyme disease, *Am J Ophthalmol* 107:77, 1989.
2. Ackermann R, Horstrup P, Schmidt R: Tick borne meningopolyneuritis (Garin-Bujadoux, Bannwarth), et al: *Yale J Biol Med* 57:485, 1984.
3. Ackermann R et al: Chronic neurologic manifestations of erythema migrans borreliosis, *Ann NY Acad Sci* 539:16, 1988.
4. Atlas E et al: Lyme myositis: muscle invasion by *Borrelia burgdorferi, Ann Intern Med* 109:245, 1988.
5. Barbour AG: Laboratory aspects of Lyme borreliosis, *Clin Microbiol Rev* 1:399, 1988.
6. Baum J et al: Bilateral keratitis as a manifestation of Lyme disease, *Am J Ophthalmol* 105:75, 1988.
7. Benach JL, Coleman JL, Golightly MG: A murine IgM monoclonal antibody binds an antigenic determinant in outer surface protein A, an immunodominant basic protein of the Lyme disease spirochete, *J Immunol* 140:265, 1988.
8. Bertuch AW, Rocco E, Schwartz EG: Eye findings in Lyme disease, *Conn Med* 51:151, 1987.
9. Bertuch AW, Rocco E, Schwartz EG: Lyme disease: ocular manifestations, *Ann Ophthalmol* 20:376, 1988.
10. Bialasiewicz AA et al: Bilateral diffuse choroiditis and exudative retinal detachments with evidence of Lyme disease, *Am J Ophthalmol* 105:419, 1988.
11. Blaumhackl U et al: Neurological manifestations of *Borrelia burgdorferi* infections: the enlarging clinical spectrum, *Zentralbl Bakteriol Mikrobiol Hyg [A]* 263:334, 1986.
12. Boutros A, Rahn E, Nauheim R: Iritis and papillitis as a primary presentation of Lyme disease, *Ann Ophthalmol* 22:24, 1990.
13. Centers for Disease Control: Lyme disease—Connecticut, *MMWR* 37:1, 1988.
14. Clark JR et al: Facial paralysis in Lyme disease, *Laryngoscope* 95:1341, 1985.
15. Dlesk A et al: Prevalence of Lyme seropositivity by indirect immunofluorescent antibody assay in normal adult individuals from an endemic area, *Arthritis Rheum* 31(Suppl):98, 1988 (abstract).
16. Dlesk A et al: Lyme serologies by indirect fluorescent antibody assay and enzyme-linked immunosorbent assay in normal residents from an endemic area, *Arthritis Rheum* 31(Suppl):98, 1988 (abstract).
17. Duray PH, Johnson RC: The histopathology of experimentally infected hamsters with the Lyme disease spirochete, *Borrelia burgdorferi, Proc Soc Exp Biol Med* 181:263, 1986.
18. Duray PH, Steere AC: Clinical pathologic correlations of Lyme disease by stage, *Ann NY Acad Sci* 539:65, 1988.
19. Farris BK, Webb RM: Lyme disease and optic neuritis, *J Clin Neuro Ophthalmol* 8:73, 1988.
20. Flach AJ, Lavoie PE: Episcleritis, conjunctivitis, and keratitis as ocular manifestations of Lyme disease, *Ophthalmology* 97:973, 1990.
21. Fox GM, Heilskov T, Smith JL: Cogan's syndrome and seroreactivity to Lyme borreliosis, *J Clin Neuro Ophthalmol* 10:83, 1990.
22. Glauser TA, Brennan PJ, Galetta SL: Reversible Horner's syndrome and Lyme disease, *J Clin Neuro Ophthalmol* 9:225, 1989.
23. Gustafson R, Svenungsson B, Unosson-Hallnas K: Optic neuropathy in *Borrelia* infection, *J Infect* 17:187, 1988.
24. Halperin JJ, Volkmann DJ, Wu P: Central nervous system abnormalities in Lyme neuroborreliosis, *Neurology* 41:1571, 1991.
25. Hanrahan JP et al: Incidence and cumulative frequency of endemic Lyme disease in a community, *J Infect Dis* 150:489, 1984.
26. Hunter EF et al: Evaluation of sera from patients with Lyme disease in FTA-Ab test for syphilis, Sex Transm Dis 13:232, 1986.
27. Jacobson DM: Neuro-ophthalmic aspects of Lyme disease, *Ophthalmol Clin North Am* 4:463, 1991.
28. Jacobson DM, Frens DB: Pseudotumor cerebri syndrome associated with Lyme disease, *Am J Ophthalmol* 107:81, 1989.
29. Jacobson DM, Marx JJ, Dlesk A: Frequency and clinical significance of Lyme seropositivity in patients with isolated optic neuritis, *Neurology* 41:706, 1991.
30. Johnson RC, Marek N, Kodner C: Infection of Syrian hamsters with Lyme disease spirochetes, *J Clin Microbiol* 20:1099, 1984.
31. Kauffmann DJH, Wormser GP: Ocular Lyme disease: case report and review of the literature, *Br J Ophthalmol* 74:325, 1990.
32. Kornmehl EW et al: Bilateral keratitis in Lyme disease, *Ophthalmology* 96:1194, 1989.
33. Kuiper H, Koelman JH, Jager MJ: Vitreous clouding associated with Lyme borreliosis, *Am J Ophthalmol* 108:453, 1989.
34. Lesser RL et al: Neuro-ophthalmic manifestations of Lyme disease, *Ophthalmology* 97:699, 1990.
35. Luger SW, Krauss E. Serologic tests for Lyme disease, *Arch Intern Med* 150:761, 1990.

36. MacDonald AB: Lyme disease: a neuro-ophthalmologic view, *J Clin Neuro Ophthalmol* 7:185, 1987.
37. MacDonald AB: Ambiguous serologies in active Lyme borreliosis, *J Clin Neuro Ophthalmol* 8:79, 1988.
38. Magnarelli LA: Quality of Lyme disease tests, *JAMA* 262:3464, 1989.
39. Magnarelli LA, Anderson JF, Johnson RC: Cross-reactivity in serologic tests for Lyme disease and other spirochetal infections, *J Infect Dis* 156:183, 1987.
40. Millner M et al: Lyme borreliosis in children: a controlled clinical study based on ELISA values, *Eur J Pediatr* 148:527, 1989.
41. Orlin SE, Lauffer JL: Lyme disease keratitis, *Am J Ophthalmol* 107:678, 1989.
42. Oteo JA et al: Lyme disease and uveitis, *Ann Intern Med* 112:883, 1990.
43. Pachner AR, Steere AC: The triad of neurologic manifestations of Lyme disease: meningitis, cranial neuritis, and radiculoneuritis, *Neurology* 35:47, 1985.
44. Pizzarello LD et al: Temporal arteritis associated with *Borrelia* infection, *J Clin Neuro Ophthalmol* 9:3, 1989.
45. Raucher HS et al: Pseudotumor cerebri and Lyme disease: a new association, *J Pediatr* 107:931, 1985.
46. Reik LR: *Lyme disease and the nervous system*, pp 57, 59, New York, 1991, Thieme Medical Publishers.
47. Reik L, Burgdorfer W, Donaldson JO: Neurologic abnormalities in Lyme disease without erythema chronicum migrans, *Am J Med* 81:73, 1986.
48. Reik L et al: Neurologic abnormalities of Lyme disease, *Medicine* 58:281, 1979.
49. Russell H et al: Enzyme-linked immunosorbent assay and indirect immunofluorescence assay for Lyme disease, *J Infect Dis* 149:465, 1984.
50. Ryberg B: Bannwarths syndrome (lymphocytic meningoradiculitis) in Sweden, *Yale J Biol Med* 57:499, 1984.
51. Schechter SL: Lyme disease associated with optic neuropathy, *Am J Med* 81:143, 1986.
52. Schmid GP: The global distribution of Lyme disease, *Rev Infect Dis* 7:41, 1985.
53. Schmutzhard E, Pohl P, Stanek G: Involvement of *Borrelia burgdorferi* in cranial nerve affection, Zentralbl Bakteriol Mikrobiol Hyg [A] 263:338, 1986.
54. Schwartz BS et al: Antibody testing in Lyme disease: a comparison of results in four laboratories, *JAMA* 262:3431, 1989.
55. Seidenberg KB, Leib ML: Orbital myositis with Lyme disease, *Am J Ophthalmol* 109:13, 1990.
56. Smith JL et al: The prevalence of Lyme disease in a nonendemic area, *J Clin Neuro Ophthalmol* 9:148, 1989.
57. Steere AC et al: The early clinical manifestations of Lyme disease, *Ann Intern Med* 99:76, 1983.
58. Steere AC et al: Unilateral blindness caused by infection with the Lyme disease spirochete, *Borrelia burgdorferi, Ann Intern Med* 103:382, 1985.
59. Steere AC et al: Longitudinal assessment of the clinical and epidemiologic features of Lyme disease in a defined population, *J Infect Dis* 154:295, 1986.
60. Stiernstedt G et al: Clinical manifestations of *Borrelia* infections of the nervous system, *Zentralbl Bakteriol Mikrobiol Hyg [A]* 263:289, 1986.
61. Stiernstedt G et al: Clinical manifestations and diagnosis of neuroborreliosis, *Ann NY Acad Sci* 539:46, 1988.
62. Tonjes W et al: Akute multifokale plakoide pigment epitheliopathie mit entzundlichem liquor befund. Sonderform einer Borreliose? *Dtsch Med Wochenschr* 114:793, 1989.
63. Weder B, Wiedesheim P, Matter L: Chronic progressive neurological involvement in *Borrelia burgdorferi* infection, *J Neurol* 234:40, 1987.
64. Winterkorn JMS: Lyme disease: neurologic and ophthalmic manifestations, *Surv Ophthalmol* 35:191, 1990.
65. Winward KE, Smith JL: Ocular disease in Caribbean patients with serologic evidence of Lyme borreliosis, *J Clin Neuro Ophthalmol* 9:65, 1989.
66. Winward KE et al: Ocular Lyme borreliosis, *Am J Ophthalmol* 108:651, 1989.
67. Wong T: The onset of bilateral uveitis in an elderly man with fever, headache, and rash, *Ophthalmic Surg* 20:154, 1989.
68. Wu G et al: Optic disc edema and Lyme disease, *Ann Ophthalmol* 18:252, 1986.
69. Zaidman GW: Episcleritis and symblepharon associated with Lyme keratitis, *Am J Ophthalmol* 109:487, 1990.
70. Zierhut M, Kreissig I, Pickert A: Panuveitis with positive serological tests for syphilis and Lyme disease, *J Clin Neuro Ophthalmol* 9:71, 1989.

13 Neurologic Aspects of North American Lyme Disease

Louis Reik, Jr.

Nervous system abnormalities in what we now call Lyme disease were reported first in Europe where painful radiculoneuritis and meningoencephalitis accompanying erythema migrans (EM) and following a tick bite were described 70 years ago.[26] Other European reports of neurologic disease associated with EM followed, and tickborne meningopolyneuritis or Bannwarth's syndrome was well-known there by the early 1970s.[41] But the delineation of similar nervous system abnormalities in North American patients bitten by ticks awaited the description of Lyme disease by Steere and colleagues later in the decade.[60,70,78]

The accelerating pace of research that followed these reports expanded our view of the spectrum of nervous system disease caused by *Borrelia burgdorferi*, and we recognize now that Lyme disease is the cause of a wide range of treatable neurologic abnormalities. We also know that although the character of these abnormalities is similar in patients infected with *B. burgdorferi* on both continents, differences do exist. The focus in this chapter is on clinical characteristics of nervous system involvement in North American Lyme disease.

Both the peripheral (PNS) and central nervous systems (CNS) can be involved in Lyme disease, either singly or in combination, and neurologic illness can begin either early or late during disseminated infection. Generally speaking, the patterns of nervous system involvement in early and late disease differ, and dividing these neurologic abnormalities into early and late occurring syndromes provides a useful framework for understanding their clinical features, even though there can be considerable overlap.

NEUROLOGIC FEATURES OF EARLY LYME DISEASE*

Nervous system involvement complicates early Lyme disease in about 20% of North American

---

*Unless stated otherwise, the data in this section are derived from References 7, 8, 11, 12, 14, 16, 19, 20, 22, 23, 27, 28, 39, 42, 43, 52, 60, 61, 65, 69-71, 74, 77, 82, and 88, which encompass 206 North American cases of Lyme disease with early neurologic involvement.

patients, both children and adults, with the symptoms often beginning soon after illness onset and sometimes while EM is still present. Headache, neck stiffness, lethargy, and even mild encephalopathy are common in patients with EM, especially those who have multiple secondary skin lesions. Among European patients with localized EM, as many as 25% may have pleocytosis.[50] In North America, the cerebrospinal fluid (CSF) of such patients usually is said to be normal, however, and it is not known whether these early neurologic symptoms are a direct result of nervous system infection.

More typically, neurologic signs and symptoms develop later in early disseminated disease, weeks to months after illness onset, usually after EM has resolved. The most common abnormalities are lymphocytic meningitis accompanied by cranial and peripheral radiculoneuropathies and, less commonly, parenchymal CNS involvement (meningopolyneuritis or Bannwarth's syndrome).

Neurologic symptoms of early disease usually debut in summer, particularly in July or August, but can begin in any month. They begin most often 2 to 4 weeks (range, 2 days to 5 months) after EM (present in up to 80% of cases). No more than 40% of patients recall an antecedent tick bite. When both are present, the tick bite usually precedes EM by 1 to 2 weeks. Additional systemic signs and symptoms characteristic of early disseminated disease are present in two thirds: fatigue, fever, myalgia, nausea, vomiting, arthralgia, and arthritis are most common.

Central nervous system abnormalities

Meningitis. Meningitis is the single most common abnormality in patients with neurologic involvement in early disseminated disease, 80% to 90% of whom have pleocytosis at the time of evaluation (Fig. 13–1). Among North American patients with Lyme disease and pleocytosis, about 85% are symptomatic.[52,61,69,70,77]

The most common symptom is headache, usually either frontal or occipital and varying in intensity from mild to disabling. Headache is present

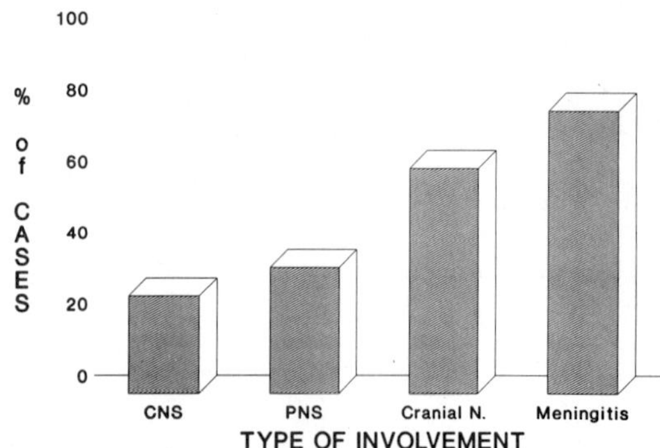

Figure 13–1 Neurologic abnormalities in 206 North American patients with Lyme disease and early neurologic involvement.

in up to 90% of patients with CSF inflammation. Mild neck stiffness accompanies the headache in about 50% of cases, as do nausea, vomiting, and low-grade fever (up to 38.5° C). Photophobia is less common (20%).[52,61,69,70,77]

Meningeal symptoms begin acutely or subacutely, usually persist for 1 to 2 months, and resolve gradually over weeks. In some cases, however, the symptoms can persist for a year or more (up to 88 weeks) fluctuating in intensity; attacks of disabling symptoms lasting several weeks alternate with similar periods of milder symptoms also lasting weeks.[60,61,69,70,77]

Although many patients with early Lyme disease and meningitis have other neurologic abnormalities, especially facial palsy, meningitis can occur alone and be the presenting feature of the illness.[8,60,78] Then Lyme disease has to be differentiated from other causes of aseptic meningitis. How often Lyme disease is the cause of aseptic meningitis in unselected cases from endemic areas in North America has not been studied, however. But in two studies from Germany, evidence for *B. burgdorferi* infection was found in 16% and 41% of children presenting with aseptic meningitis.[13,57]

Cerebrospinal fluid. The CSF pressure is usually normal, but it may be increased (up to >500 mm CSF) in as many as 20% of patients with meningitis. Lymphocytic pleocytosis of 100 to 200 cells/mm^3 (range 5 to 3750/mm^3) is typical. Cytologic examination may show plasma cells, atypical plasmacytoid cells, immunoblasts, and histiocytes with vacuolated cytoplasm in addition.[11,12,84] Although mitotic figures can be frequent and malignant lymphoma simulated, immunocytochemical staining indicates that the atypical cells in the CSF of patients with Lyme disease are polyclonal in origin.[84]

The protein level is usually increased also, typically to about 100 mg/dl (range, 8 to 400 mg/dl); increases in CSF IgG and IgM may be present as

well as oligoclonal bands of IgG. Specific anti-*B. burgdorferi* antibody is present in addition in the CSF of 75% to 100% of those with meningitis, more commonly in cases of longer duration (>3 weeks).[68,81] The CSF glucose is typically normal, but values as low as 33 mg/dl have been reported.[61]

The CSF abnormalities ultimately subside even without treatment. Cell counts peak 3 to 8 weeks after meningeal symptoms begin and remain elevated for 3 to 4 months or more. By 6 months, the cell count is usually normal. The protein content may still be increased slightly at 6 months, becoming normal thereafter. Immunoglobulin abnormalities and specific antibody can persist for years after recovery without evidence of disease progression, however.[68]

CNS parenchymal abnormalities. Twenty to 50% of North American patients with Lyme disease and menigitis may have accompanying cerebral symptoms (see Fig. 13–1).[60,61,69,70] Ordinarily mild, characteristic symptoms include somnolence, confusion, impaired memory and concentration, behaviorial change, and depression. These symptoms commonly fluctuate in intensity for weeks to months before resolving, sometimes in concert with the meningeal symptoms and sometimes independent of them. The electroencephalograms (EEGs) of most symptomatic patients are abnormal because of nonspecific slowing, either focal or generalized. Computerized tomography (CT) and magnetic resonance imaging (MRI) are typically normal, however.

More severe parenchymal involvement is less common in early disseminated disease, particularly in North America where it occurs in no more than 5% to 10% in cases. In Europe, however, severe CNS involvement is seen in 10% to 20% of cases, accompanied almost always by pleocytosis and, usually, by cranial or peripheral neuritis.[68]

Myelitis is most common,[22,60,68-70] typically an acute or subacute transverse myelitis that develops over hours to days, although it can begin more slowly with increasing deficit developing over months. Spastic paraparesis with an accompanying sensory level, usually between T_4 and T_{10}, is the most common presentation. Flaccid paraplegia, spastic quadriparesis, and lumbar and cervical sensory levels have also been reported. Bladder symptoms are common also, as is paraparesis without sensory involvement. Lhermitte's sign may be present. Lesser degrees of cord involvement produce isolated Babinski's signs and urinary abnormalities without other signs of CNS dysfunction.

More severe cerebral involvement can also occur, again almost always accompanied by pleocytosis and, often, by cranial or peripheral neuritis.[19,23,52,68-71] Symptoms typically develop over

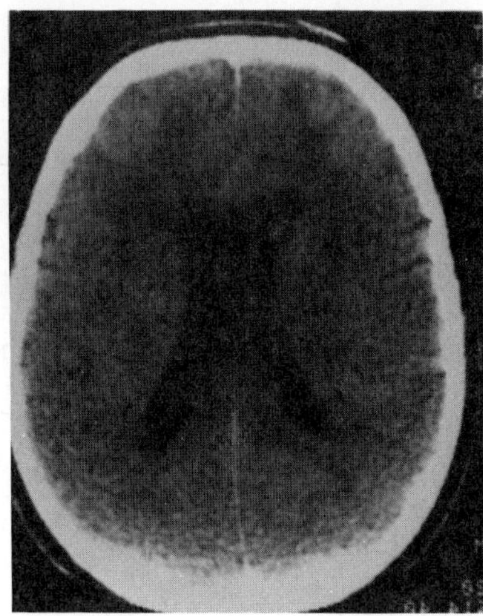

Figure 13–2 Postcontrast CT scan of a 38-year-old man with encephalitis during early disseminated Lyme disease showing extensive areas of demyelination in the frontal lobes and centrum semiovale. (Reproduced with permission from Reik L: *Lyme disease.* In Scheld WM, Whitley RJ, Durack DT, editors: *Infections of the central nervous system,* New York, 1991, Raven Press, p. 672.)

hours to days and include severe somnolence, hallucinations, paranoia, disorientation, catatonia, coma, confusion, irritability, and agitation. Seizures of a variety of types can occur also: partial complex, focal motor, and both primary and secondary generalized convulsions have been reported.[19,23,69,71]

CNS signs accompany cerebral symptoms and include hemiparesis, hemianopsia, dysphasia, alexia without agraphia, pseudobulbar palsy, Parkinson's syndrome, the locked-in syndrome, chorea, cerebellar ataxia, and Argyll Robertson pupils.[19,23,52,68-71]

The EEG in patients with severe cerebral symptoms usually shows focal or generalized slowing, and, in those with seizures, may show spikes or spike-wave complexes.* CT and MRI may be normal in spite of clear cerebral involvement.[60,61,68-70] In other cases, however, CT has shown infarct patterns in the cortex and basal ganglia, multifocal areas of white matter hypodensity (Fig. 13–2), low density contrast-enhancing areas in the cerebral cortex, and, rarely, hydrocephalus.[12,23,68,69,71] Reported MRI abnormalities have been similar, particularly multifocal areas of increased signal in the subcortical and periventricular white matter and cortex and brain stem.† Cerebral angiography in two patients with acute encephalitis has shown ev-

*References 19, 23, 52, 60, 61, 68-71.
†References 6, 22, 24, 52, 64, 68.

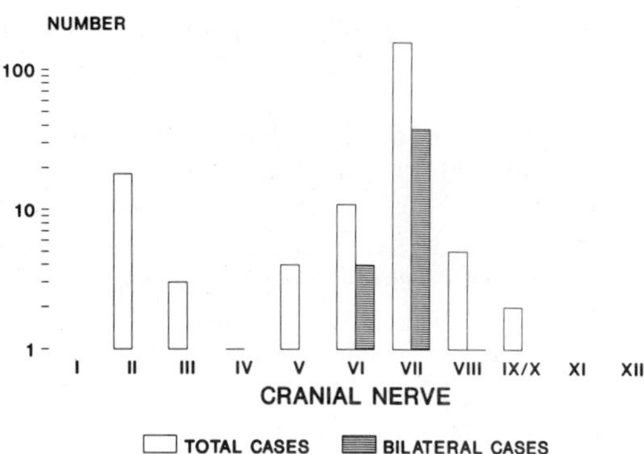

Figure 13–3 Nerves involved in 174 North American patients with cranial neuropathies during early disseminated Lyme disease.

idence for mass effect without vasculitis.[68,71]

Mild cerebral symptoms in early disseminated disease usually resolve completely, but the outcome in patients with severe parenchymal involvement is not always as favorable.[68] Residual paraparesis, tetraplegia, dementia, organic psychosis, hemiparesis, ataxia, seizures, parkinsonism, hydrocephalus, and disturbances in micturition have all been reported.[22,23,68-71,74]

Peripheral nervous system abnormalities

Cranial neuritis. About 60% of North American patients with neurologic abnormalities during early disseminated Lyme disease have cranial neuropathies (see Fig. 13–1). These are usually accompanied by pleocytosis (75% to 80%), and, frequently, by radiculoneuritis (40%). Cranial neuropathies typically begin about 3 weeks after the onset of EM in those cases where EM is present, but they can begin while the skin lesion is still present or even before it appears. Facial palsy is most common, but involvement of most of the cranial nerves has been reported, and multiple cranial neuropathies can occur.

Facial palsy. Facial palsy accounts for 80% to 90% of all cranial neuropathies in North American patients with early Lyme disease (Fig. 13–3). In one series of almost 1000 patients with Lyme disease, facial palsy developed in 10% of patients.[14]

The course of facial palsy typifies the evolution of cranial neuropathies during early Lyme disease in general. Weakness begins acutely and peaks in 1 to 2 days. When both facial nerves are affected (25%), the two sides are involved within a few days to 3 weeks of one another. Accompanying ipsilateral ear or jaw pain and facial numbness or tingling are common. Paralysis is complete in 50% to 60% of cases.[14] Nonetheless, the outcome is usually favorable, even without treatment: recovery is normally complete within 1 to 2 months. But full recovery occasionally takes longer (up to 1 year), and it may be incomplete in as many as 10% of cases.

Facial palsy can occur without other neurologic or systemic signs or symptoms and without preceding EM.[14,37,68] When facial palsy is the presenting feature of Lyme disease, confusion with idiopathic Bell's palsy is likely. Indeed, in one report from Suffolk County, New York, 6 of 22 patients with Bell's palsy had serologic evidence of exposure to *B. burgdorferi*.[37] How often *B. burgdorferi* infection is the cause of facial palsy among unselected patients from other endemic areas in North America has not been studied in detail, however,

Differentiating facial palsy due to Lyme disease from Bell's palsy is usually straightforward. Summer onset, travel to or residence in an endemic area, history of a preceding tick bite or EM, bilateral involvement, and lymphocytic pleocytosis are all helpful clues.[14,68] Moreover, specific antibody to *B. burgdorferi* is usually present in serum, and often in CSF, at the onset of paralysis.[68] Occasionally, specific antibody is not detectable at onset, but titers become elevated 4 to 6 weeks later.[37,68]

Optic neuritis. Involvement of the optic nerve is next most frequent (12% of cranial neuropathies), usually occurring in patients with other neurologic deficits.* Papilledema due to increased intracranial pressure (ICP), optic disc edema with normal ICP (optic perineuritis), optic neuritis, and ischemic optic neuropathy have all been reported. Recovery of vision is likely, but permanent visual loss and field defects, optic atrophy, and afferent pupillary defects can result.

Like facial palsy, optic neuritis can occur alone as the presenting feature of Lyme disease. In one study from Marshfield, Wisconsin,[43] 4 of 20 consecutive patients with new onset of optic neuritis had antibody reactivity against *B. burgdorferi*. CSF from three of the four was examined: two had CSF pleocytosis (27 and 47 cells/mm³), and the third had intrathecal synthesis of specific antibody without pleocytosis. Optic nerve function of all four patients improved after antibiotic therapy.

The diagnosis of Lyme disease should be considered in cases of isolated optic neuritis from endemic areas, therfore. Those due to Lyme disease can be differentiated from idiopathic optic neuritis and optic neuritis due to multiple sclerosis in the same manner that facial palsy due to Lyme disease can be distinguished from Bell's palsy.

Nerves III, IV, and VI. Paralysis of the extraocular muscles occurs in about 10% of patients with cranial neuropathies during early Lyme disease. Abducens palsy is most common (7%) and is bilateral about 35% of the time.* Third nerve palsy is next in frequency (3%).[12,69,70] Involvement of the fourth nerve is rare (<1%).[69] The onset is acute or subacute over hours to a day or two, and diplopia is the only symptom. Recovery is usually complete within 1 or 2 months.

Nerve V. Trigeminal nerve involvement accounts for 2% to 3% of cranial neuropathies.[7,70] The usual symptoms are pain, numbness, and paresthesias. Sensory signs are less frequent. Spontaneous improvement within 1 or 2 months is typical.

Nerve VIII. The eighth nerve is also involved in about 3% of cases of cranial neuropathy.[17,27,52,69,70] Hearing loss, sometimes bilateral, is most common, but vertigo also occurs. Permanent hearing loss has been reported.[52]

Nerves IX to XII. Abnormalities of the ninth and tenth nerves are rare (1% of cases).[52,61,70] Involvement of nerves XI and XII has been reported from Europe but not from North America.[68]

Radiculoneuritis. Radiculoneuritis develops in about 35% of patients with early neurologic involvement (see Fig. 13–1), usually accompanied by pleocytosis (85%) and cranial neuropathy (70%).

The first symptoms are severe radicular pains, paretheSias, or hyperesthesias that begin a mean of 1 month after a tick bite or EM (range, 1 week to 9 months).† The pains begin acutely or subacutely, usually on the trunk or proximal limbs, and reach a maximum in hours to a few days. More diffuse discomfort, typically localized under the scapulae or over the spine, often accompanies the radicular pain. Once established, the pain typically persists for weeks (range, 6 weeks to 3 months) before resolving spontaneously.

Pain is followed by neurologic signs within 1 to 4 weeks (range, days to 3 months). Motor weakness develops in two thirds and is typically asymmetric and focal or multifocal: nerves, nerve roots, and plexus are all involved, either singly or in combination. The weakness begins gradually and can progress over days to weeks, sometimes to atrophy, as separate extremities are affected in turn. Arm weakness and leg weakness are equally frequent. Common clinical patterns are mononeuritis simplex and multiplex, motor radiculitis in the extremities, and lumbosacral and brachial plexitis. Less common patterns of motor weakness include motor neuropathy without pleocytosis, weakness without preceding pain, paralysis of the diaphragm,

---

*References 7, 8, 17, 22, 42, 43, 52, 65, 69, 74, 88.

*References 7, 12, 22, 52, 60, 61, 65, 69, 70.
†References 7, 12, 20, 60, 61, 68-70.

and paralysis of the abdominal wall muscles.[16,68]

More generalized weakness can occur also, and even in patients with localized weakness there may be widespread depression of tendon reflexes suggesting a more generalized neuropathy. Moreover, tetraparesis can occur in early Lyme disease, and at least two cases of a Guillain-Barré–like syndrome in North American patients with Lyme disease have been reported. In one, the clinical picture was typical of Guillain-Barré syndrome (GBS), but there was an accompanying pleocytosis.[82] In the other, clinical, electrophysiologic, and CSF findings were typical of GBS; anti-*B. burgdorferi* antibody was present in serum and CSF; and the weakness resolved after plasmapheresis and antibiotic therapy.[39]

Actual sensory loss, as opposed to sensory symptoms, also follows pain by 1 to 4 weeks, ultimately developing in about 50% of patients with radiculoneuritis. The pattern of loss is usually dermatomal and most often cervical or lower thoracic, although any dermatome may be involved. Less frequently, sensation is lost in a nerve distribution or distally and symmetrically, particularly in the legs.

Electrophysiologic testing of patients with radiculoneuritis usually indicates axonal degeneration in both distal nerves and nerve roots.[7,60,61,68-70,82] Typical abnormalities include mild prolongation of distal motor and sensory latencies with only mild slowing of sensory and motor nerve conduction velocities (NCVs). Sensory potentials and compound action potentials may be decreased in amplitude. F waves are prolonged in about 50%. The most common electromyographic abnormalities are denervation potentials and neurogenic interference patterns in a nerve or root distribution. Less commonly, denervation potentials are absent and motor conduction velocities are slowed to 20 to 30 m/sec, indicating demyelination.[60,61,68,74,82]

Both sensory loss and motor weakness in patients with radiculoneuritis usually resolve spontaneously and completely within 2 months. Residual hypoesthesia is rare, but residual motor weakness and atrophy can occur.

Myositis

Myalgias are common among patients with early disseminated Lyme disease (40%), and muscle tenderness, stiffness, and cramping also occur (4%); but weakness is rare.[79] Although it is not certain how often these symptoms actually result from muscle inflammation, myositis does occur.

Symptoms begin 1 week to 6 months after a tick bite or EM, either acutely or gradually. Myalgias, muscle swelling and tenderness, and stiffness are most common, weakness is less so. Muscle involvement may be diffuse or localized, symmetric or asymmetric, proximal or distal. Fever, chills, anorexia, malaise, headache, nausea, and vomiting may be present in addition.*

Serum creatine kinase (CK) may be normal or increased (up to several thousand international units). Electromyography shows short-duration, low-amplitude polyphasic potentials; positive sharp waves; and fibrillation potentials. The usual finding on muscle biopsy is an interstitial myositis with perivascular lymphoplasmacytic infiltration of the perimysium and interstitium. *B. burgdorferi* has been identified between the muscle fibers with special stains. Gallium-67 imaging may show uptake of radiotracer in affected muscles.[3,44]

NEUROLOGIC FEATURES OF LATE LYME DISEASE

Other neurologic abnormalities, different from typical meningopolyneuritis, are characteristic of late disseminated Lyme disease (defined as beginning a year or more after illness onset), although identical syndromes occasionally do appear earlier, sometimes within months of the start of infection. Both the PNS and CNS are involved.

Central nervous system abnormalities

Progressive Borrelia encephalomyelitis. Progressive *Borrelia* encephalomyelitis is the best defined CNS disorder in late Lyme disease. Most cases have been reported from Europe where the syndrome appears to be more common,[2,68] but well-documented North American cases have been described also.†

Men and women are equally affected, and the average age of onset is 45 years.[2,68] Children are affected also, but less often than adults. In most cases, there is no history of antecedent tick bite, EM, or meningopolyneuritis; the onset of infection is not known. But in 7% of reported cases neurologic symptoms began 10 days to 19 months (median, 7 months) after a tick bite, in 5% they followed EM by 4 months to 6 years (median, 15 months), and in 14% they followed typical meningopolyneuritis by 3 months to 7 years (median, 12 months).[68]

Symptoms can begin either gradually or acutely. Once started, they do not resolve spontaneously but worsen progressively, either steadily or step-by-step with sudden worsening followed by only partial improvement before the next attack. Stroke and multiple sclerosis can be simulated, and the correct diagnosis is often delayed until symptoms have been present for months or even years. Ex-

---

*References 3, 21, 44, 45, 68, 72, 73.
†References 9, 10, 30, 53, 58, 59, 62.

traneural signs and symptoms of late Lyme disease are present and provide a clue to diagnosis in fewer than 5% of cases.[2,68]

The most common neurologic symptoms are limb weakness, gait difficulties, ataxia, bladder disturbance, speech abnormalities, visual and hearing loss, and poor memory and concentration. Meningeal symptoms are infrequent. Neurologic signs are multilevel, reflecting involvement of the brain, spinal cord, and cranial and peripheral nerves.[2,68]

Cerebral signs are most common (60% of patients) and are diffuse, multifocal, or both. Sudden focal deficits, either transient or permanent, occur in 30%. Most common are hemiparesis (15% of patients) and dysphasia (12%). Ataxia (37%), dysarthria (21%), and seizures (7%) are also common. More diffuse cerebral involvement commonly causes somnolence, confusion, poor concentration, irritability, disorientation, and impaired memory.[2,68]

Spinal cord involvement, present in 50% of cases, presents most often as progressive spastic paraparesis or quadriparesis accompanied by urinary bladder dysfunction. Sensory loss is less frequent than motor weakness, but transverse myelitis does occur.[2,68]

Typical cranial nerve abnormalities, present in 45%, are bilateral hearing loss and unilateral facial palsy. Optic nerve involvement is also common. Less often, abnormalities of nerves III, V, VI, the vestibular portion of VIII, IX, X, and XII have been reported.[2,68]

Radiculoneuritis is rare, occurring in only 8% of cases. Reported patterns include polyneuritis, mononeuritis simplex and multiplex, and radiculitis and radiculoplexitis.[2,68]

The CSF is frequently abnormal. Typical abnormalities include a pleocytosis of up to 2300 cells/mm^3 (usually 100 to 200 and mostly lymphocytes) and an increased protein of up to 1800 mg/dl (usually 100 to 200). The glucose concentration is routinely normal but may be decreased in as many as 10% of patients (values as low as 12 mg/dl). CSF IgG, IgA, and IgM may be increased, and oligoclonal IgG bands may be present. Patients often have had intrathecally concentrated anti-*B. burgdorferi* antibody.[2,68]

EEGs in patients with cerebral symptoms have shown focal or generalized slowing, bitemporal dysrhythmia with sharp waves, or no abnormality at all.[68] CT has shown infarcts in the cerebral cortex, internal capsule, and thalamus; multiple foci of cerebral and periventricular white matter hypodensity, sometimes with contrast enhancement; hydrocephalus; and cerebral atrophy with calcifications.[10,68] MRI has similarly shown infarcts in

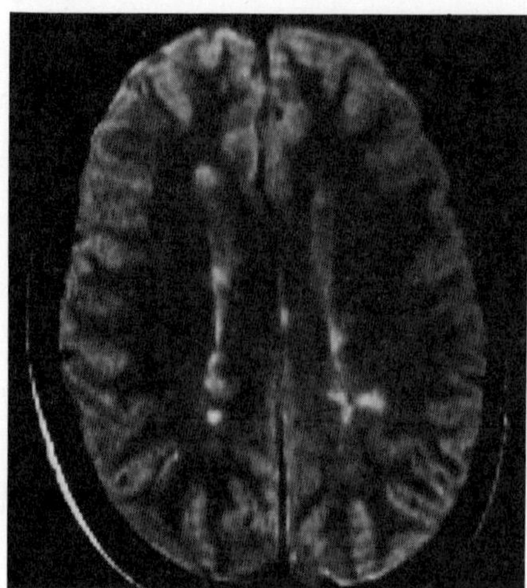

Figure 13–4 MR images of the brain of a 42-year-old woman with progressive *Borrelia* encephalomyelitis of 2 years' duration. Multiple areas of increased signal are present in the paraventricular white matter (TE 40/TR 3500). (Reproduced with permission from Reik L: *Lyme disease and the nervous system,* New York, 1991, Thieme Medical Publishers, p. 81.)

the thalamus and multiple areas of increased signal in the periventricular white matter and brain stem (Fig. 13–4).[53,58,59,62,68] Cerebral angiography in several cases,[10,68] and postmortem examination in one,[51] has suggested that these abnormalities result from vasculitis. Reported abnormalities include intracranial vessel irregularity with beading, narrowing, multiple stenoses, poststenotic dilatations, and branch occlusions. In a few patients with myelitis, MRI has shown focal or diffuse increase in signal in the cervical spinal cord.[68] In one patient, myelography demonstrated arachnoiditis.[46]

Late encephalopathy. Although the severe CNS abnormalities of progressive *Borrelia* encephalomyelitis occur uncommonly among North American patients with late Lyme disease, milder symptoms of CNS dysfunction are frequent. Affected patients experience defects in memory and concentration accompanied by profound fatigue. Both children and adults are affected.*

The symptoms begin months to years after the beginning of infection and can persist for years without treatment. Bedside tests of mental status are often abnormal, and detailed neuropsychologic testing demonstrates defects in immediate and delayed memory, the ability to learn new information, sustained attention, concentration, problem solving, perceptual-motor performance, and word finding. Mood changes (depression, irritability) are also common.[32,53]

---

*References 5, 32, 34, 36, 53, 62.

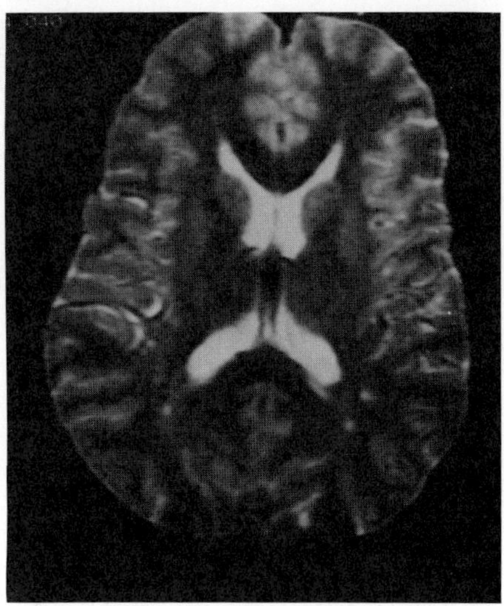

Figure 13–5 MR image of the brain of a 32-year-old man with Lyme disease and encephalopathy. There are three punctate areas of increased signal intensity in the white matter posteriorly (TE 80/TR 2500). (Reproduced with permission from Reik L: *Lyme disease.* In Scheld WM, Whitley RJ, Durack DT, editors: *Infections of the central nervous system,* New York, 1991, Raven Press, p. 676.)

Physical signs of CNS dysfunction are usually not present, but concomitant polyneuropathy is common.[53] The CSF contents are often normal, although occasional patients have lymphocytic pleocytosis,[32] and a third or more may have an elevated protein content.[53] The IgG index is also typically normal and oligoclonal bands of IgG are not present. Specific anti-*B. burgdorferi* antibody is concentrated intrathecally in 40% or more of patients, however.[32,34,53] EEG slowing is only occasionally present, and CT is usually normal. MRI, on the other hand, shows multiple punctate areas of increased signal in the cerebral white matter of 15% to 40% of those affected (Fig. 13–5).[32,34,53]

Other late CNS abnormalities

Lyme disease and multiple sclerosis. There appears to be no causal relationship between *B. burgdorferi* infection and multiple sclerosis (MS). Although clinical similarities between CNS Lyme disease and MS have led to diagnostic confusion,[68] the frequency of serum antibodies against *B. burgdorferi* is no higher among MS patients from endemic areas than among normal controls from the same areas.[15] Moreover, in seropositive patients with clinically definite MS, the antibody is not concentrated intrathecally.[32]

Lyme disease and motor neuron disease. The relationship between *B. burgdorferi* infection and motor neuron disease or amyotrophic lateral scle-

rosis (ALS) is less clear. Investigators in Wisconsin[86] and Long Island, New York,[35] found an increased prevalence of specific antibody among patients with ALS. Among ALS patients seen in Boston, Massachusetts,[55] serum immunoreactivity against *B. burgdorferi* was not present, however, nor has it been among my Connecticut patients with ALS (unpublished observation).

Latent CNS disease. The CNS abnormalities that develop during late Lyme disease often appear after a long asymptomatic interval, sometimes lasting years. The latent CNS infection occurs seem undeniable. How to test for it is less certain. Although Ackermann et al.[2] have attributed intrathecal synthesis of anti-*B. burgdorferi* antibody in asymptomatic patients who had recovered from an earlier meningopolyneuritis to latent CNS borreliosis, the presence of specific antibody in the CSF is not sufficient evidence to prove latent infection. Specific antibody can persist in the CSF for years after the successful antibiotic treatment of progressive *Borrelia* encephalomyelitis[87] or after the spontaneous resolution of meningopolyneuritis.[49] The best test for diagnosing latent CNS infection remains to be determined.

Peripheral nervous system abnormalities

Late polyneuropathy. Many North American patients with late Lyme disease also suffer from a mild, multifocal polyneuropathy. This neuropathy is distinct from meningopolyneuritis: it causes less striking signs and symptoms and does not improve spontaneously. Both children and adults are affected, and 30% to 90% of those affected may have accompanying encephalopathy.[31,32,38,53]

Sensory symptoms, usually tingling paresthesias of the extremities, are most common, occurring in as many as 50% of patients with late Lyme disease.[31,32,38,53] Often intermittent and commonly distal, the parethesias can be asymmetric and patchy. They can involve the arms, the legs, or both. The parethesias typically begin months after illness onset and have been present a year or more by the time of diagnosis.

Less often (25%), radicular pain, especially in the legs, is also present.[31,32,38,53] The radicular pain usually begins at about the same time as the paresthesias, months after the beginning of infection.

Carpal tunnel syndrome (CTS) also is present in about 25% of patients with late disease, typically developing several years after illness onset.[31,32,33,38] Those affected have acral paresthesias in the distribution of the median nerve that are exacerbated during sleep or by using the hands. The CTS is bilateral in two thirds of cases.

Physical signs of neuropathy are less frequent. Motor weakness and reflex loss are rare. Thirty to

60% of those with sensory symptoms have a mild stocking and glove distal sensory loss, however.[32,33,38,53]

Electrophysiologic testing has shown abnormalities of two or more peripheral nerves in 40% to 50% of North American patients with late disease.[32,33,38,53] The abnormalities detected indicate a patchy, multifocal, axonal neuropathy affecting both distal axons and nerve roots. Electromyography often shows denervation potentials both in proximal paraspinal and in more distal limb muscles whereas electroneurography can show mild slowing of motor or sensory NCVs, decreased sensory amplitudes, prolongation of distal motor latencies, decreased compound action potentials, and increased F wave latencies. Occasional patients have had more severe slowing of motor conduction or areas of conduction block suggestive of demyelination. Patients with Lyme disease and CTS have slowing of segmental conduction or sensory or motor NCV at the wrist.[33]

Accompanying CSF abnormalities, present in up to 70% of patients, include increased CSF protein content and intrathecal concentration of specific anti-*B. burgdorferi* antibody.[53] However, most of these patients have also had a late encephalopathy, which may affect their CSF picture. Pleocytosis is unusual but does occur.[31,53] There are usually no other laboratory abnormalities.

Neuropathy with late sclerotic skin lesions. A similar but somewhat more severe peripheral neuropathy is common among European patients with acrodermatitis chronica atrophicans (ACA) and other late sclerotic skin lesions.[1,40,48]

Twenty-five to 70% of such patients have neuropathic symptoms—paresthesias, burning dysesthesias, sharp pains, hyperesthesias, weakness, or muscle cramps.[1,40,48] Moreover, as many as two thirds may have physical signs of neuropathy in addition—reflex changes, sensory loss, muscle weakness, and atrophy. Both signs and symptoms are usually asymmetric and most marked in regions of skin involvement.[1,40,48] The clinical patterns of neuropathy that result are cutaneous mononeuropathy, distal asymmetric polyneuropathy, and distal symmetric polyneuropathy.[48]

Recorded electrophysiologic abnormalities are similar to those seen in North American patients with late Lyme disease and polyneuropathy.[40,48]

Myositis

Myositis occurs in association with ACA in late disseminated disease also,[72,73] but it has not been described yet in North American patients. The course is progressive over months, and localized weakness is the main symptom. Serum CK may be normal or modestly increased. Electromyogra-

phy has shown short-duration, low-amplitude polyphasic potentials, fibrillations, and positive sharp waves in affected muscles. Biopsies have shown both focal nodular and inclusion body myositis. Spirochetes are present in silver-stained specimens.

Pathology and pathogenesis. Neurologic abnormalities in Lyme disease likely result from both the direct effects of *B. burgdorferi* on nervous tissue and the host's response to it.

Almost certainly, meningitis is caused directly by invasion of the CSF by *B. burgdorferi*: antibiotics shorten the course,[77] and the organism has been cultured from CSF.[80] Similarly, antibiotic therapy halts the progression of parenchymal CNS abnormalities,[2] and *B. burgdorferi* has been isolated from and demonstrated histologically in brain tissue,[51,54,59] suggesting that these abnormalities also are caused directly by invasion of the brain and spinal cord.

Other evidence suggests that parenchymal CNS abnormalities in Lyme disease are caused by vasculitis.[70] The evidence includes the diffuse and multifocal pattern of these neurologic abnormalities, the occurrence of strokelike episodes in progressive *Borrelia* encephalomyelitis, accompanying CT and MRI abnormalities suggesting infarction, and cerebral angiographic changes indicating vasculitis.[66]

Indeed, autopsy examination in one fatal case of progressive encephalomyelitis did show obliterative meningovasculitis causing brainstem infarction; and spirochetes were present around subependymal vessels in the fourth ventricle.[51] Whether *B. burgdorfderi* damaged the vessels directly or the vessels were damaged secondarily by the inflammatory response to its presence is not clear, however.

CNS abnormalities in Lyme disease may arise through indirect immunopathic mechanisms in addition. Antibodies to myelin and myelin basic protein are present in CSF of some patients with neurologic abnormalities[4,25]; the CSF of some patients with radiculomyelitis contains T-cells reactive with myelin, myelin basic protein, and galactocerebrosides[56]; and CT and MRI of some patients with cerebral symptoms have shown changes consistent with demyelination.[58,68,71] Finally, serum from patients with neurologic manifestations of Lyme disease, but not those without, contains IgM antibodies that bind to normal human axons.[75]

B. burgdorferi may damage the PNS through more than one mechanism as well. Spinal radiculitis and cranial neuritis could be caused directly by spread of inflammation from the subarachnoid space to the nerve roots.[61] But involvement of the seventh nerve is often more peripheral, distal to the chorda tympani, and some patients with radiculitis do not have pleocytosis.[68] Moreover, the usual clinical pattern of multifocal and asymmetric involvement along with the usual electrophysiologic pattern of multifocal axonal injury strongly suggests that these PNS abnormalities, like their CNS counterparts, are caused by vasculopathy.[66,68,70] Examination of sural nerve biopsies from Lyme disease patients with various neuropathies (meningopolyneuritis,[85] late polyneuropathy,[31] and the neuropathy accompanying ACA[48]) confirms this suggestion: all show similar epineurial perivasculitis with occasional luminal thrombosis.

Yet in other cases, electrophysiologic tests indicate demyelination.[29,61,82] Whether axonal injury and demyelination in Lyme disease both result from the same vasculopathy is not clear, however. The presence of antibodies to myelin and myelin basic protein in serum and CSF of patients with neurologic abnormalities[4,25] and the presence of T-cell lines in their CSF reactive to peripheral myelin[56] suggest that indirect immunopathic mechanisms may also be involved.

DIAGNOSIS OF NERVOUS SYSTEM LYME DISEASE

Nervous system Lyme disease should be considered in any patient with chronic lymphocytic meningitis or meningoencephalitis, especially if there are accompanying cranial or peripheral neuropathies or radiculoneuropathies. But Lyme disease is also possible in patients with a variety of other neurologic abnormalities (Table 13–1).

When other cardinal features of Lyme disease (EM, ACA, lymphocytoma, Lyme arthritis, or myocarditis) accompany these abnormalities, the diagnosis is straightforward. When the neurologic abnormalities occur alone, then travel to or residence in an edemic area, history of an antecedent tick bite, or summer onset are epidemiologic clues.

Table 13–1 Neurologic syndromes that may be associated with Lyme disease

Early	Late
CNS abnormalities	
Acute aseptic meningitis	Progressive encephalomyelitis
Acute purulent meningitis*	Focal encephalitis
Chronic lymphocytic meningitis	Cerebral vasculitis
Recurrent meningitis	Stroke
Acute meningoencephalitis	Multiinfarct dementia
Acute focal encephalitis	Leukoencephalitis
Encephalomyelitis	Brainstem encephalitis
Leukoencephalitis	Hydrocephalus
Acute cerebellar ataxia	Late encephalopathy
Acute Parkinson's syndrome	Cerebellar ataxia
Hydrocephalus	Transverse myelitis
Seizure disorder	Progressive spastic paraparesis or quadriparesis
Acute transverse myelitis	? Motor neuron disease
Subacute myelitis	
? Syringomyelia*	
PNS abnormalities	
Painful radiculitis	Meningoradiculitis
Plexitis or radiculoplexitis	Radiculoplexitis
Mononeuritis simplex/multiplex	Progressive radiculoneuritis
Sensory radiculopathy	Mononeuritis simplex/multiplex
Distal symmetric polyneuritis	Distal axonopathy
?Guillain-Barré syndrome	ACA-associated neuropathy
Cauda equina syndrome	Neuropathy associated with morphea and LSA†
Cranial mononeuritis or polyneuritis (especially Bell's palsy)	Carpal tunnel syndrome
Ulnar nerve entrapment*	Cranial neuritis (especially nerves VII and VIII)
Carpal tunnel syndrome	
Muscle abnormalities	
Interstitial myositis	Focal nodular myositis

Reproduced with permission from Reik L: *Lyme disease and the nervous system,* New York, 1991, Thieme Medical Pub., p. 106.
*Evidence from only a few or single case reports.
†Lichen sclerosis et atrophicus.

Additional, but nonspecific, laboratory clues in early disease include elevation of the erythrocyte sedimentation rate, increase in the serum IgM concentration, and presence of serum cyroglobulins.[70]

Once suspected on clinical or laboratory grounds, the diagnosis can be confirmed by demonstrating an immune response to *B. burgdorferi*. The serum level of IgG anti-*B. burgdorferi* antibody is usually raised by the time the nervous system is involved in early Lyme disease, whereas the level of specific IgM antibody may or may not be.[80] The IgG titer is similarly high in patients with late nervous system involvement, but IgM titers then are typically normal.[2,34]

But no serologic measurement, regardless of titer, accurately reflects disease activity or predicts response to treatment. The presence of serum immunity to *B. burgdorferi* is not sufficient to diagnose nervous system infection, because seropositivity can represent mere coincidental exposure to the organism of a patient with some other neurologic illness.[68]

The measurement of CSF antibody titer can aid the diagnosis in neurologic cases. CSF analysis demonstrates intrathecal synthesis of IgG anti-*B. burgdorferi* antibody in approximately 90% of patients with early nervous system involvement,[81] including some whose serum antibody tests are negative, typically those with symptoms of 3 or fewer weeks' duration.[83] Intrathecal synthesis is frequently demonstrable in patients with progressive *Borrelia* encephalomyelitis as well.[2,81] But it is less frequent (30% to 40%) among North American patients with late encephalopathy, and it is rare among patients with late polyneuropathy alone.[34,81]

The clinical diagnosis of definite Lyme disease involving the nervous system can be made, therefore, when there is a compatible neurologic abnormality (see Table 13–1) without other cause and at least one of the following: (1) a history of well-documented (physician-diagnosed) EM, (2) history or presence of lymphocytoma, (3) presence of ACA, (4) serum *and* CSF reactivity or CSF reactivity alone against *B. burgdorferi*, (5) both other organ system involvement typical of Lyme disease and raised titers of specific serum antibody, or (6) seroconversion or four-fold rise in titer of paired serum specimens (Table 13–2).[67,68] Cases in which all these criteria are not fulfilled may still represent Lyme disease, but the diagnosis is then not certain, and other diagnoses should be considered before antibiotic treatment is prescribed.[68]

TREATMENT AND RESPONSE

Antibiotic regimens for the treatment of Lyme disease with nervous system involvement are outlined in Chapters 18 and 19.

When patients with early neurologic involvement do receive antibiotic therapy, meningismus, radicular pain, and systemic symptoms begin to improve within days.[47,63,76,77] Recovery from peripheral motor weakness is usually slower, often taking weeks, and is sometimes incomplete. Although mild CNS symptoms typically resolve completely after treatment, more severe deficits may only stabilize or improve partially.[76,77] CSF cell counts are routinely lower by the end of therapy. However, it may take months for pleocytosis to resolve completely, and CSF protein may remain elevated for a year or more.[63,76,77]

Table 13–2 Diagnostic criteria for Lyme neuroborreliosis

Definite neuroborreliosis

Compatible neurologic abnormality without other cause and one or more of the following:

(1) History of well-documented EM

(2) Presence of ACA or lymphocytoma

(3) Serum *and* CSF immunoreactivity, or CSF reactivity alone, against *B. burgdorferi* by ELISA or immunoblot

(4) Both other organ system involvement typical of Lyme disease (for example, Lyme arthritis) and serum immunoreactivity to *B. burgdorferi*

(5) Seroconversion or fourfold rise in titer of antibody to *B. burgdorferi* between acute and convalescent sera

Probable neuroborreliosis

Compatible neurologic abnormality without other cause and serum immunoreactivity to *B. burgdorferi*

Possible neuroborreliosis

Compatible neurologic abnormality without other cause and tick bite or travel or residence in an endemic area

---

Adapted from Reik L: *Lyme disease.* In Scheld WM, Whitley RJ, Durack DT, editors: *Infections of the central nervous system,* New York, 1991, Raven Press, p. 678.

Progressive *Borrelia* encephalomyelitis also responds to parenteral antibiotic therapy with resolution of pleocytosis and reduction of CSF protein content within 3 months.[2,47] Clinical signs usually only stabilize or regress incompletely after treatment, however. Total recovery is rare.[68]

In most cases of late encephalopathy, CNS symptoms abate slowly after antibiotic therapy.[18,32,53] Little change is seen during the course of treatment itself, and maximum improvement can take 6 months.

In patients with late polyneuropathy, paresthesias resolve within 3 to 6 months after antibiotic treatment, as do the electrophysiologic abnormalities.[31-33,38,53] Radicular pain and symptoms of CTS are relieved in only about half of those treated, however. As with its North American counterpart, the neuropathy associated with ACA also responds to antibiotic therapy.[40,48]

Treated patients with interstitial myositis are rid of pain and weakness within a month or two,[68] those with focal nodular myositis are rid of pain within several months.[73]

REFERENCES

1. Aberer E et al: Neuroborreliosis in morphea and lichen sclerosus et atrophicus, *J Am Acad Dermatol* 19:820, 1988.
2. Ackermann R et al: Chronic neurologic manifestations of erythema migrans borreliosis, *Ann NY Acad Sci* 539:16, 1988.
3. Atlas E et al: Lyme myositis: muscle invasion by *Borrelia burgdorferi*, *Ann Intern Med* 109:245, 1988.
4. Baig S, Olsson T, Link H: Predominance of *Borrelia burgdorferi* specific B cells in cerebrospinal fluid in neuroborreliosis, *Lancet* 2:71, 1989.
5. Belman AL et al: Neurological involvement in pediatric Lyme disease, *Ann Neurol* 26:476, 1989.
6. Belman AL et al: Brain MRI abnormalities in children infected by *B. burgdorferi*, *Neurology* 41(Suppl 1):180, 1991.
7. Bertuch AW, Rocco E, Schwartz EG: Lyme disease: ocular manifestations, *Ann Ophthalmol* 20:376, 1988.
8. Boutros A, Rahn E, Nauheim R: Iritis and papillitis as a primary presentation of Lyme disease, *Ann Opthalmol* 22:24, 1990.
9. Broderick JP, Sandok BA, Mertz LE: Focal encephalitis in a young woman 6 years after the onset of Lyme disease: tertiary Lyme disease? *Mayo Clin Proc* 62:313, 1987.
10. Brogan GX, Homan CS, Viccellio P: The enlarging clinical spectrum of Lyme disease: Lyme cerebral vasculitis, a new disease entity, *Ann Emerg Med* 19:572, 1990.
11. Case records of the Massachusetts General Hospital, *N Engl J Med* 311:172, 1984.
12. Case records of the Massachusetts General Hospital, *N Engl J Med* 319:1654, 1988.
13. Christen H-J et al: Facial palsy and aseptic meningitis caused by *Borrelia burgdorferi*: report on an ongoing prospective study in childhood, presented at the Fourth International Conference on Lyme Borreliosis, June 18-21, 1990, Stockholm, Sweden.
14. Clark JR et al: Facial paralysis in Lyme disease, *Laryngoscope* 95:1341, 1985.
15. Coyle PK: *Borrelia burgdorferi* antibodies in multiple sclerosis patients, *Neurology* 39:760, 1989.
16. Daffner KR, Saver JL, Biber MP: Lyme polyradiculoneuropathy presenting as increasing abdominal girth, *Neurology* 40:373, 1990.
17. Dattwyler RJ, Halperin JJ: Failure of tetracycline therapy in early Lyme disease, *Arthritis Rheum* 30:448, 1987.
18. Dattwyler RJ et al: Treatment of late Lyme borreliosis—randomised comparison of ceftriaxone and penicillin, *Lancet* 1:1191, 1988.
19. Diringer MN, Halperin JJ, Dattwyler RJ: Lyme meningoencephalitis: report of a severe, penicillin-resistant case, *Arthritis Rheum* 30:705, 1987.
20. Donaldson JO, Lewis RA: Lymphocytic meningoradiculitis in the United States, *Neurology* 33:1476, 1983.
21. Duray PH, Steere AC: Clinical pathologic correlations of Lyme disease by stage, *Ann NY Acad Sci* 539:65, 1988.
22. Farris BK, Webb RM: Lyme disease and optic neuritis, *J Clin Neuro Ophthalmol* 8:73, 1988.
23. Feder HM, Zalneraitis EL, Reik L: Lyme disease: acute focal meningoencephalitis in a child, *Pediatrics* 82:931, 1988.
24. Fernandez RE et al: Lyme disease of the CNS: MR imaging findings in 14 cases, *AJNR* 11:479, 1990.
25. Garcia-Monco JC, Coleman JL, Benach JL: Antibodies to myelin basic protein in Lyme disease, *J Infect Dis* 158:667, 1988.
26. Garin C, Bujadoux C: Paralysie par les tiques, *J Med Lyon* 71:765, 1922.
27. Glasscock ME et al: Lyme disease: a cause of bilateral facial paralysis, *Arch Otolaryngol* 111:47, 1985.
28. Glauser TA, Brennan PJ, Galetta SL: Reversible Horner's syndrome and Lyme disease, *J Clin Neuro Ophthalmol* 9:225, 1989.
29. Graf M et al: Electrophysiologic findings in meningopolyneuritis of Garin-Bujadoux-Bannwarth, *Zentralbl Bakteriol Mikrobiol Hyg [A]* 263:324, 1986.
30. Halperin JJ: Lyme encephalomyelitis, *Neurology* 41(Suppl 1):217, 1991.
31. Halperin JJ et al: Lyme disease: cause of a treatable peripheral neuropathy, *Neurology* 37:1700, 1987.
32. Halperin JJ et al: Nervous system abnormalities in Lyme disease, *Ann NY Acad Sci* 539:24, 1988.
33. Halperin JJ et al: Carpal tunnel syndrome in Lyme borreliosis, *Muscle Nerve* 12:397, 1989.
34. Halperin JJ et al: Lyme neuroborreliosis: central nervous system manifestations, *Neurology* 39:753, 1989.
35. Halperin JJ et al: Immunologic reactivity against *Borrelia burgdorferi* in patients with motor neuron disease, *Arch Neurol* 47:586, 1990.
36. Halperin JJ et al: Lyme borreliosis-associated encephalopathy, *Neurology* 40:1340, 1990.
37. Halperin JJ et al: Lyme borreliosis in Bell's palsy, *Neurology* 40(Suppl 1):342, 1990.
38. Halperin JJ et al: Lyme neuroborreliosis: peripheral nervous system manifestations, *Brain* 113:1207, 1990.
39. Herskovitz S, Berger A, Swerdlow M: Guillain-Barré syndrome associated with Lyme borreliosis, *Neurology* 40(Suppl 1):342, 1990.
40. Hopf HC: Peripheral neuropathy in acrodermatitis chronica atrophicans (Herxheimer), *J Neurol Neurosurg Psychiatry* 38:452, 1975.
41. Hörstrup P, Ackermann R: Durch Zecken übertragene Meningopolyneuritis (Garin-Bujadoux-Bannwarth), *Fortschr Neurol Psychiatr* 41:583, 1973.
42. Jacobson DM, Frens DB: Pseudotumor cerebri syndrome associated with Lyme disease, *Am J Ophthalmol* 107:81, 1989.
43. Jacobson DM, Marx JJ, Dlesk A: Frequency and clinical significance of Lyme seropositivity in patients with isolated optic neuritis, *Neurology* 41:706, 1991.

44. Kengen RAM et al: Scintigraphic evaluation of Lyme disease: gallium 67 imaging of Lyme myositis, *Clin Nucl Med* 14:728, 1989.

45. Kirsch M et al: Fatal adult respiratory distress syndrome in a patient with Lyme disease, *JAMA* 259:2737, 1988.

46. Kohler J et al: Chronic central nervous system involvement in Lyme borreliosis, *Neurology* 38:863, 1988.

47. Kohlhepp W, Oschmann P, Mertens H-G: Treatment of Lyme borreliosis: randomized comparison of doxycycline and penicillin G, *J Neurol* 236:464, 1989.

48. Kristoferitsch W et al: Neuropathy associated with acrodermatitis chronica atrophicans: clinical and morphological features, *Ann NY Acad Sci* 539:35, 1988.

49. Krüger H et al: Meningoradiculitis and encephalomyelitis due to *Borrelia burgdorferi*: a follow-up study of 72 patients over 27 years, *J Neurol* 236:322, 1989.

50. Kuiper H et al: Evidence of asymptomatic nervous system involvement in localized erythema migrans, presented at the Fourth International Conference on Lyme Borreliosis, June 18-21, 1990, Stockholm, Sweden.

51. Kuntzer T et al: *Borrelia* rhombencephalomyelopathy, *Arch Neurol* 48:832, 1991.

52. Lesser RL et al: Neuro-ophthalmologic manifestations of Lyme disease, *Ophthalmology* 97:699, 1990.

53. Logigian EL, Kaplan RF, Steere AC: Chronic neurologic manifestations of Lyme disease, *N Engl J Med* 323:1438, 1990.

54. MacDonald AB, Miranda JM: Concurrent neocortical borreliosis and Alzheimer's disease, *Hum Pathol* 18:759, 1987.

55. Mandell H et al: Lack of antibodies to *Borrelia burgdorferi* in patients with amyotrophic lateral sclerosis, *N Engl J Med* 320:255, 1989.

56. Martin R et al: *Borrelia burgdorferi*-specific and autoreactive T-cell lines from cerebrospinal fluid in Lyme radiculomyelitis, *Ann Neurol* 24:509, 1988.

57. Millner M et al: Lyme borreliosis in children: a controlled clinical study based on ELISA values, *Eur J Pediatr* 148:527, 1989.

58. Pachner AR: *Borrelia burgdorferi* in the nervous system: the new "great imitator," *Ann NY Acad Sci* 539:56, 1988.

59. Pachner AR, Duray P, Steere AC: Central nervous system manifestations of Lyme disease, *Arch Neurol* 46:790, 1989.

60. Pachner AR, Steere AC: Neurologic findings of Lyme disease, *Yale J Biol Med* 57:481, 1984.

61. Pachner AR, Steere AC: The triad of neurologic manifestations of Lyme disease: meningitis, cranial neuritis, and radiculoneuritis, *Neurology* 35:47, 1985.

62. Pachner AR, Steere AC: CNS manifestations of third stage Lyme disease, *Zentralbl Bakteriol Mikrobiol Hyg [A]* 263:301, 1986.

63. Pfister H-W et al: Cefotaxime vs penicillin G for acute neurologic manifestations in Lyme borreliosis: a prospective randomized study, *Arch Neurol* 46:1190, 1989.

64. Rafto SE et al: Biopsy-confirmed CNS Lyme disease: MR appearance at 1.5T, *AJNR* 11:482, 1990.

65. Raucher HS et al: Pseudotumor cerebri and Lyme disease: a new association, *J Pediatr* 107:931, 1985.

66. Reik L: *Borrelia burgdorferi* infection: a neurologist's perspective, *Ann NY Acad Sci* 539:1, 1988.

67. Reik L: *Lyme disease*. In Scheld WM, Whitley RJ, Durack DT, editors: *Infections of the central nervous system,* New York, 1991, Raven Press.

68. Reik L: *Lyme disease and the nervous system,* New York, 1991, Thieme Medical Publishers.

69. Reik L, Burgdorfer W, Donaldson JO: Neurologic abnormalities in Lyme disease without erythema chronicum migrans, *Am J Med* 81:73, 1986.

70. Reik L et al: Neurologic abnormalities of Lyme disease, *Medicine* (Baltimore) 58:281, 1979.

71. Reik L et al: Demyelinating encepahlopathy in Lyme disease, *Neurology* 35:267, 1985.

72. Reimers CD et al: Myositis associated with *Borrelia burgdorferi*-infection, presented at the Fourth International Conference on Lyme Borreliosis, June 18-21, 1990, Stockholm, Sweden.

73. Reimers CD et al: Myositis caused by *Borrelia burgdorferi*: report of four cases, *J Neurol Sci* 91:215, 1989.

74. Schechter SL: Lyme disease associated with optic neuropathy, *Am J Med* 81:143, 1986.

75. Sigal LH, Tatum AH: Lyme disease patients' serum contains IgM antibodies to *Borrelia burgdorferi* that cross-react with neuronal antigens, *Neurology* 38:1439, 1988.

76. Sköldenberg B et al: Treatment of Lyme borreliosis with emphasis on neurological disease, *Ann NY Acad Sci* 539:317, 1988.

77. Steere AC, Pachner AR, Malawista SE: Neurologic abnormalities of Lyme disease: successful treatment with high-dose intravenous penicillin, *Ann Intern Med* 99:767, 1983.

78. Steere AC et al: Erythema chronicum migrans and Lyme arthritis: the enlarging clinical spectrum, *Ann Intern Med* 86:685, 1977.

79. Steere AC et al: The early clinical manifestations of Lyme disease, *Ann Intern Med* 99:76, 1983.

80. Steere AC et al: The spirochetal etiology of Lyme disease, *N Engl J Med* 308:733, 1983.

81. Steere AC et al: Evaluation of the intrathecal antibody response to *Borrelia burgdorferi* as a diagnostic test for Lyme neuroborreliosis, *J Infect Dis* 161:1203, 1990.

82. Sterman AB, Nelson S, Barclay P: Demyelinating neuropathy accompanying Lyme disease, *Neurology* 32:1302, 1982.

83. Stiernstedt GT et al: Diagnosis of spirochetal meningitis by enzyme-linked immunosorbent assay and indirect immunofluorescent assay in serum and cerebrospinal fluid, *J Clin Microbiol* 21:819, 1985.

84. Szyfelbein WM, Ross JS: Lyme disease meningopolyneuritis simulating malignant lymphoma, *Mod Pathol* 1:464, 1988.

85. Vallat JM et al: Tick-bite meningoradiculoneuritis: clinical, electrophysiologic, and histologic findings in 10 cases, *Neurology* 37:749, 1987.

86. Waisbren BA et al: *Borrelia burgdorferi* antibodies and amyotrophic lateral sclerosis 2:332, 1987.

87. Weder B et al: Chronic progressive neurologic involvement in *Borrelia burgdorferi* infection, *J Neurol* 234:40, 1987.

88. Wu G et al: Optic disc edema and Lyme disease, *Ann Ophthalmol* 18:252, 1986.

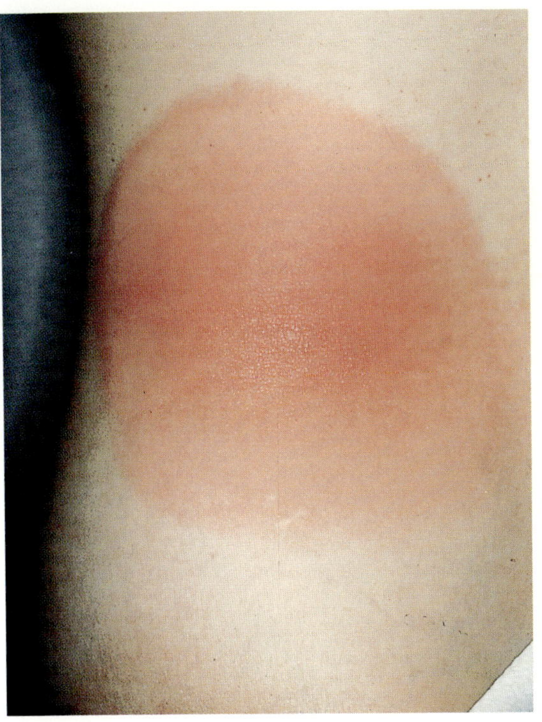

Color Plate 1 Erythema migrans presenting as an erythematous, annular plaque.

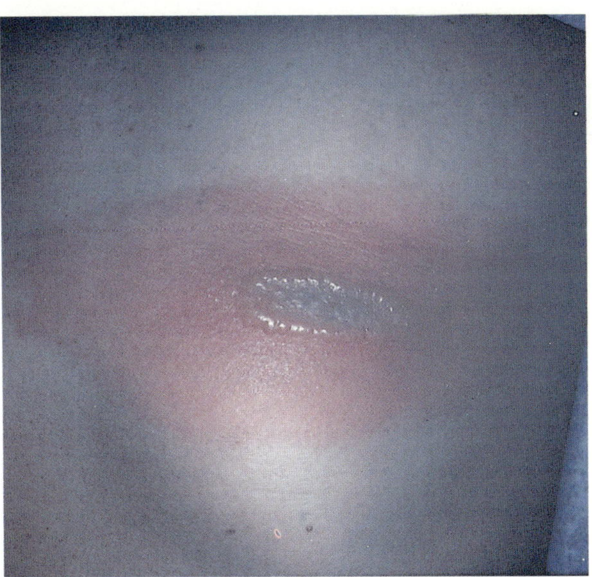

Color Plate 2 Erythema migrans with an annular, vesicular, central portion.

Color Plate 3 An erythema migrans lesion with a triangular configuration also demonstrating a red annular central portion separated from the peripheral erythema by clinically normal skin.

Color Plate 4 A large plaque of erythema migrans which attained a size of 30 × 33 cm in 21 days. (From Berger BW et al: Use of an autologous antigen in the serologic testing of patients with erythema migrans of Lyme disease, *J Am Acad Dermatol* 18:1243, 1988.)

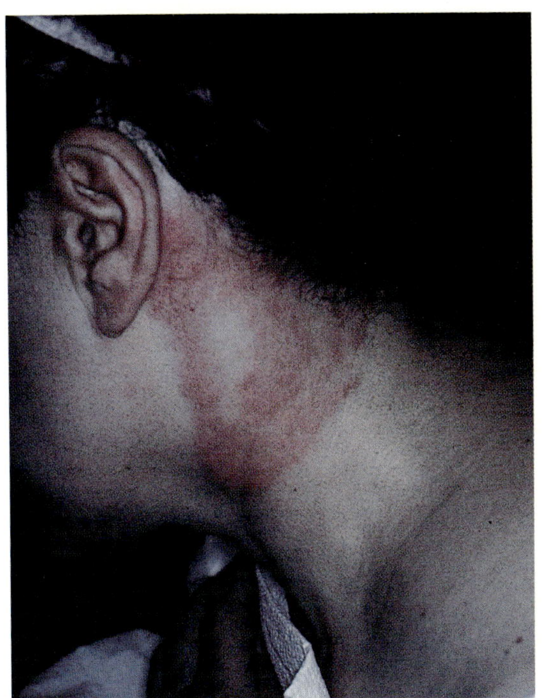

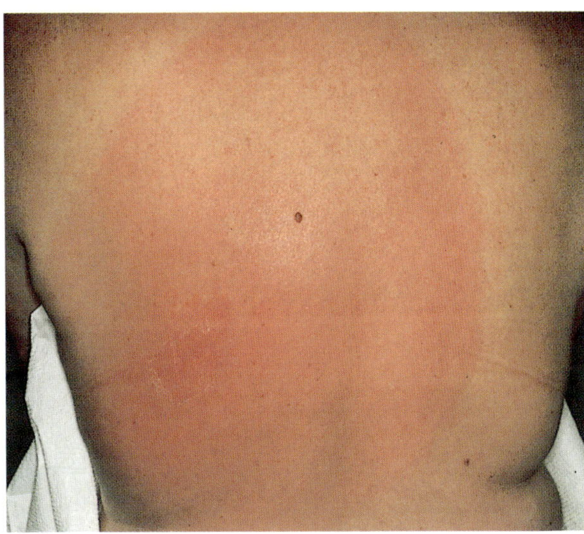

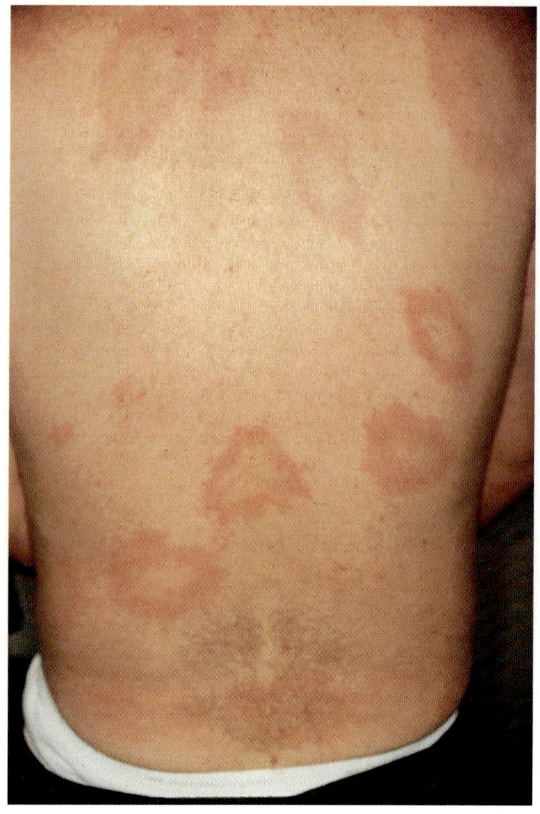

Color Plate 5 Erythema migrans appearing in multiplicity. (From Berger BW, Dermatologic manifestations of Lyme disease, *Rev Infect Dis* 11:S1475, 1989.)

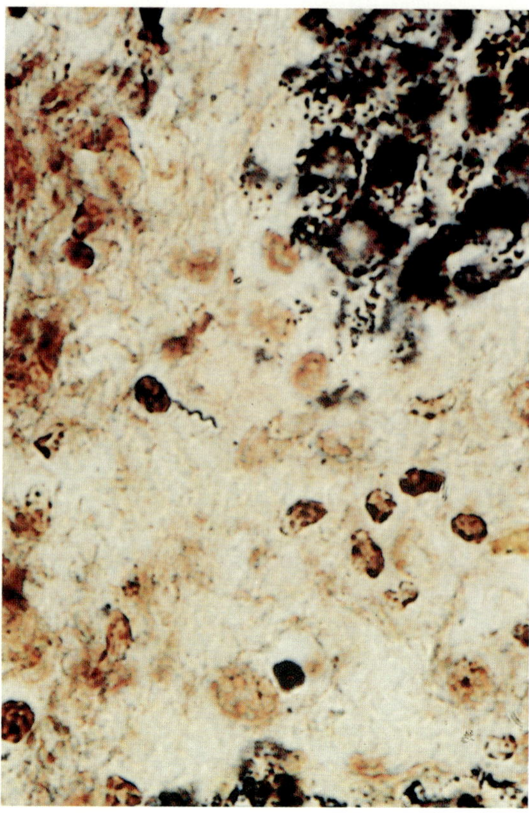

Color Plate 6 Warthin-Starry staining demonstrating *Borrelia burgdorferi* in the papillary dermis of a skin biopsy specimen obtained from an erythema migrans lesion. (From Berger BW et al: Isolation and characterization of the Lyme disease spirochete from the skin of patients with erythema chronicum migrans, *J Am Acad Dermatol* 3:444, 1985.)

Color Plate 7 Indirect immunofluorescence demonstrating *Borrelia burgdorferi* in a myocardial biopsy. Reproduced with permission. (From Vlay SC et al. Ventricular tachycardia associated with Lyme carditis, *American Heart J* 121:1559-1560, 1991.)

Color Plate 8 Term placenta with random typical spirochete organisms (*Borrelia burgdorferi*). (Courtesy of Dr. Cynthia Kaplan.)

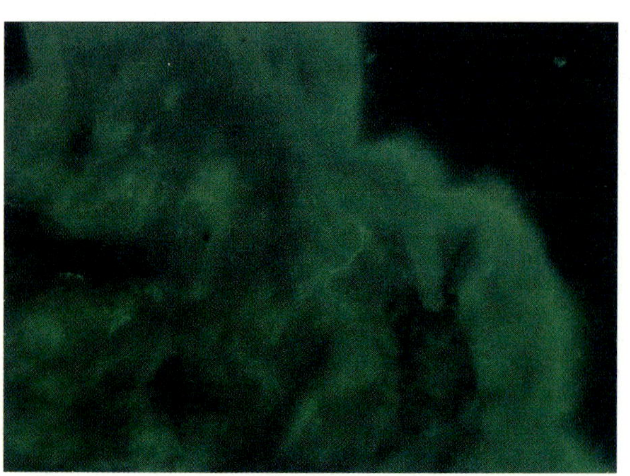

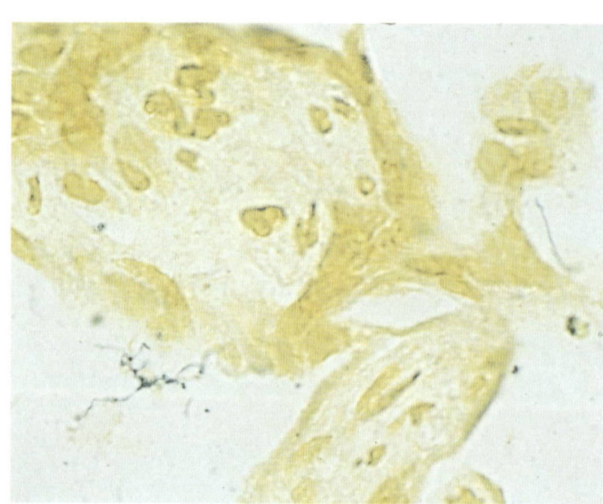

Diagnosis

14 Antibody Assays

Marc G. Golightly

It is well known that *Borrelia burgdorferi* infection can produce a wide spectrum of clinical manifestations that can be confused with many other disease entities (see Section II, Clinical Aspects). Therefore, in many cases, the clinical differential is often complex.[16,37-39] This clinical complexity has resulted in a heavy reliance on the laboratory to provide diagnostic evidence for infection or exposure to *B. burgdorferi*. Ideally, culture or isolation of the organism would be the definitive laboratory confirmation of infection. In many bacterial diseases, this is the "gold standard" and is relatively easily accomplished. Unfortunately, isolation, culture, and identification of *B. burgdorferi* is a low yield procedure, may be invasive (that is, skin biopsy)* and, therefore, is not of general diagnostic utility. There has been a report of a higher success rate of culturing these organisms from blood of patients with early Lyme.[30] However, most of these patients were seropositive and the length of time required to culture the organism may be several weeks or longer. Therefore, this method, with some exceptions, is also not likely to be diagnostically useful. The main value of culture at this time is to provide a source of culture confirmed cases that can be used to refine and test the clinical criteria and laboratory diagnostic tests for Lyme disease. In some cases, it has also been used for retrospective evidence of active infection (although a negative culture does not rule out infection). Alternatively, other antigen detection systems have been proposed. These include the polymerase chain reaction (PCR) to detect *B. burgdorferi* deoxyribonucleic acid (DNA).[33] Although it has not yet been extensively clinically evaluated, as a research tool this is a powerful technique. However, without a U.S. Food and Drug Administration (FDA) approved clinical diagnostic PRC kit, it is doubtful that the technology will be able to be performed by common hospital or diagnostic laboratories for some time even if it does prove diagnostically useful. Another antigen detection assay examines the

urine for excreted *B. burgdorferi* antigens as an indication of Lyme borreliosis.[4,7] Although this appears to work in animal models, in humans this test has not proven useful. More work and clinical studies need to be performed in this area as well. These and other antigen assays are discussed in Chapter 17.

Unlike most other bacterial infections, the detection of antibodies to the organism is the most common available method for diagnostic evidence of Lyme borreliosis. Specifically, these include the enzyme-linked immunosorbent assay (ELISA), the indirect immunofluorescent assay (IFA), and the western blot (immunoblot). Unfortunately, in light of what is often being asked of these assays, they are far from ideal with respect to sensitivity and specificity. This becomes evident considering the indiscriminant ordering of these tests without consideration for clinical history and presentation. Even the most ideal assay has difficulties when used as a screening test with disregard for the clinical history. However, when these tests are used prudently with careful integration of the patient's symptoms and clinical history, they can provide useful information that complements the clinician's diagnostic skills.

The general humoral antibody response to *B. burgdorferi* is well characterized. However, it is extremely complex and individually variable (especially with regard to the response against the individual spirochete antigens). In general, the specific IgM response peaks between 3 and 6 weeks after the onset of symptoms. Typically, the specific IgM gradually decreases in most patients. In some patients, the IgM titers may remain high throughout the course of the disease.[10,11] The reason for this is unclear although these IgM responses were shown to be directed against different antigens from those of the early IgM response. However, this would not be able to be differentiated by the standard IFA or ELISA methods. The response to the antigens recognized late is individually variable and not predictable. Early in the course of the disease, the primary antibody response (both IgM and

---

*References 5, 6, 19, 22, 39, 40.

115

IgG) is usually to the 41-kD spirochetal flagellin antigen.[3,8,11,20] Unfortunately, this antigen is not species specific and has marked amino acid sequence homology with other microbial flagellin.[9] Many other *B. burgdorferi* antigens have reported to cross-react with other bacterial antigens and include the 17, various 55 to 60, and 72-kD proteins among others.[11,20,24] This cross-reactivity is important to the understanding of biologic false-positives and proper interpretation of serologic tests. However, there are several *B. burgdorferi* proteins that seem to be more specific for Lyme borreliosis (OspA 31 kD, OspB 34 kD). The response to these proteins is quite variable, usually occurring late in disease, if at all. Therefore, it becomes clear that although these antibody assays may correctly identify an antibody response to *B. burgdorferi* antigens, the presence of antibodies reactive to *B. burgdorferi* may not be specific for Lyme disease. Many normal, apparently healthy people have low levels of antibodies that cross-react with the 41-kD antigen as well as some of the other common bacterial antigens (how to deal with this is discussed in detail later in this chapter). Like most secondary IgG responses, it lags the IgM response and generally increases to peak levels during the arthritic symptoms. The specific IgG may remain detectable for years like IgG responses to many infectious organisms. In addition, a stable positive ELISA titer *after* treatment does not necessarily indicate treatment failure or continued presence of the spirochete, and additional treatment should not be based on this. This variability among different individuals and stage of disease may account for some of the variability noted among different commercial kits, because the antigen targets used in these kits vary. Also typical of most serologic tests to infectious organisms is the fact that a negative antibody test early in the course of the disease does not rule out the disease. This is especially true of early Lyme borreliosis where the sensitivity at the low end is questionable.[15,21,26,36] If early, acute Lyme borreliosis is suspected, another sample should be drawn 4 to 8 weeks later. Ideally, the acute and convalescent sample should be run together.[32] (The full interpretation and proper utilization of these tests are discussed in following sections of this chapter.)

ANTIBODY METHODS

As previously stated, the detection of antibodies to *B. burgdorferi* is the most common commercial method used to obtain laboratory evidence of past or present exposure to the organism. It should be emphasized that the diagnosis of Lyme borreliosis is primarily clinical. The role of the clinical laboratory should be *only* secondary or confirmatory

and not the sole diagnostic criterion. The first common serologic method to be used for Lyme borreliosis was IFA, followed shortly thereafter by various forms of ELISA. Unfortunately, both of these assays have been plagued with unrealistic diagnostic expectations as well as other problems. It has become apparent that many of these problems are due to the misinterpretation and misuse (inappropriate ordering) of these tests. In addition, there have been serious questions relating to the performance and quality of various test kits. As a result, there has been a need for additional laboratory data to confirm this often questioned information. To this end, the western blot or immunoblot has been used. Unfortunately, because of the individuality of the humoral response and the reactivity to common antigens, the western blot cannot take the same role as it has in human immunodeficiency virus (HIV) as a "confirmatory" test. However, this is not to say that the western blot is without diagnostic value. It can be extremely useful under certain conditions, which will be discussed.

Indirect immunofluorescent assays (IFA)

The Lyme IFA is typical of most IFA assays for infectious agents. It has all the performance problems normally encountered with this type of assay, plus some of its own. In this assay, the organism is fixed to a microscope slide by various methods, which differ with the manufacturer. The patient's sera is added, followed by washes and incubation with the secondary fluorescent antihuman antibody. This methodology is ideal for low volume testing. No special equipment is required (except for fluorescence microscope), and experienced Lyme laboratories have found it to be quite accurate.[27,34] In fact, it is reported that some biologic false-positives can be distinguished in the IFA by the pattern of fluorescence. Some patients with rheumatic diseases have been reported to give false-positive ELISAs.[29] However, an astute laboratory using an IFA may pick this up as a beaded pattern of fluorescence. This staining pattern does not appear to be restricted to the Lyme IFA, because the FTA-Abs (fluorescent treponemal antibody absorption) test for syphilis has also been reported to give a beaded appearance with some patients with various connective tissue diseases, including systemic lupus erythematosus (SLE).[28] It is fortunate that in syphilis diagnostics there is another test based on another antibody system (the VDRL or RPR), and the FTA-Abs is not totally relied on.

Although the Lyme IFA in theory may have some advantages, in practice many routine diagnostic laboratories have had problems. The IFA has done and continues to do poorly in New York State proficiency tests.[19] This poor performance may be the result of a combination of problems: (1) As mentioned, there is a degree of experience required and common to all IFA procedures; there is subjectivity in the reading or scoring of the tests. (2) There is manufacturer variability, which most likely reflects the different ways the spirochetes are grown, the slides prepared, and the serum treated before testing. Although some of these problems may be addressed, it is unlikely (using the fluorescent antinuclear antibodies [ANA] test as a model example) that the subjectivity problem will resolve with time.

Enzyme-linked immunosorbent assays (ELISA)

ELISA has been replacing IFA in many diagnostic serologies, and Lyme borreliosis is no exception. ELISA (unlike IFA) is ideal for high-volume testing and, if the kit comes as strip wells, low-volume testing can also be performed. The subjectivity in reading is eliminated because results are indicated colorimetrically and read on a microtiter plate spectrophotometer. The results are generally quantitative and on a continuous scale. ELISA methods have generally done better than IFA in the New York State Lyme proficiency tests.[19] However, recently, many ELISAs also performed poorly.[31] There is still great variability in the results from different laboratories using different ELISA test kits.[10,25,36] Generally, it has been demonstrated that there is a specific lack of sensitivity for patients with early Lyme disease, whereas patients with late Lyme disease were more reliably identified. We have evaluated the status of seven commercial Lyme borreliosis kits for their ability to detect antibody to *B. burgdorferi* in patients with different stages of clinically diagnosed Lyme borreliosis.[17,18] The sera from patients with a clinical history of Lyme borreliosis at different stages with and without antibiotic treatment were examined, as well as sera from individuals without clinical evidence of Lyme borreliosis. It was demonstrated that during the very early stages of Lyme borreliosis (EM rash apparent less than 1 week) all tests were negative. At a slightly later time period (EM apparent 1 to 2 weeks), there was a large variation in test results ranging from >66% positive to 0% positive. This extreme variation may represent the different philosophies in the antigens used for coating the microtiter plates. Because there are many cross-reactive antigens, some companies have elected to purify or enrich certain antigens in an attempt to make the assay more specific. Unfortunately, this is often at the expense of sensitivity. In addition, because the humoral response to *B. burgdorferi* is so individual, it is possible that some patients may be missed if the primary antigens that they respond

to are absent or in low concentration. On the other hand, enrichment of other antigens such as the common flagellar 41-kD antigen may increase sensitivity at the expense of specificity. Still others use unpurified sonicates of the organism under the assumption that this more closely reflects the antigen proportions that are seen in vivo. During the later stages of the disease course, all tests improved in their ability to detect *B. burgdorferi* specific antibodies; however, there was still a large range in the performance of these kits (from >97% to <37% positive).[17,18] In healthy individuals without Lyme borreliosis, the rate of false-positivity was low. These results demonstrate that improvement of the majority of commercially available diagnostic Lyme borreliosis kits is required, and that these tests are especially poor (high false-negatives) in the diagnosis of early disease. An adjunct test certainly would be helpful.

Western blot or immunoblot

Many clinicians have begun using the western blot or immunoblot as an alternative to or in conjunction with the above tests for the reasons discussed above. The western blot also detects antibody but is technically more involved and has been traditionally used as a research tool to characterize the different antigens of *B. burgdorferi* and the antibody responses to each.[11,14,20] However, it can be and has been commercialized for the general clinical diagnostic laboratory.

It has been suggested that immunoblotting is more sensitive and specific than previously used ELISA methods for diagnosing early Lyme disease. However, this is not always the case and the reputation of the western blot in HIV testing as the "gold standard" or "confirmatory test" method does not presently hold for Lyme borreliosis. The major problem with the western blot for Lyme disease is in the extremely subjective interpretation and lack of standardization. How does one interpret the presence of reactivity to common antigens (41 kD, 50 to 72 kD)? At what level of reactivity does one call a band positive? Grodzicki and Steere found that 45% of healthy people had IgG antibodies (and no IgM antibodies) that bound to three or less polypeptides (mostly to the 41-kD but sometimes also to 25-, 31-, 34-, or 66-kD proteins).[20] Furthermore, normal healthy people are usually not the samples that are seen in the clinical diagnostic situation. When hospitalized patients (not those with Lyme disease) were examined, both IgG and IgM antibodies were found in a significant number. When considering the diagnosis of Lyme borreliosis, various autoimmune diseases, chronic fatigue (possibly Epstein-Barr virus [EBV] or other viral illness), other spirochetal diseases, and many other entities should be included in the clinical differential. Golightly et al.[19] has examined people with no clinical diagnosis of Lyme disease but who had some of these other diseases that entered into the clinical differential diagnosis and diseases that caused a humoral expansion and might be expected to give rise to false-positives. It was demonstrated that patients with various autoimmune diseases (rheumatoid arthritis and systemic sclerosis), acute EBV infection, polyclonal increases in immunoglobulin (acquired immunodeficiency syndrome [AIDS]), sicca syndrome, fever of unknown origin (FUO), and chronic nephritis all had significant bands with both IgG and IgM. Most of these blots would be considered positive even by the most strict criteria. The problem becomes how to discriminate Lyme borreliosis from other illness and how to standardize interpretation of the Lyme western blot. The patient's history and presentation are absolutely required to assign a significance and to interpret properly a western blot result. Without this information, the usefulness of the western blot is limited at best. When the western blot is useful and its interpretation are considered below. Other problems plaguing the western blot is the lack of standardization of the procedure. Differences in procedures have been noted in dilution of patient sera, concentration of antigen used, strain of antigen, dilution of secondary antibody, the use and concentration of different blocking solutions, and even incubation times. Complicating the issue further is the fact that different *B. burgdorferi* strains occur naturally in different parts of the world[2] and may elicit different antibody responses. This makes a universal criteria for the reactivity of a western blot based on subjective interpretations and unstandardized procedure inappropriate.

INTERPRETATIONS

With all of these problems, it is not a simple matter to decide which tests to run, by whom, and how to interpret the results. Pure statistics, without knowing the laboratory, would dictate that the ELISA would be the method of choice. However, as mentioned, a good experienced laboratory using an IFA can give high quality results equal to an ELISA. To whom the tests are sent is also very difficult because the site performance depends on the test kit being used (which often changes) and the general quality of the laboratory. It is the opinion of this author that the best way of picking a diagnostic kit or performance institution is to test the contenders against several clinically defined early Lyme disease cases and several patients with diseases other than Lyme disease. The Centers for Disease Control (CDC) is establishing a bank of case-defined serum for this purpose. After these

concerns have been addressed, one is left with how to interpret the results obtained.

The evaluation of Lyme disease serology has many similarities to serologies for other infectious diseases; a negative result *early* in the disease course does not rule out the disease. All serologic tests will be negative if the specimen is taken too early (that is, before antibody is made). However, in Lyme borreliosis where the sensitivity of many commercial kits at the low end is so variable,[10,15,26,36] this is especially true. If early Lyme borreliosis is suspected clinically and the initial test form a reputable laboratory is negative, a second specimen should be taken in 3 to 4 weeks if laboratory confirmation is sought and clinically required. It should be noted, as stated in previous chapters, that the diagnosis of classical Lyme borreliosis is *clinical* and treatment should not be withheld until a positive laboratory test is obtained. In fact, the second specimen may not seroconvert to positive if antibiotic treatment is started promptly based on clinical diagnosis at presentation.[39] In this case, the failure to seroconvert is meaningless because it neither confirms nor disproves the clinical diagnosis. In those cases when the clinical diagnosis is less certain and the decision not to treat is made, the negative *second* specimen does have value and provides support against Lyme disease as the diagnosis. Positives in early Lyme disease are generally low level positives (especially if a polyvalent antisera is being used). Assays determining separate anti-*B. burgdorferi* IgG and IgM antibodies should be interpreted with caution with respect to IgM = acute and IgG = convalescent. As previously mentioned, this correlation does not always hold.

A negative serology is useful and evidence against Lyme borreliosis as a diagnosis when the clinical symptoms and history are consistent with those found in late or chronic Lyme disease (arthritis and so forth). Most Lyme kits do not have problems with these specimens because they are generally high titer.[1,19] This includes those with chronic late symptoms *recently* treated with antibiotics because the titers may remain positive for years despite successful treatment. It should be noted that negative, low level, or decreasing Lyme titers, although not common in untreated chronic Lyme disease, can occur.[1,23,35] In addition, occasionally a patient presents with symptoms consistent with Lyme borreliosis and the history reveals that close to the onset of symptoms the patient was treated with short-term antibiotics usually for an unrelated reason (for example, dental work). In this case, a negative serology is inconclusive. Some of these patients, although lacking a detectable humoral response, may exhibit a cell-mediated immune (CMI) response to *B. burgdorferi*.[12,13,41] Overall, the CMI is expensive, unstandardized, and not extremely specific or sensitive. Unless there is a specific clinical reason to perform such testing, it should probably be avoided except as a research tool. This assay is discussed further in Chapter 15. Some seronegative patients may have low levels of antibodies, formed within immune complexes. Complexed antibody, and the problem of seronegativity in general, are covered in greater depth in Chapter 25.

The interpretation of positive results must also be subjected to the same caution and integration of clinical data. With the occasional exceptions mentioned above, low-level positive or borderline results should be consistent with the clinical symptoms and suspicion of *early* Lyme borreliosis to be taken as good evidence for infection, whereas *late* Lyme borreliosis usually is associated with a high titer serology. If the clinical symptoms are more consistent with those commonly associated with chronic or late Lyme disease, or are vague but chronic in nature and low positive or borderline results are obtained, then other diseases within the clinical differential should be thoroughly examined as a possible reason for the positive ELISA. These low positives and borderline results have the highest probability of being biologic false-positives (polyclonal B cell expansion, viral disease, autoimmunity, syphilis, and so forth) especially when the clinical picture does not match the expected results. In these cases, a western blot is **sometimes** helpful if no clinical decision can be made. However, the interpretation of the western blot results is unstandardized and great expertise is required to attach correct significance to them. Very often the western blot result just adds to the uncertainty of the clinical impression. In contrast, a patient with clinical symptoms similar to those found in primary early disease with a high titer Lyme serology is unusual and suspect. A past or recurrent infection should be considered as a possible cause of this inconsistency. The issue of a new reinfection or a recurrence of a past infection is one in which standard serologies are of little help.

Unfortunately, there is tremendous pressure to rely heavily on the laboratory for serologic evidence of exposure or infection by *B. burgdorferi*. Although there are many reasons for this, it does not negate the necessity to integrate the clinical data with the serologic results because the diagnosis of Lyme borreliosis is, in fact, *clinical*. The serologic results *cannot* be properly interpreted without this integration and may be meaningless if an attempt is made to do so. As with most serologic laboratory tests, a positive result on an apparently healthy person (that is, a screening test without

clinical indication) will most likely be a false-positive. Lyme serologies are no exception. Unfortunately, because of the pressure on physicians and the laboratory, these tests (including those that are still in the research phases and not yet clinically proven) are often used as screening tests for Lyme borreliosis even when there is no history of exposure or symptomatology. If these tests are to be used effectively, clinical skills must be relied on to eliminate testing those patients that do not fit the clinical criteria for Lyme disease and, at the very least, eliminate testing on healthy people with no significant risk factors. Proper clinical screening will effectively increase the prevalence of Lyme borreliosis in the patients being tested. The end result is that the predictive value of a positive test indicating actual disease will increase. However, due to the nature of the antibody response, positive results must still be reviewed critically with regards to expected results for stage of disease and potential confounding diseases. When the serologies are used properly and their limitations are taken into account, they can be a useful adjunct to the physician's clinical skills.

REFERENCES

1. Barbour AG: Laboratory aspects of Lyme borreliosis, *Clin Microbiol Rev* 1(4):399, 1988.
2. Barbour AG, Heiland RA, Howe TR: Heterogeneity of major proteins in Lyme disease borrelia: a molecular analysis of North American and European isolates, *J Infect Dis* 152:484, 1985.
3. Barbour AG et al: Antibodies of patients with Lyme disease to components of *Ixodes dammini* spirochete, *J Clin Invest* 72:504, 1983.
4. Benach JL, Coleman JI, Golightly MG: A murine IgM monoclonal antibody binds an antigenic determinant in outer surface protein A, an immunodominant basic protein of the Lyme disease spirochete, *J Immunol* 140:265, 1988.
5. Benach JL et al: Spirochetes isolated from the blood of two patients with Lyme disease, *N Engl J Med* 30:740, 1983.
6. Berger BW, Clemmensen OJ, Ackerman AB: Lyme disease is a spirochetosis. A review of the disease and evidence for its cause, *Am J Dermatopathol* 5:111, 1983.
7. Bosler EM, Schulze: The prevalence and significance of *Borrelia burgdorferi* in the urine of feral reservoir hosts, *Zentralbl Bakteriol Mikrobiol Hyg [A]* 263:40, 1986.
8. Coleman JL, Benach JL: Isolation of antigenic components from the Lyme disease spirochete: their role in early diagnosis, *J Infect Dis* 155:756, 1987.
9. Coleman JL, Benach JL: Identification and characterization of an endoflagellin antigen of *Borrelia burgdorferi*, *J Clin Invest* 4:322, 1989.
10. Craft JE, Grodzicki RL, Steere AC: Antibody response in Lyme disease: evaluation of diagnostic tests, *J Infect Dis* 149:79, 1984.
11. Craft JE et al: Antigens of *Borrelia burgdorferi* recognized during Lyme disease. Appearance of a new immunoglobulin M response and expansion of the immunoglobulin G response late in the illness, *J Clin Invest* 7:934, 1986.
12. Dattwyler RJ et al: Seronegative Lyme disease: dissociation of specific T- and B-lymphocyte responses to *Borrelia burgdorferi*, *N Engl J Med* 319:1441, 1989.

13. Dressler F, Yoshinari M, Steere A: The T-cell proliferative assay in the diagnosis of Lyme disease, *Ann Internal Med* 115:533, 1991.

14. Fister RD et al: Comparative evaluation of three products for the detection of *Borrelia burgdorferi* antibody in human serum, *J Clin Microbiol* 27:234, 1989.

15. Golightly M: Diagnosis of Lyme borreliosis, *Diag Clin Testing* 27:39, 1989.

16. Golightly M, Dattwyler R: Lyme disease vs. rheumatic disease, *Immunopathology* 10:4, 1986.

17. Golightly MG, Soirez L, Viciana A: Variability in Lyme borreliosis testing among commercial diagnostic kits. 1990, IV International Conference on Lyme Borreliosis, Stockholm, Sweden.

18. Golightly MG, Thomas J, Soirez L: Reliability of commercial diagnostic kits for the detection of antibodies to *Borrelia burgdorferi*. In preparation.

19. Golightly MG, Thomas JA, Viciana AL: The laboratory diagnosis of Lyme borreliosis, *Lab Med* 21:299, 1990.

20. Grodzicki RL, Steere AC: Comparison of immunoblotting and indirect enzyme-linked immunosorbent assay using different antigen preparations for diagnosing early Lyme disease, *J Infect Dis* 157(4):790, 1988.

21. Halperin JJ et al: Lyme neuroborreliosis: central nervous system manifestations, *Neurology* 39:753, 1989.

22. Johnston YE et al: Lyme arthritis—spirochetes found in synovial microangiopathic lesions, *Am J Pathol* 11:26, 1985.

23. Lavoie PE, Lane RS, Murray RH: Seronegative Lyme borreliosis in three Californians with late manifestations, *Arthritis Rheum* 30(4):S36, 1987.

24. Luft B et al: Specificity of human B-cell responses of immunodominant antigens of *Borrelia burgdorferi*, *Ann NY Acad Sci* 539:39, 1988.

25. Luger S, Krauss E: Serologic tests for Lyme disease: interlaboratory variability, *Arch Intern Med* 150:761, 1990.

26. Magnarelli LA: Quality of Lyme disease tests, *JAMA* 262:3464, 1989.

27. Magnarelli LA et al: Comparison of an indirect fluorescent-antibody test with an enzyme-linked immunosorbent assay for serological studies in Lyme disease, *J Clin Microbiol* 20:11, 1984.

28. McKenna C et al: The fluorescent treponemal antibody absorbed (FTA-ABS) test beading phenomenon in connective tissue diseases, *Mayo Clin Proc* 48:545, 1973.

29. Muhlemann M, Wright D, Black C: Serology of Lyme disease, *Lancet* 1:553, 1986.

30. Nadelman RB, Pavia CS: Isolation of *Borrelia burgdorferi* from the blood of seven patients with Lyme disease, *Am J Med* 21, 1990.

31. New York State Department of Health Proficiency Tests 1990, 1991.

32. NIH State of the Art Conference, Diagnosis and Treatment of Lyme Disease, *Clinical Courier* 9:1, 1991.

33. Rosa PA, Schwan TG: A specific and sensitive assay for the Lyme disease spirochete *Borrelia burgdorferi* using the polymerase chain reaction, *J Infect Dis* 160:101, 1989.

34. Russell H et al: Enzyme-linked immunosorbent assay and indirect immunofluorescence assay for Lyme disease, *J Infect Dis* 149:465, 1984.

35. Schutzer S et al: *B. burgdorferi* specific antibody in circulating immune complexes in seronegative Lyme disease, *Lancet* 1:312, 1990.

36. Schwartz BS et al: Antibody testing in Lyme disease. A comparison of results in four laboratories, *JAMA* 262:3431, 1989.

37. Steere AC et al: Lyme arthritis: an epidemic of oligoarticular arthritis in children and adults in three Connecticut communities, *Arthritis Rheum* 20:7, 1977.

38. Steere AC et al: Erythema chronicum migrans and Lyme arthritis—the enlarging clinical spectrum, *Ann Intern Med* 6:65, 1977.

39. Steere AC et al: The spirochetal etiology of Lyme disease, *N Engl J Med* 30:733, 1983.

40. Waldo ED, Sidhu GS: The spirochete in erythema chronicum migrans, *Am J Dermatopathol* 5:125, 1983.

41. Zoschke D, Skemp A, Defosse D: Lymphoproliferative responses to *Borrelia burgdorferi* in Lyme disease, *Ann Intern Med* 114:285, 1991.

15 Cellular Immune Assays

David J. Volkman

Lyme borreliosis has become a recognized national and worldwide illness.[4,6,31,32] Lyme disease has been reported in 46 states, in most eastern and western European countries, in several former Soviet republics, and in China. It is endemic along the northeastern Atlantic coast and in parts of Europe. Although as many as two thirds of affected individuals present with a characteristic spreading, circular erythema migrans (EM) rash,[7,28] the reliable diagnosis of this infection has remained problematic.[16,19,23,29,34]

The EM rash may be unrecognized or mistaken for another annular dermatosis. Even in endemic areas of the United States, such as eastern New York and Connecticut, EM went unrecognized by most physicians until the early 1980s. In children, the rash can be totally missed, occurring in the scalp area or other unobserved locations, and the disease is only suspected months later when the child has frank arthritis.[24,31] Moreover, the serum test for antibodies against *Borrelia burgdorferi* has been plagued until recently by high false-negatives, false-positives, and lack of reproducibility.[16,19,23,29] Serum tests using immunofluorescent assays against whole *Borrelia* spirochetes resulted in high background fluorescence and low sensitivity in detecting true positives.[8,29] Most commercial laboratories have switched to the more accurate enzyme-linked immunosorbent assay (ELISA) method for measuring specific antibody levels. Results nationally have become much more consistent and comparable to results from reliable university laboratories such as SUNY, Stony Brook, and Yale University (unpublished data).

However, a major problem with the serodiagnosis of Lyme disease remains. As in syphilis, early antibiotic therapy blocks infected individuals from developing sustained humoral immunity and often renders them seronegative within 3 months of treatment. Even in individuals treated with doses of antibiotics inadequate to eradicate infection, the development of a strong *Borrelia*-specific antibody response can be blocked.[12] Thus, chronic Lyme borreliosis may occur in patients with negative serology and a history of antibiotic exposure early in infection. Although these patients represent a minority of individuals with Lyme disease (estimated at less than 5% of our clinic cases), they, nonetheless, are a difficult and significant diagnostic problem. Accurately detecting true Lyme borreliosis in these patients remains an important goal in the clinical laboratory because correct diagnosis and subsequent therapy can cure their often debilitating signs and symptoms.

Cellular immune responses are commonly used in clinical medicine to assess prior or continuing infection by a pathogenic microbe both by skin tests for delayed type hypersensitivity (DTH), such as the tuberculin test or tests for T-cell anergy, and by in vitro assays. Microbial infections such as Lyme borreliosis usually trigger both a humoral and cell-mediated immune (CMI) response. The antibody response to *B. burgdorferi* and its constituents is well described.[3,9,11] A vigorous cellular response with stimulation indices (SI) above 20 was described by Dattwyler et al.[10] These responses were found to be mediated by T lymphocytes, to be monocyte-dependent, and to be stimulated best by whole or particulate *Borrelia* antigen rather than by soluble antigens from disaggregated spirochetes.[11] Others have subsequently demonstrated *Borrelia*-specific T-cell responses in cerebrospinal fluid (CSF) and synovial mononuclear cells.[25,30] The precise assay conditions, the sensitivity and specificity of the assay, and the ontogeny and duration of *Borrelia*-specific T cell proliferative responses are described in this review.

ASSAY CONDITIONS

The T-cell receptor on *B. burgdorferi*-specific T cells recognizes small *Borrelia* peptides in the context of either class I or class II major histocompatibility antigens on the surface of antigen-presenting cells (APC). An optimum assay for T-cell reactivity would be extremely sensitive in detecting every person exposed to the causative *Borrelia* on the one hand, and highly specific in being positive only in people truly having had Lyme disease on the other hand. However, T-cell immune responses vary among different individuals and different microbial stimuli. The assay is further complicated by the large number of antigens in the *Borrelia* bacteria and their homology to similar antigens in other bacteria. Thus, the assay is designed to detect the majority of CMI-positive individuals while optimizing the specificity of a positive test.

The following assay is similar to those previously described.[10-12]

Peripheral blood

Heparinized peripheral blood is obtained from donors to be tested. Although freshly drawn blood is desirable, comparable results have been obtained using blood drawn up to 24 hours previously. If blood is shipped from another site, it should be transported at ambient temperature to avoid monocyte clumping, which occurs at temperatures around 4° C.

Lymphocyte proliferation

Mononuclear cells (MNC) are isolated as previously described[5] from the heparinized peripheral blood by Ficoll-Hypaque density sedimentation (Ficoll-Paque, Pharmacia, Piscataway, NJ). Proliferative responses are assessed by culturing MNC in RPMI-1640 (GIBCO, Grand Island, NY), 10% heat-inactivated human AB serum, and antibiotics (penicillin/streptomycin) in flat-bottomed, 96-well microtiter dishes. Cells are cultured at a density of 2×10^5 cells per well in the presence of antigens. Cultures are incubated for 7 days and 1 μCi per well of ^{3}H-thymidine is added for the last 16 hours of culture. Replicate cultures are done in quadruplicate, and results are expressed as mean values $\pm$ the standard deviations.

Several points should be made regarding the precise culturing conditions. First, the medium consists of 10% heat-inactivated human AB serum. The use of human serum results in substantially lower background proliferation than using xenogeneic serum such as fetal calf serum, which contains foreign antigens against which there are small T-cell responses. Human serum also provides higher stimulation with *Borrelia* or tetanus toxoid antigens. Second, much of the proliferation observed is due to recruitment of nonspecific T cells, not to the proliferation of the small number of *Borrelia*-specific cells activated within the first 4 days of incubation. Thus, cultures can be pulsed with ^{3}H-thymidine at either 5, 6, or 7 days. Six days was determined to be a point at which vigorous proliferation could be observed, but background stimulation remained low. Finally, although radioactive measurement of proliferation is convenient, other measures of proliferation such as the colorimetric method using the tetrazolium salt MTT[14] are equally valid.

B. burgdorferi antigens

The antigens used to assay for cell-mediated responses are critical. Fortunately, in Lyme disease the pathogenic organism is readily available, can be grown in liquid cultures, and can be isolated from different regions of the world.[1-3] However, *B. burgdorferi* is a bacteria, and high concentrations of this antigen are often stimulatory to MNC, either directly, through superantigens, or through cross-reactive antigens. Moreover, cultures of *Borrelia*, grown in rich medium,[1,32] are sometimes contaminated with nonborrelial organisms. This potentially further stimulates high background.

The most common laboratory-adopted strain of *B. burgdorferi* is B31 obtained from the ATCC (ATCC 35210, Rockville, MD). The *Borrelia* is grown at 32° C in BSK-II medium as previously described.[1,2] Different batches of the bacteria are screened in blastogenesis assays to determine which induces good responses in Lyme-immune donors but stimulates low backgrounds in nonimmune subjects. *Borrelia* are counted using darkfield phase contrast microscopy, resuspended in medium at 10^9 spirochetes per ml, and stored at $-70°$ C

Table 15–1 Proliferative response to increasing amount of whole *B. burgdorferi*

Donor	Medium	*B. burgdorferi* 2×10^4	2×10^5	2×10^6	TT*	PWM†
Control						
1	106‡	393	1,601	658	3,129	91,655
2	573	1,499	2,260	2,845	911	168,197
Lyme borreliosis						
1	385	121,378	67,063	24,502	7,135	222,535
2	279	31,484	42,828	15,949	3,418	145,678

*Tetanus toxoid used at 10 μg/ml.
†Pokeweed mitogen used at 1:200 dilution of stock.
‡Mean dpm of quadruplicate determinations.

until use. Other strains of spirochetes can be handled in a similar manner.

Proliferative responses are measured using a range of concentrations of *Borrelia*. MNC are cultured in flat-bottomed 96-well microtiter plates containing 200 μL per well of medium and whole *Borrelia* at concentrations of 10^5, 10^6, and 10^7 organisms per ml. Either whole *Borrelia* or sonicated *Borrelia* can be used. Of note, isolated soluble *Borrelia* proteins used in initial studies by some investigators proved to be a poor blastogenic stimulus when compared to whole or sonicated *Borrelia*.[11] When soluble and particulate antigens are compared in the same donor, particulate antigens are often 5 to 10 times more stimulatory.

Table 15–1 shows the proliferative responses of two seropositive donors with a history of EM. Also shown is the response of two normal, seronegative donors with no history of EM or an illness suggestive of Lyme disease. In addition, the responses to a recall antigen, tetanus toxoid, and a polyclonal mitogen, pokeweed mitogen, are shown for comparison. The mitogen response establishes the viability of the mononuclear cells being assayed. Pokeweed mitogen is used because it gives a sustained proliferative response measurable at 6 days when the cells are pulsed with thymidine in contrast to phytohemagglutinin, which gives peak proliferative responses at 2 days and falls off rapidly thereafter.

SPECIFICITY AND SENSITIVITY

Many antigenic structures are preserved among the various spirochetes and even among more distantly related bacteria.[15,17,27] Close homologies have been found in the flagella-associated spirochetal proteins[15,18,27,36] and in heat shock proteins from diverse sources.[17,26,33] The T-cell receptor recognizes small peptides in association with self HLA tissue antigens, and, as specific T cells proliferate in response to Lyme borreliosis, it is likely that some of the peptides that T cells recognize are shared among different microbial organisms. In addition, the T-cell repertoire is smaller than that of B cells, and the fine recognition may be less specific.

Table 15–2 shows the mean blastogenic response of four donors with a history of EM and specific serum antibodies indicative of previous *B. burgdorferi* exposure to different strains of *B. burgdorferi* (North American [B31 and IDS] and European [IRS]), along with responses to *B. hermsii*. Table 15–3 shows the response of four other Lyme donors to *Treponema pallidum* (all donors were negative for syphilis-specific serology). From these data, it is apparent that people immunized with *B. burgdorferi* also show a vigorous T-cell reactivity to other spirochetes. In individuals with syphilis and no known exposure to *B. burgdorferi*, a similar T-cell reactivity to both organisms is usually seen (data not shown). Thus, T-cell reactivity in Lyme disease shows similar cross-reactivity with other spirochetes as that seen with antibody tests that also cross-react strongly between spirochetes.[3,22,35]

Also shown in Table 15–2 is that different strains of *B. burgdorferi* may elicit varying blastogenic responses. The donors tested all contracted Lyme disease in the Northeast, the source of the two isolates, B31 and IDS (*Ixodes dammini* strain). These strains elicit the strongest proliferative re-

Table 15–2 T-cell responses to related *Borrelia*

Subject	Medium	B31	IDS	IRS	*B. hermsii*
Control	306*	470	658	454	886
Lyme disease					
(*n* = 4)	824	26,326	35,385	15,012	5,827

*Data represent mean ^{3}H-thymidine incorporation (dpm) (16-hr pulse at the end of incubation) of triplicate cultures incubated in the presence of 10^5 spirochetes/well for 6 days. MNC cultured at a density of 2×10^5/well.

Table 15–3 T-cell cross-reactivity between *B. burgdorferi* and *T. pallidum*

Donor	*B. burgdorferi*			*T. pallidium*		
	2×10^4	2×10^5	2×10^6	2×10^4	2×10^5	2×10^6
Control						
(*n* = 2)	459*	853	1,228	371	378	852
Lyme borreliosis						
(*n* = 4)	52,825	48,388	21,838	1,601	6,558	26,145

*Mean dpm of quadruplicate determinations.

sponse, whereas the European strain is less stimulatory and *B. hermsii* is the least potent antigen. *T. pallidum* also stimulates people with negative VDRL tests but who were previously infected with *B. burgdorferi*. This is shown in Table 15–3. Higher amounts of *T. pallidum* are required to stimulate peak MNC responses than *B. burgdorferi*, and the levels of response are substantially lower. Cross-reactivity is also seen in the opposite direction. MNC from people with positive syphilis serology often also have a blastogenic response to *B. burgdorferi* (unpublished data). In addition, because humans often carry commensal treponemes among their oral flora, previous oral infections may immunize individuals to spirochetal antigens and give a false-positive assay for CMI. Thus, spirochetes, in general, cross-stimulate CMI responses in Lyme-exposed individuals, and cross-stimulation against *B. burgdorferi* can be observed in patients infected with other spirochetes. The CMI is less specific and generally less sensitive than serologic assays being positive (SI > 20) in only approximately two thirds of seropositive donors.[12]

ONTOGENY AND PERSISTENCE OF T-CELL RESPONSES

Cell-mediated responses due primarily to T lymphocytes arise early in infection. As shown in Table 15–4, these responses are often evident at the time of EM rash, usually occurring 1 to 3 weeks after infection. In contrast, humoral responses mediated by B lymphocytes are typically negative at this point.[8,9,11,34] As infection proceeds, IgG antibody responses appear and T-cell responses persist. If antibiotic therapy is given early during the infection, the load of spirochetes is dramatically reduced and antibodies either never develop or disappear by 3 to 4 months after treatment. However, even doses of antibiotics insufficient to completely eradicate Lyme borreliosis can render the patient seronegative. A proportion of these inadequately treated patients clearly go on to chronic illness with frank arthritis or neurologic sequelae, although

these represent only a small minority of Lyme patients seen in endemic areas (1% to 3%). These patients often retain their CMI reactivity to *Borrelia* despite being seronegative.[12,21,37] These data are summarized in Table 15–4.

Given a history of an EM rash, early antibiotic exposure, and objective evidence of chronic disease consistent with Lyme disease, a positive CMI can confirm *Borrelia* exposure and provide a strong rationale for aggressive therapy. However, given a poor history of *B. burgdorferi* exposure or the absence of antibiotic therapy, even a positive CMI is unlikely to point to Lyme borreliosis as a diagnosis.

Both T- and B-cell responses persist after effective antibiotic therapy. Their persistence is often a function of the length of time a person was infected with *B. burgdorferi* before antibiotic therapy. Patients with more chronic infections generally have more persistent anti-*B. burgdorferi* antibody levels and more persistent T-cell responses after eradication of the infecting bacteria.

SUMMARY AND CONCLUSIONS

CMI responses after infection with *B. burgdorferi* are largely due to antigen-specific T cells and can be reliably measured. This observation has been confirmed in several laboratories.[13,21] Although a few reports have cited the lack of specificity and sensitivity of proliferative assays against *Borrelia*, these assays have, indeed, been characterized by poor responses in known patients and similar low-level responses in putative controls[38] and should not detract from the positive data in regard to lymphoproliferative assays reported by others.[12,13,21]

T-cell responses are observed early in infection, often at the EM rash stage preceding the development of specific antibodies, and generally persist for some time after therapy with antibiotics. A small percentage of people initially treated with inadequate levels of antibiotics may go on to develop chronic Lyme disease but typically have a negative serologic test for anti-*Borrelia* antibodies. These patients, especially those with persistent in-

Table 15–4 Ontogeny of T cell responses to *B. burgdorferi* infection

Donors	*n*	SI[†]	SEM[‡]	mean dpm[§]	Reference
			Borrelia* responses		
Negative control	17	3.1	0.5	2,932	Dattwyler et al[12]
EM	9	46.1	15.2	36,270	Volkman et al[33]
Seropositive Lyme	18	15.8	3.2	17,543	Dattwyler et al[12]
Seronegative Lyme	17	17.8	3.3	19,455	Dattwyler et al[12]

*Peak blastogenic responses to *B. burgdorferi* spirochete at 2×10^3 to 2×10^5.
†Stimulation index (dpm-stimulated)/(dpm-unstimulated).
‡Standard error of the mean.
§dpm-disintegration per minute.

fection, often retain their CMI responses, which can provide the sole objective evidence of *Borrelia* exposure.[12,21]

However, the measurement of CMI responses has several limitations. T-cell blastogenic responses to *B. burgdorferi* cross-react with other spirochetes, including *T. pallidum*. Thus, patients exposed to treponemes may also show T-cell responses to *B. burgdorferi*. Because of the bacterial nature of the antigen used in the Lyme CMI, background stimulation in normal, uninfected controls is also higher than that observed with simply protein antigens. These high backgrounds are observed especially at higher antigenic concentrations. Different cultures of *B. burgdorferi* also differ in their properties of inducing specific and nonspecific proliferation. Batches must be screened for low background and high specific stimulation.

A recent report claiming to show the lack of specificity of the *Borrelia* CMI assay[38] instead highlighted the pitfalls of CMI measurement and the importance of carefully selecting the nature and the concentration of the antigen used. These investigators could find no significant difference in the CMIs between Lyme disease patients and their normal controls using 10^6 organisms per microculture. Rather than investigating antigens and concentrations at which Lyme patients could be reliably distinguished from normal controls, for example, at the 2×10^4 concentration used in other studies,[11,12] the authors concluded that their assay was ambiguous.

Finally, a real drawback of assaying *Borrelia*-specific T-cell blastogenesis is that significant CMI responses are not as sensitive as antibody measurement in Lyme disease. In the absence of antibiotic therapy, more than 95% of individuals become seropositive within 6 weeks after a Lyme EM rash. In contrast, even in seropositive patients with chronic Lyme borreliosis, only approximately two thirds have CMIs significantly above control levels.[12]

The utility of the T-cell assay is twofold. First, CMI responses represent the only established method to indicate spirochete exposure in those rare patients with a history compatible with Lyme disease but whose early antibiotic exposure has rendered them seronegative. Hopefully, direct methods of documenting the presence of *B. burgdorferi* such as polymerase chain reaction (PCR) technology will be available in the future.[20] When used appropriately, the CMI method can provide useful information, but it can never replace the direct demonstration of the organism to document disease. Second, T-cell responses against whole *B. burgdorferi* and against constituent antigens can be readily measured. This allows investigators to determine which antigens elicit strong T-cell responses in natural infection and which peptides are most important in this response. The development of effective vaccines will depend on the ability to measure accurately these T-cell responses to candidate immunogens.

ACKNOWLEDGMENTS

This work was supported by Grant R01-AI 29008 from the United States Public Health Service.

REFERENCES

1. Barbour AG: Isolation and cultivation of Lyme disease spirochetes, *Yale J Biol Med* 57:521, 1984.
2. Barbour AG et al: Isolation of a cultivable spirochete from *Ixodes ricinus* ticks in Switzerland, *Curr Microbiol* 8:123, 1983.
3. Barbour AG et al: A *Borrelia*-specific monoclonal antibody binds to a flagellar epitope, *Infect Immun* 52:549, 1986.
4. Benach JL, Bosler EM, editors: Lyme disease and related disorders, *Ann NY Acad Sci* 539:1, 1988.
5. Böyum A: Isolation of mononuclear cells and granulocytes from human blood, *Scand J Clin Lab Invest* 21(Suppl 97):77, 1968.
6. Burgdorfer W et al: Lyme disease—a tick-borne spirochetosis? *Science* 216:1317, 1982.
7. Case definitions for public health surveillance, Lyme disease. *MMWR* 39:19, 1991.
8. Craft JE, Grodzicki RL, Steere AC: Antibody response in Lyme disease: evaluation of diagnostic tests, *J Infect Dis* 149:789, 1984.
9. Craft JE et al: Antigens of *Borrelia burgdorferi* recognized during Lyme disease. Appearance of a new immunoglobulin M response and expansion of the immunoglobulin G response late in the illness, *J Clin Invest* 78:934, 1986.
10. Dattwyler RJ et al: Cellular immune responses in Lyme disease, *Zentralbl Bakteriol Mikrobiol Hyg* 263:151, 1986.
11. Dattwyler RJ et al: Specific immune responses in Lyme borreliosis. Characterization of T cell and B cell responses to *Borrelia burgdorferi*, *Ann N Y Acad Sci* 539:93, 1988.
12. Dattwyler RJ et al: Seronegative Lyme disease: dissociation of specific T- and B-lymphocyte responses to *B. burgdorferi*, *N Engl J Med* 319:1441, 1989.
13. Dressler F, Yoshinari NH, Steere AC: The T-cell proliferative assay in the diagnosis of Lyme disease, *Ann Intern Med* 115:533, 1991.
14. Ferrari M, Fornasiero MC, Isetta AM: MTT colorimetric assay for testing macrophage cytotoxic activity in vitro, *J Immunol Methods* 131:165, 1990.
15. Gassman GS et al: Nucleotide sequence of a gene encoding the *Borrelia burgdorferi* flagellum, *Nucleic Acid Res* 17:3590, 1989.
16. Grodzicki RL, Steere AC: Comparison of immunoblotting and indirect enzyme-linked immunosorbent assay using different antigen preparations for diagnosing early Lyme disease, *J Infect Dis* 157:790, 1988.
17. Hansen K et al: Immunochemical characterization of and isolation of the gene for a *Borrelia burgdorferi* immunodominant 60-kilodalton antigen common to a wide range of bacteria, *Infect Immun* 56:2047, 1988.
18. Jiang W et al: Mapping the major antigenic domains of the native flagella antigen of *B. burgdorferi*, *J Clin Micro* (in press).
19. Kaell AT et al: Positive Lyme serology in subacute bacterial endocarditis: a study of four patients, *JAMA* 264:2916, 1990.

20. Keller TL, Halperin JJ, Whitman M: PCR detection of *B. burgdorferi* DNA in cerebrospinal fluid of Lyme neuroborreliosis patients, *Neurology* 42:32, 1992.
21. Krüger H et al: Long-term persistence of specific T- and B-lymphocyte responses to *B. burgdorferi* following untreated neuroborreliosis, *Infection* 18:263, 1990.
22. Luft BJ et al: Human B cell responses against immunodominant antigens of *Borrelia burgdorferi, Ann NY Acad Sci* 539:398, 1988.
23. Luger SW, Krauss E: Serologic tests for Lyme disease. Interlaboratory variability, *Arch Intern Med* 150:761, 1990.
24. Lyme disease—Connecticut, *MMWR* 15;37(1):1, 1988.
25. Pachner AR et al: Antigen-specific proliferation of CSF lymphocytes in Lyme disease, *Neurology* 35:1642, 1985.
26. Polla B: A role for heat shock proteins in inflammation? *Immunol Today* 9:134, 1988.
27. Pullesen L, Hindersson P: Cloning and sequencing of a *Treponema pallidum* gene encoding a 31.3 kilodalton endoflagellar subunit, FlaB2, *Infect Immun* 57:2166, 1989.
28. Rahn DW, Malawista SE: Lyme disease: recommendations for diagnosis and treatment, *Ann Intern Med* 114:472, 1991.
29. Schwartz BS et al: Antibody testing in Lyme disease. A comparison of results in four laboratories, *JAMA* 262:3431, 1989.
30. Sigal LH et al: Proliferative responses of mononuclear cells in Lyme disease. Reactivity to *Borrelia burgdorferi* antigens is greater in joint fluid than in blood, *Arthritis Rheum* 29:761, 1986.
31. Steere AC et al: Erythema chronicum migrans and Lyme arthritis, *Ann Intern Med* 86:685, 1977.
32. Steere AC et al: The spirochetal etiology of Lyme disease, *N Engl J Med* 308:733, 1983.
33. Van Eden W et al: Cloning of the mycobacterial epitope recognized by T-lymphocytes in adjuvant arthritis, *Nature (London)* 331:171, 1988.
34. Volkman DJ, Dattwyler RJ: Immunodiagnosis and treatment of Lyme borreliosis, *Resident & Staff Physician* 117:59, 1989.
35. Volkman DJ et al: Characterization of an immunoreactive 93 kd core protein of *B. burgdorferi* with a human IgG monoclonal antibody, *J Immunol* 146:3177, 1991.
36. Wallich R et al: The *Borrelia burgdorferi* flagellum-associated 41 kilodalton antigen (flagellin): molecular cloning, expression, and amplification of the gene, *Infect Immun* 58:1711, 1990.
37. Wilske B et al: Antigenic variability of *B. burgdorferi, Ann NY Acad Sci* 539:126, 1988.
38. Zoschke DC, Skemp AA, Defosse DL: Lymphoproliferative response to *B. burgdorferi* in Lyme disease, *Ann Intern Med* 114:285, 1991.

16 Nucleic Acid Detection of *Borrelia burgdorferi* Infection

Jesse L. Goodman

Because Lyme disease is difficult to diagnose, there is a great deal of interest in the potential role of newly developed nucleic acid amplification and detection techniques in the diagnosis of *Borrelia burgdorferi* infection. Although no such methodologies are presently of proven or practical diagnostic use, their promise remains great. The purpose of this chapter is to review these methodologies, the preliminary results available, and the potential uses of nucleic acid based strategies in improving both the diagnosis and understanding of Lyme disease.

The limitations of current standard diagnostic serologic tests for human Lyme disease have been discussed in other chapters (see Chapters 14 and 25). Problems include the common delay of up to several months after infection until seroconversion occurs, the blunting of antibody responses by appropriate antimicrobial therapy, false-positive tests due to apparent cross-reacting antigens, particularly in the presence of polyclonal B cell responses, and interlaboratory variation in testing. In addition, some people with later manifestations of Lyme disease may remain nonreactive in standard serologic testing. Finally, the full spectrum of manifestations of human Lyme disease is unknown, and it is possible that a variety of new or nonspecific manifestations could be related to *B. burgdorferi* infection, a concern often raised by both physicians and patients. Direct isolation of *B. burgdorferi* has been difficult due both to the complex growth requirements and slow growth of the organism, and, presumably, the low numbers of organisms present in biologic specimens. This combination of a variable serologic response with inability to cultivate the organism routinely has made the direct detection of spirochetal proteins or nucleic acids an area of interest. The detection of antigenic protein components of the spirochete is discussed elsewhere (see Chapter 17). This chapter reviews the preliminary literature concerned with detection of *B. burgdorferi* nucleic acids. Such methods can be roughly divided into those that use biologic samples

to attempt to detect existing nucleic acids directly by hybridization with a nucleic acid probe and other far more sensitive methods that use various amplification techniques to increase the amount of the chosen target sequence in the specimen.

DIRECT DETECTION OF *B. BURGDORFERI* NUCLEIC ACIDS

Direct detection methods have major advantages in terms of simplicity. The only requirements are that one have a probe able to hybridize to specific nucleic acid sequences of the target. Most often, this probe is cloned deoxyribonucleic acid (DNA) labeled with radioactive isotope, which is then hybridized to nucleic acids from the specimen, which were extracted and fixed to a membrane support. Such methods, unfortunately, are relatively insensitive, requiring thousands of target molecules for detection even with the most highly radiolabeled probe and have, therefore, in general, been useful only in studies in which relatively large numbers of infecting organisms are likely to be present. In such settings, direct hybridization may provide a more rapid method than culture. In addition to detection, genetic hybridization methods also offer potentially simpler or more specific identification of organisms. For such reasons, Schwan and Barbour[26] used cloned DNA fragments from the outer surface protein A (OspA) of *B. burgdorferi* as radiolabeled probes for detecting *Borrelia* nucleic acids affixed to membranes. Using <1-kb subclones from OspA, the authors were able to detect approximately ten thousand organisms. They noted weak cross-hybridization with *B. hermsii*, a causative agent of relapsing fever, and only weak hybridization with one German *B. burgdorferi* isolate. In a subsequent publication, the same laboratory reported using a 500-bp subclone from the same 49-kb linear plasmid encoding OspA, which hybridized to 10 different *B. burgdorferi* strains without significant cross-hybridization to *B. hermsii*.[28] In addition, using a larger subclone from the 49-kb plasmid that cross-hybridized to both *B.*

hermsii and *B. parkeri*, the authors were able to detect approximately 3000 spirochetes. Simpson et al[29] also examined the specificity of hybridization using cloned sequences from multicopy supercoiled plasmids of *B. burgdorferi* and identified repeated DNA sequences specific for *B. borgdorferi*. Finally, in the process of developing a DNA amplification assay, our laboratory cloned a chromosomal sequence of *B. burgdorferi*, Ly-1, and studied its use as a probe in direct hybridization.[6] This 3.7-kb clone specifically detected from 10 to 100 pg of *B. burgdorferi* DNA corresponding to approximately 5,000 to 50,000 spirochetes.

In summary, probes useful for direct hybridization of *B. burgdorferi* have been developed and can be used to detect directly thousands of spirochetes. Such numbers of spirochetes are unlikely to be present in most obtainable diagnostic specimens although such direct hybridization assays might be adaptable to detect high copy number ribonucleic acid (RNA) sequences. The development of newer techniques that amplify extremely small numbers of target sequences before their detection has provided a new impetus to efforts of molecular detection of *B. burgdorferi*.

NUCLEIC ACID AMPLIFICATION
Overview of the polymerase chain reaction

The best characterized nucleic acid amplification technique is the polymerase chain reaction (PCR). The basic PCR procedure is illustrated in Fig. 16–1. The reaction requires knowledge of flanking DNA sequences defining opposite ends of a fragment in the target DNA or RNA. Synthetic oligonucleotides complementary to these sequences are used to anneal to opposite ends of the target sequence and serve as primers for new DNA synthesis. The target, usually, as on the right hand side of Fig. 16–1, a double-stranded DNA sequence, is melted into its single strands, usually at 95° C *(A)*. This reaction is carried out in a mixture containing an excess of the synthetic oligonucleotide primers, which then anneal to opposite ends of the target sequence on both disassociated strands as the reaction is cooled *(B)*. These short stretches of reassociated double-stranded DNA provide a template for a thermostable DNA polymerase to synthesize, from nucleotides contained in the solution, a new strand complementary to the DNA for the fragment defined *(C)*. The temperature of annealing (step B) critically affects the specificity of binding. Thus, at temperatures near the temperature for disassociation of perfectly matched oligonucleotide sequences, binding is highly specific and only perfectly matched target DNA will bind to primers. At lower temperatures, binding may occur with partially mismatched DNA reducing the specificity

of the priming. Typical temperatures for annealing range from 37° C to 72° C depending on the sequence and the specificity of annealing desired. Traditionally, the PCR contains a separate third step (C) during which the temperature is raised to 72° C, optimal for the function of the heat stable Taq DNA polymerase to act in extending the newly synthesized strand. However, it may be possible for annealing and extension steps to be combined and performed at the same temperature. In any event, the net result of binding of primers to the original two strands of the target DNA molecule and the action of Taq polymerase in synthesizing complementary strands is to provide, at the end of the synthesis step, a doubling of the number of DNA strands initially present. This cycling process is repeated with melting of the two copies into four DNA strands (D), annealing of additional primers to those strands (E), and synthesis of an additional four complementary strands (F), yielding four double-stranded molecules at the end of the second cycle. Repetitive thermal cycling is generally performed in a computer-controlled, automated heating and cooling block, usually from 25 to 40 times, providing a theoretical amplification power from an initial single target molecule to over a billion molecules after 30 cycles. Although a number of factors contribute to a reduction in the efficiency of the PCR reaction, including a plateauing of amplification at high target levels, greater than a millionfold amplifications of single molecules can be routinely achieved, resulting in a final quantity of amplified product that is usually detectable by traditional methods such as gel electrophoresis and hybridization.[24]

It is also possible to use PCR-based technologies to amplify and detect a specific RNA target in a sample. The detection of RNA has potential advantages and unique uses. First, in the cases of either mRNAs of actively transcribed genes or of structural ribosomal RNAs, there may be hundreds to thousands of copies present per organism as compared to a single DNA copy, potentially greatly facilitating detection. In addition, detecting active RNA expression allows one to ascertain viability of an organism and study expression of specific genes. Potential problems with RNA detection include the relatively high lability and susceptibility of RNA to environmentally ubiquitous nucleases and the possibility that active gene expression may not be present in all infections and/or tissues. A typical approach to using PCR to detect RNA is shown in the left-hand portion of Fig. 16–1. In an initial reverse transcriptase (RT) reaction, the RT enzyme is primed with a properly oriented primer and catalyzes the synthesis of a DNA strand complementary to the RNA target. This reaction con-

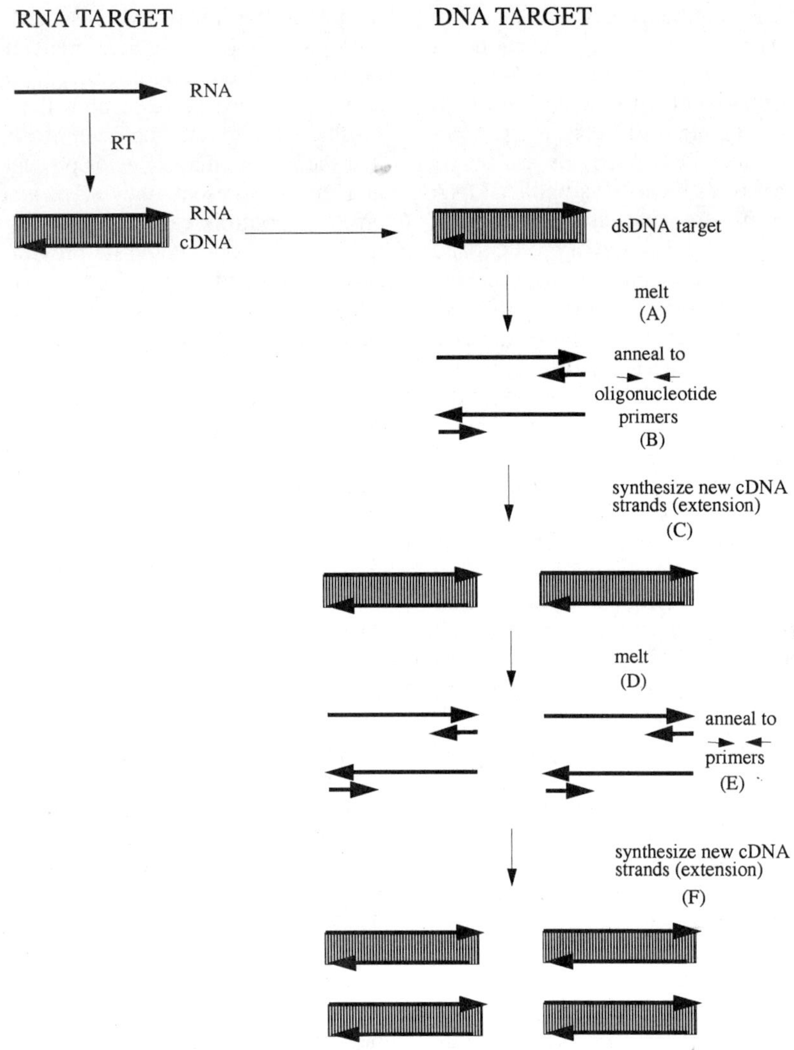

Figure 16–1 Schematic representation of the polymerase chain reaction (PCR) for DNA (right) and for RNA (reverse transcriptase [RT] PCR, left).

taining the newly synthesized complementary DNA molecule is then subjected to the DNA PCR as described.

PCR problems and potential solutions

To interpret and evaluate studies that use PCR methodologies, it is helpful to understand some of the more common problems that may arise.

False positive results. The most serious problem is in the technique's power to detect only one copy not only of real target (true positive) but also of contaminating DNA or RNA (false positive) in a specimen. Thus, if a laboratory grows the organism in question, has cloned its DNA, or uses high positive controls, contamination of samples becomes likely. The PCR process causes contamination problems by routinely generating millions of copies of newly synthesized target sequence, called "amplicons," which may contaminate and be detected in subsequent PCR reactions. For example, if 10^7 amplicons were present in one 100-μl reaction tube of amplified DNA, only 1 μl would contain 10^5 copies of a perfectly matched sequence, any one of which could result in a false-positive PCR if inadvertently added to subsequent reactions. Thus, if $1/10^5$ μl of sample were to be spread by contact or aerosolization to a subsequent PCR reaction, a false-positive could occur. This type of problem has led to almost universal difficulties with contamination in laboratories using the PCR when methods of detection have been optimized to detect very low copy numbers. It is critical that multiple negative controls containing no added target sequences be processed and subjected to amplification similarly to and simultaneously with any clinical samples. This allows the detection of contamination but will not eliminate the problem. It also is critical that laboratories practicing PCR employ complete separation of areas where samples are processed and PCR reactions are set up (pre-PCR) from areas where either amplified DNA or target organisms are present (post-PCR).[13] Along with this physical separation of pre-PCR and post-PCR events, the use of pipettes with disposable pistons and tips or aerosol barrier tips is essential. In addition, a number of specific methods have recently been devised to help control the amplicon problem. Ultraviolet (UV) radiation of the reaction tubes before addition of target samples generally eliminates low-level contamination of reaction components,[25] but, because the target must be added to the tube after UV treatment, this may not totally eliminate contamination. Other methods focus on modification of amplicons so that they cannot be reamplified in subsequent reactions. One available approach is the incorporation of dUTP into the PCR product and subsequent modification with the enzyme UNG to produce a nonamplifiable template. Another method performs PCR in the presence of psoralens compounds followed by UV treatment to produce sufficient damage to the DNA product to preclude further amplification.[11] Such approaches hold great promise in reducing the problem of amplicon contamination.

In addition to false-positive results due to contamination, false-positivity may occur due to amplification of nucleic acid sequences from other organisms or human DNA that share enough homology to anneal to the PCR primers used. Gel electrophoresis to demonstrate a proper sized amplified product and hybridization of the product to an internal oligonucleotide probe can add a great deal of specificity to the results, and such controls are essential in the characterization of new PCR assays.

False-negative results. Although false-positive results are the most obvious problem in PCR, failure to detect a microbial pathogen may also occur despite the presence of nucleic acids from the organism in the original sample. DNA or RNA may actually be lost during sample preparation procedures such as extraction. The most common reason for false-negative results is, however, the presence of substances that inhibit the PCR. Such inhibitors have been found in a variety of tissues and fluids, most notably blood and urine. Therefore, direct PCR on these materials often yields false-negatives, and careful attention to sample preparation is required. Nucleic acid extraction procedures using organic solvents or chaotropic agents reduce this problem but may not always eliminate it. The

nature of the inhibitory substances involved and the optimization of sample preparation methodologies for different biologic specimens are undefined. Thus, before assuming that negative PCR results are correct, one needs to be certain both that there were nucleic acids present in the sample and that, if present, they were amplifiable. Two types of controls can be employed. First, an unrelated gene that should be present in the sample can be amplified as a positive control. For example, it should be possible to amplify conserved human genes such as beta globin or actin from samples such as blood or urine normally containing cellular material. This controls for both the presence of target DNA in the sample (preparation) and for its ability to be amplified (inhibitors). The problem with this type of control is that sufficient human DNA may not always be present to amplify easily. Another type of control involves the actual addition to the sample of an excess of one of these conserved human molecules or of some unrelated target DNA for which effective PCR primers are available. Whatever approach is taken, such controls to rule out false-negatives are important before accepting a negative PCR study as definitive. A final source of apparent false-negatives is, instead, actually a failure of the primers used to detect the organism. This can occur as a result of unsuspected genetic diversity of the microorganism in which the sequences complementary to the primers are not sufficiently conserved. For example, in studies using OspA-based primers, *B. burgdorferi* isolates from geographically diverse sources have failed to be amplified.[21] This type of problem illustrates the importance of characterizing PCR primers well for their ability to amplify diverse isolates of *B. burgdorferi*.

Applications of PCR to detection of *B. burgdorferi* infection

General. A number of laboratories are involved in developing and using different primer and PCR systems for *B. burgdorferi*. These PCR systems have been characterized to various degrees with respect to their specificity and ability to amplify diverse *B. burgdorferi* strains. The published information and uses of the primer pairs are summarized in Table 16–1. A number of other PCR systems are becoming available, and publications should be forthcoming. It should be emphasized that few studies report optimizing parameters of the PCR reaction, which may be critical in determining sensitivity and specificity, most notably magnesium and primer concentrations. The target sequences used include those encoded on plasmids, such as OspA, and a variety of chromosomal sequences both from known genes such as flagellin,

Table 16–1 Published PCR primers for *B. burgdorferi:* characteristics and studies performed

Targets	Strains +/# tested	Sensitivity	Specificity*	Published use/results	Comments	Reference
Chromosomal						
Clone "2H1"	17/18	≤ 50 fg	− (Amplify Bh†)	None		23
"Derived strain G-2 se- quences"	31/31	ND	+	None	Study suggests 2 genetic classes of Bb†	22
Flagellin‡						
"Fla1" (121-149) "Fla3" (291-320)	ND	ND	− (Amplify other bor- relia)	Detection in pre- served ticks		20
"F1" (52-73), "F3" (823-842)	18/18	2-20 spirochetes	− (Amplify other bor- relia, Bb specific probe)	Detection in in- fected gerbils		14
16S rDNA (77-bp fragment locus not specified)	5/5 Bb 7/7 Bh	ND	− (Amplifies other borrelia, Bb spe- cific probe)	Detection in pre- served ticks		20
Clone "Ly-1"	9/9	≤ 5 spirochetes ≤ 10 fg		4/9 human urine + from "late" Lyme disease		6
Plasmid						
OspA‡						
"A1" (301-323) "A2" (929-946)	7/10 (− isolates from Germany, CA, NY)	ND	ND	None		20, 21
"A2" (301-323) "A4" (788-812)	ND	ND	ND	Detection of Bb in ticks	Equivalent to DFA§	20, 21
"SN1" (306-331) "SN2" (450-426)	1/1	50 fg	+	None		19
"Osp-A₁," (360- 385) "Osp-A₂" (640-688)	10/10‖	10 spirochetes	+	1/15 blood + from seroposi- tive dogs	? No DNA extrac- tion	17
"N1" (334-356), "N2" (362-381), "C1" (874-894), "C2" (693-713)#	5/5	ND	+	2/5 human EM sera +	No controls Nested primers for N1, N2	9

*Negative with *B. hermsii* +/− other organisms.
†Bh = *B. hermsii*, Bb = *B. burgdorferi*.
‡Nucleotide positions as in published OspA sequence[3] or flagellin sequence.[5]
§DFA = Direct fluorescent antibody microscopy.

‖No German strains tested.
#Internal nested primers.
ND = Not done, or not reported.

from DNA of unknown function, as well as from sequences encoding ribosomal RNA. A potential advantage of using plasmid encoded sequences would be if such sequences were present in high copy numbers per cell, but so far there is little evidence that this is the case for most *B. burgdorferi* plasmids. Another potential advantage would ensue if plasmid DNAs were shed in vesicles in vivo, a finding suggested by one immune electron microscopic study.[4] A potential disadvantage of plasmid-encoded sequences would occur if they were either highly variable among strains or not maintained stably either in ticks or during animal infection as compared with stable chromosomal sequences such as flagellin.[5] As mentioned, such instability is suggested by preliminary data concerning OspA. No definitive data suggest the superiority of one type or set of PCR primers. It may, therefore, be best for research studies to employ both plasmid and chromosomal targets and to, where possible, aim for detection of more than one target sequence. Unlike plasmid DNA, ribosomal RNAs should be present in high copy numbers and, if and when sensitive and specific primers are designed, may prove quite useful.

In addition to issues of primer choice and characterization, it is still unclear which sample types may be useful targets for nucleic acid amplification and during which manifestations of Lyme disease. It appears that spirochetemia sufficiently intense to yield positive blood cultures occurs in early Lyme disease, but uncommonly.[18] In addition, the few studies performed in animal models suggest that spirochetemia is usually a transient event early in infection.[7] Thus, although available data do not rule out the possibility that recurrent bouts of spirochetemia may occur, detection of bloodborne spirochetes may be most likely early in infection while skin rash and/or febrile symptoms are present. Given the known tropism of other spirochetes (for example, leptospires) for the urinary tract and the demonstration that infected mice[27] and hamsters[7] have persistent *B. burgdorferi* bladder infection, urine is a potential target for Lyme disease. There have also been preliminary observations of *B. burgdorferi* antigens in human urine.[4,10] Other obvious targets for gene amplification would include cerebrospinal fluid (CSF) in cases of neurologic involvement, joint fluid in arthritis, and, where indicated, skin and other tissue (for example, endomyocardium) biopsies. The organism has been cultivated commonly from skin lesions[2] as well as from some CSF samples, but rarely from joint fluid or other tissues. This may reflect low numbers of organisms, poor viability, and/or insensitive culture methods. Unfortunately, with the exception of blood and urine, such fluids and tissues are not often available from patients. Just as the best general methods for sample preparation for PCR have not been defined, optimal methods for concentrating and extracting organisms from body fluids are unknown. Despite such limitations in background information, efforts to define the frequency of body fluid or tissue involvement in human and animal infection are underway.

PCR in human and animal infections. Given the accessibility of urine as a diagnostic fluid, and the findings discussed above of persistent bladder infections in reservoir rodent hosts, our laboratory undertook PCR diagnostic studies on urine samples from humans with later manifestations of Lyme disease.[6] These studies were performed on frozen stored samples from a highly selected group of individuals believed by experienced clinicians to have Lyme disease. Nine patient and four control subject urines were evaluated using PCR with the Ly-1-based chromosomal primers. As shown in Fig. 16–2, a Southern transfer of an electrophoresed agarose gel hybridized to an internal oligonucleotide probe, strong positive signals were seen in samples from patients, 3, 7, and 10, and a faintly positive signal in patient sample 8. All positive signals were present in a repeated study. Thus, four

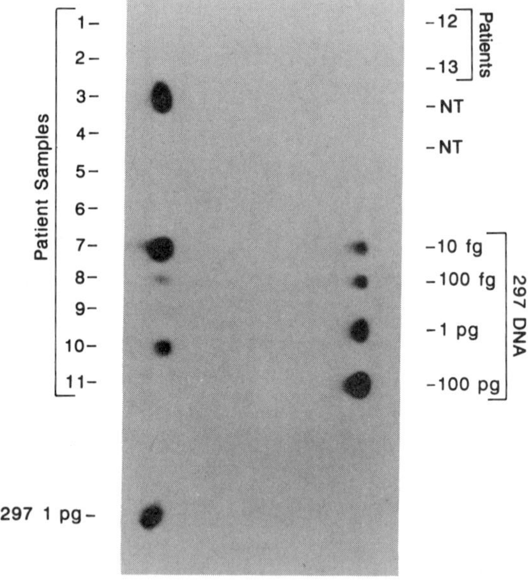

Figure 16–2 PCR-amplified products from Lyme disease and control patient urines (samples 1 through 13) and no target (NT) and positive controls (*B. burgdorferi* strain 297, 10 fg-100 pg). Southern hybridization to an internal oligonucleotide probe. (Reproduced from Goodman JL et al: Molecular detection of persistent *Borrelia burgdorferi* in the urine of patients with active Lyme disease, *Infect Immunol* 59:269, 1991, with permission of the American Society of Microbiology).

of nine patient samples were positive, but all six control PCR reactions (urine samples 2, 11, 12, and 13 and two PCR reaction tubes to which no target DNA was added [NT]) were negative. By extrapolation from the positive controls, we roughly estimated that from less than 50 to greater than 5000 genomes per milliliter may have been originally present in the positive patient urines. These PCR-positive patients were all either untreated or undertreated, from endemic areas, and had significant arthritic or neurologic findings. Furthermore, all were seroreactive, although one was borderline, by IgG ELISA. Three of the four had a subsequent complete response to appropriate antibiotic therapy, whereas one had chronic neurologic deficits that did not clearly respond. Of the five PCR-negative patients felt to have Lyme disease, four were clearly seropositive and one was borderline by IgG ELISA. These PCR-negative patients had already received appropriate intravenous antimicrobial therapy but, in four of five instances, had persistent symptoms. Although this study is preliminary and involved retrospectively collected and analyzed patient samples, it suggests that spirochetes or spirochetal fragments may be found in the urine of some patients with active later forms of Lyme disease.

Beyond this report, published data concerning studies of human samples are very limited. Guy and Stanek[9] recently reported performing PCR using OspA-based primers on five serum samples from people with erythema migrans. Two of five people had positive serum PCRs reported, but no controls are mentioned. A second round of PCR with internal "nested" primers was used, a procedure that may add sensitivity but is particularly likely to lead to contamination and false-positives. Another report, published as a letter,[12] noted detection of an amplified flagellin gene fragment from CSF of 5 of 6 patients with definite neuroborelliosis, but from 0 of 10 controls. Finally, Stephen Malawista of Yale University has found that the joint fluids from an unknown proportion of people with active synovitis who have clinical and serologic evidence for Lyme disease may be positive for *B. burgdorferi* DNA by PCR (unpublished data). Although exciting and promising, these initial human studies have involved retrospectively obtained and stored samples, have been performed nonblinded, and could not employ recently developed methods of rendering amplicons nonamplifiable. Therefore, the true sensitivity or specificity of such testing remains to be determined.

Animal studies are also preliminary. Lebech and colleagues[14] reported on the amplification of a portion of the flagellin gene from experimentally infected gerbils. They found that 21 of 24 (88%)

organs (kidney, spleen, or urinary bladder) from infected animals but none of 9 organs from uninfected animals were PCR positive. All 17 culture-positive and 4 of 7 culture-negative organs were PCR positive. Whether this reflects a greater sensitivity of PCR compared to culture or whether the PCR-positive, culture-negative samples may represent contamination is uncertain, but the results demonstrate that PCR can be used to detect *B. burgdorferi* in the tissues of infected animals with results at least comparable to culture. One other published PCR study involving animals has been reported. Malloy et al[17] used OspA primers on whole blood from 15 *B. burgdorferi* seropositive dogs and on urine from 2 of these dogs and found only one positive specimen (blood) among these 17 samples. These specimens apparently were not processed by extraction, and it is, therefore, possible that inhibitory substances interfered with the PCR. In addition, the specificity of canine serology is unclear, as reflected by a 50% or greater seropositivity rate even among asymptomatic canines in endemic areas.[16]

PCR in studies of vectors. The traditional way to establish whether ticks are carrying *B. burgdorferi* has been either to use immunofluorescence or to perform culture. The adaptation of PCR to studying ticks for infection with *B. burgdorferi*[20,21] has demonstrated a sensitivity of spirochete detection at least similar to an immunofluorescent assay. In addition, PCR has the advantage of not requiring the presence of viable organisms and can be performed on preserved specimens. Thus, archival tick specimens, stored in ethanol and saved in the Harvard Museum of Comparative Zoology and the Rocky Mountain Laboratory Collection of the Smithsonian Institute, could be examined for evidence of *B. burgdorferi*. Positive results were obtained from 13 of 97 *Ixodes dammini* specimens examined and suggested that *B. burgdorferi* was present in the United States at least 2 to 3 decades before the recognition of the clinical entity of Lyme disease.[20]

Other amplification methods

Although PCR is the best characterized method for gene amplification, there is an ongoing proliferation of other methods to allow detection of rare nucleic acid target sequences. For example, the transcript amplification system (TAS or 3SR, 8) uses either an RNA or DNA target to synthesize DNA intermediates that contain a promoter for T7 RNA polymerase. The intermediates are used as templates for synthesis of multiple RNA copies of the original molecule, which are again subjected to reverse transcription of new intermediary molecules. Potential specificity problems of the TAS exist as a result of the relatively low annealing temperature required to not inactivate currently available RNA polymerases. Other methods include the ligase chain reaction[1] involving multiple sequential ligations of immediately adjacent primers specifically bound to targets, and the Q-beta replicase system,[15] which uses a bacterial phage RNA polymerase coupled to a specific probe, which is then replicated after binding to target sequences. Additional methods to amplify or detect signals are under investigation but beyond the scope of this discussion. Both the PCR and other assays may potentially be adapted to automated formats using direct detection systems. Thus, if *B. burgdorferi* nucleic acids do prove to be useful markers for the diagnosis of Lyme disease and for monitoring clinical activity and response to treatment, there is great potential for the improvement, simplification, and development of such methods to allow their more economical, reproducible, and widespread use.

SUMMARY

Nucleic acid detection is a promising potential addition to the diagnostic and research armamentarium for Lyme disease. PCR-based methods can detect less than 10 *B. burgdorferi* organisms in biologic samples, and such detection can be carried out with a great deal of specificity. The extreme sensitivity of PCR can result in problems with false-positives. This problem can generally be controlled in a research laboratory by careful attention to controls and to laboratory technique. The application of PCR-based technology to clinically relevant issues in Lyme disease has been limited. Preliminary data indicate that PCR should be similar to or superior to culture for detecting *B. burgdorferi* in tissues of infected animals and in ticks. Such applications should be useful in studies of epidemiology and disease pathogenesis. Initial PCR studies in humans suggest that some patients with active Lyme disease may have amplifiable nucleic acids present in blood, CSF, and urine. Because sensitivity and specificity of such assays on clinical materials in various stages of Lyme disease remain undetermined, gene amplification testing for Lyme disease is currently a research technique only. When data from prospective blinded studies become available, PCR and other developing techniques for amplifying and detecting rare DNA and RNA molecules may play a useful role in diagnosis and treatment monitoring in selected clinical settings.

REFERENCES

1. Barany F: Genetic disease detection and DNA amplification using cloned thermostable ligase, *Proc Natl Acad Sci* 88:189, 1991.
2. Berger BW et al: Cultivation of *Borrelia burgdorferi* from erythema migrans lesions and perilesional skin, *J Clin Microbiol* 30:359, 1992.
3. Bergstrom S, Bundoc VG, Barbour AG: Molecular analysis of linear plasmid-encoded major surface proteins, OspA and OspB, of the Lyme disease spirochaete *Borrelia burgdorferi*, *Molec Micro* 3:479, 1989.
4. Dorward DW, Schwan TG, Garon CF: Immune capture and detection of *Borrelia burgdorferi* antigens in urine, blood, or tissues from infected ticks, mice, dogs, and humans, *J Clin Microbiol* 29:1162, 1991.
5. Gassmann GS et al: Nucleotide sequence of gene encoding the *Borrelia burgdorferi* flagellin, *Nucleic Acids Res* 17:3590, 1989.
6. Goodman JL et al: Molecular detection of persistent *Borrelia burgdorferi* in the urine of patients with active Lyme disease, *Infect Immun* 59:269, 1991.
7. Goodman JL et al: Persistent cardiac and urinary tract infections with *Borrelia burgdorferi* in experimentally infected Syrian hamsters, *J Clin Microbiol* 29:894-896, 1991.
8. Guatelli JC et al: Isothermal, *in vitro* amplication of nucleic acids by a multienzyme reaction model after retroviral replication, *Proc Natl Acad Sci USA* 87:1874, 1990.
9. Guy EC, Stanek G: Detection of *Borrelia burgdorferi* in patients with Lyme disease by the polymerase chain reaction, *J Clin Pathol* 44:610, 1991.
10. Hyde FW et al: Detection of antigens in urine of mice and humans infected with *Borrelia burgdorferi*, etiologic agent of Lyme disease, *J Clin Microbiol* 27:58, 1989.
11. Isaacs ST et al: Post-PCR sterilization: development and application to an HIV-1 diagnostic assay, *Nucleic Acids Res* 19:109, 1990.
12. Jaulhac B et al: Detection of *Borrelia burgdorferi* in cerebrospinal fluid of patients with Lyme borreliosis, *N Engl J Med* 324:1440, 1991.
13. Kwok S, Higuchi R: Avoiding false positives with PCR, *Nature* 339:237, 1989.
14. Lebech AM et al: Comparison of *in vitro* and polymerase chain reaction for detection of *Borrelia burgdorferi* in tissue from experimentally infected animals, *J Clin Microbiol* 29:731, 1991.
15. Lizardi PM et al: Exponential amplification of recombinant-RNA hybridization probes, *Bio/Tech* 6:1197, 1988.
16. Magnarelli LA et al: Clinical and serologic studies of canine borreliosis, *JAVMA* 191:1089, 1987.
17. Malloy DC, Nauman RK, Paxton H: Detection of *Borrelia burgdorferi* using the polymerase chain reaction, *J Clin Microbiol* 28:1089, 1990.
18. Nadelman RB et al: Isolation of *Borrelia burgdorferi* from the blood of seven patients with Lyme disease, *Am J Med* 88:21, 1990.
19. Nielson SL, Young KKY, Barbour AG: Detection of *Borrelia burgdorferi* DNA by the polymerase chain reaction, *Mol Cell Probes* 4:73, 1990.
20. Persing DH et al: Detection of *Borrelia burgdorferi* DNA in museum specimens of *Ixodes dammini* ticks. *Science* 249:1420, 1990.
21. Persing DH et al: Detection of *Borrelia burgdorferi* in *Ixodes dammini* ticks with the polymerase chain reaction, *J Clin Microbiol* 28:566, 1990.
22. Rosa PA, Hogan D, Schwan TG: Polymerase chain reaction analyses identify two distinct classes of *Borrelia burgdorferi*, *J Clin Microbiol* 29:524, 1991.
23. Rosa PA, Schwan TG: A specific and sensitive assay for the Lyme disease spirochete *Borrelia burgdorferi* using the polymerase chain reaction, *J Infect Dis* 160:1018, 1989.
24. Saiki RK et al: Primer-directed enzymatic amplification of DNA with a thermostable DNA polymerase, *Science* 239:487, 1987.

25. Sarkar G, Sommer SS: Shedding light on PCR contamination, *Nature* 343:27, 1990.
26. Schwan TG, Barbour AG: Efficacy of nucleic acid hybridization probes for the detection and identification of *Borrelia burgdorferi*, *Ann NY Acad Sci* 539:419, 1988.
27. Schwan T et al: The urinary bladder, a consistent source of *Borrelia burgdorferi* in experimentally infected white-footed mice, *(Peromyscus leucopus)*, *J Clin Microbiol* 26:893, 1988.
28. Schwan TG et al: Identification of *Borrelia burgdorferi* and *B. hermsii* using DNA hybridization probes, *J Clin Microbiol* 26:1734, 1989.
29. Simpson WJ, Garon CF, Schwan TG: *Borrelia burgdorferi* contains repeated DNA sequences that are species specific and plasmid associated, *Infect Immun.* 58:847, 1990.

Antigen Detection and Cerebrospinal Fluid Studies

P. K. Coyle

ANTIGEN DETECTION

Lyme disease stands in distinction to most human infections because it is extremely difficult to stain, isolate, or culture the pathogenic organism from infected body fluids and organs.[3,21,72] The diagnosis of Lyme disease is primarily a clinical one, with supportive laboratory data. The diagnosis is made when a patient shows a consistent clinical picture, in the setting of probable exposure to the etiologic agent. Exposure is generally documented by detection of specific antibodies to *Borrelia burgdorferi*. Unfortunately, there are certain problems with current antibody tests.[32,42,44,68] It is also true that detection of such antibodies only indicates that the host's immune system has been exposed to *B. burgdorferi* at some time in the past. Specific antibodies do not indicate that viable spirochetes are still present with active infection.

A better test to verify true active infection would be to look for specific *B. burgdorferi* components. Two approaches involve detection of spirochetal nucleic acids (by way of polymerase chain reaction [PCR] testing) and detection of spirochetal antigens. There is both in vitro and in vivo evidence that the *B. burgdorferi* spirochete sheds surface membrane vesicles or "blebs," which contain DNA as well as surface-associated proteins.[4,24] Such proteins could provide a source of *B. burgdorferi* antigens within various body fluid compartments. This section reviews the studies that have been carried out in this area, as well as the potential role of antigen detection in Lyme disease.

Antigen assays

B. burgdorferi antigens have been detected in the blood, cerebrospinal fluid (CSF), and urine of both humans and animals.[5,14,17,23,34] A variety of tests have been used, including several types of enzyme-linked immunosorbent assay (ELISA), Western (immuno) blot, and electron microscopy (Table 17–1). The antigens detected have included the 41-kD flagellin, which is a major spirochetal protein but one that is not *B. burgdorferi*-specific, as well as the 31-kD outer surface protein A (OspA),

the 34-kD outer surface protein B (OspB), and an 83-kD membrane vesicle-associated protein. These latter proteins are *B. burgdorferi*-specific, although not all organism strains express OspB.

In the first report of successful detection of *B. burgdorferi* antigens, monoclonal antibodies were used in a Western immunoblot assay to stain OspA in the urine of infected hamsters.[5] Animals were infected by intraperitoneal injection of spirochetes, and urine was collected at multiple time points over the next 3 days. Urine was found to contain intact OspA during the entire 3-day period. The authors interpreted their data as consistent with the OspA antigen being shed into urine, rather than representing a breakdown product of the organism. This would go along with the very high frequency of persistent bladder infection that occurs when animals are experimentally inoculated with *B. burgdorferi*.[25] The authors speculated that detection of antigen might prove diagnostically useful for human Lyme disease.

A subsequent study looked at urine samples collected from patients with early and late Lyme disease, as well as from mice that had been experimentally infected with *B. burgdorferi*.[34] Monoclonal antibodies to OspA, OspB, and flagellin were used to examine urine proteins in a standard Western blot assay, as well as a dot blot ELISA. In the dot blot ELISA, urine proteins were first vacuum concentrated onto nitrocellulose membranes within microtiter wells. Urine was probed with the monoclonal antibodies, followed by enzyme-conjugated anti-mouse antibodies. The assay was developed and read as a typical ELISA. *B. burgdorferi* antigens were detected in the urines collected from 10 patients with early and late Lyme disease, but not from 10 urines collected from normal controls. The authors note that several Lyme disease patients had negative urines, but the total number of urines screened was not reported. Reactivity for urine antigens was found to be highly variable. A urine specimen might be positive for one, two, or all three spirochetal antigens. No correlation was noted between serum antibody titer to

Table 17–1 Assays used to detect *B. burgdorferi* antigens in body fluids

Technique	Body fluid	Antigen
Dot blot ELISA[34]	Urine (human, hamster, mouse)	OspA, OspB, flagellin
ELISA[14]	CSF (human)	OspA, OspB, flagellin
	Urine (human)	
Fluorescent ELISA	Urine (human)	OspA, OspB
Immune electron microscopy[17]	Blood (mouse)	Extracellular membrane
	Urine (human, dog, mouse)	vesicles
Western blot[5,14,23,34]	CSF (human)	OspA, OspB, flagellin
	Urine (human, hamster, mouse)	OspA, OspB, flagellin

B. burgdorferi and detectable urine antigens. With regard to the infected mice, OspA was detected in urine by dot blot ELISA as far out as 22 days postinfection. No later time points were examined.

In another study that looked at central nervous system (CNS) invasion by *B. burgdorferi,* monoclonal antibodies to OspA and OspB were used in a Western blot assay to probe human CSF samples.[23] The CSF was collected from five Lyme disease patients with early infection. All five patients had erythema migrans (EM) and were symptomatic with mild headache, stiff neck, and fever. All were seronegative in both CSF and blood, but were subsequently documented to develop anti-*B. burgdorferi* antibodies in convalescent serum. Three of the five CSF samples contained *B. burgdorferi* antigens.

In a later study, membrane vesicles released from *B. burgdorferi* grown in vitro were used to generate polyclonal antibodies from immunized rabbits.[17] These antibodies were affinity purified, the nonspecific Fc portion was removed, then they were coated onto electron microscope grids. The grids were incubated with urine and blood samples from Lyme disease patients and infected animals, to allow the antibodies to capture any antigens present in the samples. Bound *B. burgdorferi* antigens were probed using polyclonal antibodies to an 83-kD major extracellular protein band purified from the vesicles. These polyclonal antibodies appear to react to OspA and OspB, as well as to IgM. Flocculent antigen material was ultimately detected by electron microscopic inspection using a gold probe. Using this assay, 38 of 39 urines from Lyme disease patients were reported to contain antigenic material. Although patient histories were not detailed, the urine samples were probably collected from patients with early and late infections. Samples collected from animals infected with *B. burgdorferi* were also looked at. All urine and blood samples from mice were said to be positive, as was urine from an infected dog.

In a recent report, OspA, OspB, and flagellin were found in human CSF collected from patients infected with *B. burgdorferi* who had neurologic problems.[14] Antigens were measured using double-sandwich antigen capture ELISA and Western blot. In the ELISA, monoclonal antibodies were used to capture antigen. Bound antigens were detected using F(ab')$_2$ rabbit polyclonal antibodies against whole spirochete. By ELISA, 38 of 77 (49%) CSF specimens from *B. burgdorferi*-infected patients were positive compared to 1 of 34 (3%) control CSF. Western blot was positive for antigen in 12 of 22 (55%) CSF from *B. burgdorferi*-infected patients, compared to 0 of 11 CSF from control patients. Antigens were present in CSF from Lyme patients with both early and late infections, including some patients who had been treated with antibiotics but continued to have persistent neurologic problems.

There is one commercially available urine antigen test (3M FASTLYME urine antigen test, 3M Diagnostic Systems Inc., Calif), but its use is restricted to investigational purposes. The commercial test involves a competitive inhibition ELISA, in which sample is first incubated with enzyme-conjugated anti-OspA and OspB antibodies. The sample is tested for unbound antibody, with the generated fluorescent signal from a specimen inversely proportional to its amount of antigen. This commercial assay is under evaluation and has not yet been published in the scientific literature.

Clinical applications

The finding of detectable antigen in the body fluids of Lyme disease patients makes empiric sense. Experimental and human studies document that *B. burgdorferi* is capable of producing prolonged infections in a variety of body organs, including the brain, heart, and bladder.[23,25,53,67,71] Despite a paucity of resident spirochetes in such infected tissue, studies suggest that spirochetes may slough OspA, a major and unique *B. burgdorferi* protein, from their surfaces.[4] Membrane blebs, which contain OspA and OspB proteins, may also be continually released by the organisms.[24] Shedding of these components into adjacent body fluids such as CSF, urine, or blood would provide a continuing source of antigen. Antigen detection has proven useful for a number of human infections. Generally, detection of antigen in blood is more problematic than other body fluids because of the variety of extraneous factors that may interfere with the detection test. CSF and urine are often easier fluids to work with than blood because they are less likely to produce interference. CSF antigen detection has been used in bacterial meningitis (for agents such as *H. influenzae,* meningococcus, and pneumococcus),[27,37] viral infections (for detection of p24 HIV-1 antigen),[18] and fungal infections (for detection of cryptococcal and histoplasma polysaccharide antigens).[26,81] Urine antigen detection has been used in a variety of human infections involving *Chlamydia, Histoplasma, Legionella,* and *Plasmodium falciparum* (malaria).[39,65,69,85]

The presence of antigen does not always indicate viable organisms. After treatment, there is likely to be a lag period during which pieces of degraded killed organisms are released from sequestered tissue. As an example, cryptococcal antigen may remain present for some time after treatment despite negative cultures and negative stains, and antigen detection per se is not necessarily considered an indication for continuing antifungal treatment.[11] However, it is likely that the prolonged presence of antigen does reflect a persistent infection.

Current diagnostic role

Antigen detection tests, although promising, cannot be used to diagnose or manage Lyme disease patients. Reagents are not standardized, sufficient numbers of patients and controls have not been critically looked at, sample and assay parameters have not been optimized, and even the true significance of detectable antigens has not been determined. The urine-based commercial antigen test should only be used experimentally along with antibody results to gather data. Other antigen assays are available only in specialized research laboratories. More studies are needed to determine whether antigen detection in body fluids will prove sufficiently sensitive and economically feasible to play an important role in the diagnosis and management of Lyme disease.

CEREBROSPINAL FLUID STUDIES

The CSF compartment consists of 120 to 150 ml of fluid contained in the subarachnoid and intraventricular spaces.[20] CSF is made continuously,

circulates within and around the brain and spinal cord, and then drains into the blood system. The entire volume of CSF is completely regenerated four times daily, so that the 10 to 20 ml removed during standard lumbar puncture are regenerated within an hour. Normal CSF parameters are well known (Table 17–2). Conditions such as diabetes mellitus or spinal disk disease produce an increase in CSF protein, so that such associated medical disorders in a given person need to be taken into account when evaluating their CSF results. The normal CSF parameters also change somewhat for the extremes of age. In neonates, for example, normal CSF appearance, cell count, protein, and glucose ranges differ from those of children and adults.[27] However, most cases of suspected Lyme disease occur beyond the neonatal period, and the values in Table 17–2 can be applied to analyze CSF results.

CSF is in direct contact with the extracellular brain microenvironment as well as the outer and inner surfaces of the brain and its lining meninges. When these areas are involved in a generalized inflammatory process such as infection, CSF is usually abnormal. Except in instances when there is a focal brain lesion (such as abscess), CSF should be routinely obtained when a neurologic infection is suspected. Meningitis, which involves inflammatory cells infiltrating meninges, typically produces high CSF cell counts. As a rule, bacterial infections result in a neutrophil pleocytosis, and viral infections result in a mononuclear (lymphocyte, monocyte) pleocytosis. CSF glucose is usually unaffected by viral infections but is decreased by bacterial infections. All neurologic infections tend to increase CSF protein due to blood-brain barrier damage. Increased CSF pressure may occur with infection but is a nonspecific abnormality. When the neurologic infection primarily involves brain or spinal cord parenchyma (encephalitis or myelitis) rather than the meninges, the increase in CSF cells is much more variable. Infections of the peripheral nerve or muscle do not produce any CSF changes. The one exception is when there is involvement of spinal nerve roots. This area is close enough to the CSF compartment that a significant inflammatory process will affect CSF parameters.

CSF abnormalities in European Lyme disease

There is an extensive literature on CSF changes in neurologic Lyme disease.* However, these reports are based on European cases. European strains of *B. burgdorferi* differ from North American strains. They appear to be more neurotropic. In contrast to the United States, European Lyme disease is

---

*References 1, 2, 8, 30, 31, 33, 46, 66, 70, 76, 79, 82.

Table 17–2 Normal CSF parameters

CSF studies	Normal values
Routine studies	
WBC count (cells/mm³) and differential	≤5 (85% lymphocytes, 15% neutrophils)
Protein (mg/dl)	15-45
	30-60 (over age 60)
Glucose (mg/dl)	45-80 (0.6 of blood glucose)
Pressure (mm)	≤200
Frequent studies	
Cultures	No growth
Cytology	Scattered WBC
IgG index; intrathecal IgG production (mg/day)	≤0.7; <3.3
Oligoclonal bands	Negative
Stains (acid fast, Gram's, India ink)	Negative
VDRL	Nonreactive
Occasional studies	
Myelin basic protein	Negative
Specific antibodies	± (Proportionate to serum levels)
Intrathecal production of specific antibodies	Absent
Specific antigens	Negative

mainly neurologic. The most frequent neurologic involvement seen in Europe is Bannwarth's syndrome or lymphocytic meningoradiculitis.[33,66] This syndrome is associated with marked CSF inflammatory changes in virtually 100% of patients. These changes include a mononuclear pleocytosis; intrathecal IgG, IgM, and IgA production; intrathecal production of specific anti-*B. burgdorferi* antibodies, including IgG, IgM, and IgA antibodies; oligoclonal IgG and IgM bands; and elevated protein. The pleocytosis includes plasma cells as well as lymphocytes and monocytes. Cell count averages around 100 to 300 cells/mm³ but may be over a thousand. Protein averages around 135 mg/dl but may be as high as 1300. In some European patients, anti-*B. burgdorferi* antibodies have been detected in CSF even though blood serology was negative.[76] Despite treatment and clinical recovery, CSF oligoclonal bands may persist for at least 16 months.[30] Intrathecal antibody production (particularly IgG) also may persist for prolonged periods even after successful treatment.[31] When examined in vitro, CSF cells from patients are continuing to secrete anti-*B. burgdorferi* antibodies for many months despite antibiotic treatment.[1] The marked CSF inflammatory changes are not confined to Bannwarth's syndrome but are also seen in late encephalomyelitis cases and patients with unusual syndromes attributed to their *B. burgdorferi* infection.* Even patients with isolated Bell's palsy show a high incidence of CSF abnormalities.[7,51,64] In fact,

the European literature suggests that neurologic Lyme disease is almost always accompanied by CSF changes.[30,31,46,70]

Despite this almost universal association with inflammatory changes, there have been occasional European cases where *B. burgdorferi* has been cultured from noninflammatory CSF.[57-59] However, this is clearly exceptional, and most neurologic Lyme disease patients reported from Europe have CSF abnormalities that may be quite marked. It is important to keep in mind that this European experience, which makes up an extensive part of the literature on Lyme disease, is somewhat different from the North American experience.[41]

Indications for lumbar puncture

CSF should be examined as part of the evaluation for suspected neurologic Lyme disease. Because it is not known how often silent seeding of the CNS occurs in Lyme disease, and because peripheral and central neurologic involvement may coexist, even patients with purely peripheral nervous system syndromes should probably have CSF studies. In addition, patients with known Lyme disease, but without obvious neurologic involvement, should undergo lumbar puncture if they have headache or stiff neck. There are three main reasons to look at CSF: to aid diagnosis, to determine therapy, and to document baseline abnormalities. Infection with *B. burgdorferi* may be asymptomatic, and in endemic areas positive serologies are found in a significant proportion of the population. Abnormal CSF in a seropositive person helps confirm that a

---

*References 6, 38, 47-49, 78, 80, 83.

neurologic syndrome is due to *B. burgdorferi*, rather than an unrelated cause. Seeding of the CNS is also generally accepted as an indication for parenteral rather than oral antibiotic treatment. Isolated facial nerve (Bell's) palsy, for example, may be a peripheral or central neurologic manifestation of Lyme disease. Abnormal CSF in such a case would be an indication for parenteral antibiotics. Finally, documentation of the extent of CSF abnormalities provides a baseline from which subjective improvement may be confirmed by objective improvement in CSF. Abnormal CSF parameters should improve with therapy, although certain immune reactions may persist within the intrathecal compartment for years. Repeat CSF analysis becomes particularly critical when treated patients complain of persistent postinfectious problems that may or may not reflect ongoing infection. Documentation of normal CSF mitigates against an ongoing infection.

CSF diagnostic studies

The routine CSF studies indicated in Table 17–3 should be sent at the time of lumbar puncture for suspected neurologic Lyme disease. If more than one lumbar puncture is performed on a given patient, these routine studies should generally be repeated, with the exception of the VDRL. Once

Table 17–3 CSF tests for suspected Lyme disease

Routine studies
WBC count
Protein
Glucose
Pressure
Anti-*B. burgdorferi* antibodies
Intrathecal anti-*B. burgdorferi* antibody production (CSF Lyme antibody index)
VDRL
Intrathecal IgG production or IgG index
Oligoclonal bands
Cytology

Occasional studies
Cultures (bacterial, tuberculosis, fungal)
Cryptococcal antigen
Latex agglutination
Myelin basic protein
Stains (Gram's, acid fast, India ink)

Experimental studies
Specific and nonspecific immune complexes
B. burgdorferi antigens
B. burgdorferi nucleic acid (PCR)
B. burgdorferi cultures
Autoantibodies, autoreactive T cells

---

syphilis is ruled out as a confounding reason for false-positive Lyme serology, there is no need to repeat a CSF VDRL on subsequent spinal taps. The most helpful routine CSF study is intrathecal anti-*B. burgdorferi* antibody production (the CSF Lyme antibody index). Unfortunately, as discussed below, a number of patients do not show such antibody production, and a negative result cannot be used to rule out neurologic Lyme disease. Among these routine studies, abnormalities that particularly suggest Lyme disease include a mild mononuclear pleocytosis, a mildly increased protein concentration, and the presence of plasma cells on cytologic screening.

Occasionally, other CSF diagnostic studies need to be sent as well. When a meningitis patient is evaluated, it is important to rule out other infections with specific cultures, antigens, and staining studies. The release of myelin basic protein into CSF does not occur in Lyme disease but is often associated with acute relapses of multiple sclerosis.[12] This CSF study may be helpful in distinguishing multiple sclerosis from neurologic Lyme disease in a patient who presents with optic neuritis. Most multiple sclerosis patients show elevated IgG index and oligoclonal bands in their CSF, which are unusual findings in North American Lyme disease. They also typically lack intrathecal production of anti-*B. burgdorferi* antibodies.

The experimental CSF studies listed in Table 17–3 are not routinely available. CSF immune complexes have been reported in 70% of patients with neurologic syndromes attributed to *B. burgdorferi* infection.[13] This includes patients with classic neurologic Lyme disease syndromes (meningitis, cranial neuropathy, radiculoneuropathy, chronic encephalopathy) as well as patients with atypical, but otherwise unexplained syndromes (intractable headaches and stiff neck, acute confusional states, and benign intracranial hypertension with papilledema). Immune complexes may be present in the setting of otherwise normal CSF parameters, including cell count, protein, and glucose, and without detectable intrathecal production of anti-*B. burgdorferi* antibodies. When these CSF immune complexes were isolated and examined, almost 60% were *B. burgdorferi*-specific. They contained IgG, and occasionally IgM and IgA, directed against the spirochete. Specific CSF IgM complexes have only been found in patients with neurologic syndromes of less than 1 month's duration. In one patient, CSF samples obtained 11 days apart showed clearance of specific IgM complexes coincident with neurologic recovery. There was no change in any other CSF parameter. The role of CSF immune complexes in the pathogenesis of neurologic Lyme syndromes remains to be elucidated, however. Another experimental CSF test, detection of spirochetal antigens, is discussed above. PCR is being evaluated in a number of centers, and it has been applied to detect *B. burgdorferi* nucleic acids in CSF.[16,36,41a] There are two basic problems with the use of PCR in Lyme disease.[56,84] The first problem is the lack of assay standardization. PCR is extremely susceptible to contamination, with false-positive results. Quality control in the laboratory is crucial, and no commercial PCR assay should be used currently to diagnose Lyme disease. The second problem is the lack of data on whether positive PCR in Lyme disease indicates viable organisms and active infection. PCR is so sensitive that nucleic acid from a single organism can be detected. It is not clear whether single organisms, either living or dead, could be shed harmlessly into CSF over a period of time in patients who have been successfully treated for neurologic Lyme disease.

Culture of *B. burgdorferi* from CSF has occasionally been successful.[57,59,74] However, culture requires special media and prolonged incubation periods of many weeks.[3] Successful culture also requires experienced laboratory personnel. Most clinical microbiology laboratories are not equipped to culture *B. burgdorferi,* and attempts are successful less than 10% of the time. Even in the best of hands, culture positivity (for blood from recently infected patients) is only 21%.[50]

Finally, several studies have reported detection of CSF autoantibodies, and CSF cells secreting autoantibodies, to myelin basic protein.[2,22,80] CSF T cells have also been noted that were reactive to autoantigens including central and peripheral myelin, cardiolipin, and galactocerebroside.[45] These immunologic studies are of great interest but are available only at a few research centers.

Intrathecal anti-*B. burgdorferi* antibody production (CSF Lyme antibody index)

This test is currently considered the best routine CSF assay for neurologic Lyme disease. It is much more meaningful than measuring specific antibody in CSF, which may simply reflect passive diffusion or leak of blood antibody. The intrathecal assay instead measures local brain compartment synthesis of spirochete-specific antibodies.

The test is carried out on paired CSF and serum samples, and several techniques are used. One technique involves a specialized antibody-capture ELISA.[31,75] When the antibody response is greater in CSF than serum, intrathecal antibody production is said to be present. This method requires no prior standardization of the CSF and serum samples but is technically more cumbersome than a regular ELISA. A second technique normalizes CSF and serum to the same IgG concentration, then runs the paired samples for anti-*B. burgdorferi* antibodies by routine ELISA.[29] When the CSF Lyme antibody index (CSF optical density/serum optical density) is greater than 1, local CSF antibody production is said to be present. A third technique measures spirochete-specific IgG or IgM in paired CSF and serum using serial dilutions, as well as the total CSF and serum IgG or IgM.[82] When the ratio of specific to total immunoglobulin in CSF compared to serum is greater than 1, intrathecal antibody production is said to be present.

Intrathecal anti-*B. burgdorferi* antibody production is helpful when positive, because it strongly suggests CNS invasion by the spirochete. However, a negative result does not rule out neurologic Lyme disease. In addition, this assay is not interpretable if CSF and serum are negative for anti-*B. burgdorferi* antibodies in a routine assay.

The occurrence of CSF anti-*B. burgdorferi* antibodies in the absence of serum antibodies has been rare in North American patients.[28] There are four circumstances in which it might occur: (1) early infection, with a more vigorous rising antibody response in CSF than blood; (2) inadequate antibiotic treatment soon after infection, with a consequent blunting of the peripheral antibody response; (3) treated Lyme disease, where a prior positive blood antibody titer has now become negative; (4) an immune abnormality.

CSF findings in specific neurologic syndromes

Meningitis. By definition, all patients with Lyme meningitis must have a CSF pleocytosis at some point in time. In North American studies, cell counts range from 5 to 3750 WBC/mm^3, with a median count in the range of 110 to 170 cells.* One recent series reported a median count of only 11 WBC for Lyme meningitis, but the duration of symptoms was prolonged in a third of these cases and it was unclear whether they had received prior antibiotics.[28] There is a mononuclear cell predominance (lymphocytes and monocytes) of 40% to 100% (median 93%). The CSF cells may also include plasma cells, atypical lymphocytes, and immunoblasts. Compared to blood cells, CSF cells from Lyme meningitis patients are enriched for lymphocytes that are reactive to *B. burgdorferi*.[55] This is not surprising, because Lyme meningitis is due to spirochete invasion of the CNS; *B. burgdorferi* has been isolated from the CSF of meningitis patients.[74] CSF protein is elevated in 15% to 53% of meningitis patients. The range is 8 to 400 mg/dl, with median values in different series rang-

---

*References 15, 28, 54, 61, 62, 75.

ing from 26 to 79. Protein tends to be higher in patients with associated spinal nerve root involvement (radiculitis). CSF glucose is generally normal; less than 15% of meningitis patients have CSF glucose values under 45 mg/dl. The CSF profile is that of an aseptic meningitis. There is a single case report in the European literature of Lyme meningitis presenting with a septic picture (low glucose and a high neutrophil WBC count in the thousands).[9] CSF pressure is generally normal but is more likely to be increased in children with meningitis. An elevated IgG index or IgG intrathecal synthesis rate is present in only 40% to 46% of North American series, and oligoclonal bands are present in only 46%. CSF myelin basic protein and VDRL are consistently negative. In North American series, intrathecal anti-*B. burgdorferi* antibody production (CSF Lyme antibody index greater than 1) is found in 73% to 92% of cases. Intrathecal anti-*B. burgdorferi* antibodies may consist solely of IgG, IgM, or IgA isotype. In fact, in one study of meningitis patients, intrathecal anti-*B. burgdorferi* IgA was found to be the most frequent isotype.[75] There is generally a fairly rapid response to antibiotics. In one series of 12 patients, 10 days into treatment the mean CSF count had fallen from 153 ± 154 WBC (82% mononuclear) to 54 ± 32 WBC (83% mononuclear); protein had decreased from 70 ± 59 mg/dl to 53 ± 47 mg/dl; and glucose remained unchanged (54 ± 10 mg/dl to 56 ± 9 mg/dl).[73] In another patient, 10 days of antibiotics reduced the cell count from 273 to 41 WBC/mm³, and the protein value decreased from 90 to 46 mg/dl. CSF glucose increased from 44 to 66 mg/dl.[15]

Encephalopathy. Only 4% to 5% of patients with the late subacute encephalopathy show CSF pleocytosis.[28,40,75,77] It is low grade, almost always less than 40 WBC/mm³. Protein is increased in 17% to 46%. In one series of 12 patients, protein values ranged from 51 to 106 mg/dl, with a median value of 79. In another series of 41 patients, protein ranged from 15 to 58 mg/dl, with a median value of only 32. Elevated IgG index or intrathecal IgG production occurs in less than 5%. Intrathecal anti-*B. burgdorferi* antibody production is present in less than 50%. These patients do not have oligoclonal bands, detectable myelin basic protein, reactive VDRL, or decreased CSF glucose. After treatment, CSF protein tends to fall, but the CSF Lyme antibody index often remains unchanged.

Encephalomyelitis. In 45 North American patients with encephalomyelitis attributed to Lyme disease, 40% had a mononuclear CSF pleocytosis.* Although the WBC count ranged from 0 to 1830

*References 10, 19, 28, 40, 52, 63.

cells, the median cell count in the largest series was only 2. CSF protein is elevated in 33% and ranges from 11 to 481 mg/dl, with a median value around 40. Increased IgG index or intrathecal IgG production is present in only 28%, and oligoclonal bands are present in 29%. The CSF Lyme antibody index is elevated in only 41%. CSF myelin basic protein and VDRL are negative. CSF glucose was low in a single patient.

Isolated cranial neuropathy. Cranial nerve palsy may be the clinical presentation of an occult meningitis. When such patients show an elevated CSF cell count, they are generally included in the Lyme meningitis group. Cranial neuropathy can also occur with normal CSF. Most often, patients have Bell's palsy, but involvement of other cranial nerves (such as II; III; IV and VI; V; VIII; IX and X) also occurs. Intrathecal anti-*B. burgdorferi* antibody production is noted in 10% or less of patients with cranial neuropathy without meningitis.[28,29] In three patients with recent *B. burgdorferi* infection and a new optic neuritis who underwent lumbar puncture, two had a CSF pleocytosis of 27 and 47 cells.[35] None had increased CSF protein, IgG, or oligoclonal bands. Two of three had an increased CSF Lyme antibody index.

Neuropathy. The mild axonal polyneuropathy noted with late Lyme disease is typically associated with completely normal CSF, unless there is an associated encephalopathy.[29,40,75] In rare cases, oligoclonal bands, increased IgG index, and mild intrathecal anti-*B. burgdorferi* antibody production have been reported. Just as is true for isolated cranial neuropathy, radiculoneuritis may be the clinical presentation of meningitis with CSF findings as noted above. Occasionally, radicular involvement occurs in the setting of normal CSF.

Does normal CSF exclude neurologic Lyme disease?

CSF findings of a mononuclear pleocytosis, elevated protein, and intrathecal anti-*B. burgdorferi* antibody production indicate neurologic infection by *B. burgdorferi*. Such patients should be given a course of parenteral antibiotics that penetrate the blood-brain barrier. Once the patient is treated, CSF abnormalities should show improvement on repeat examination, although certain immune markers as well as increased protein may remain present in the CSF for months to years.

The difficulty arises in the patient with neurologic problems and normal CSF, who is seropositive to *B. burgdorferi*. As reviewed above, CSF is generally normal in neurologic Lyme disease involving the peripheral nervous system (polyneuropathy, and certain cases of spinal nerve root and cranial nerve involvement). Even in CNS Lyme disease, CSF abnormalities in North American patients have been variable except for meningitis patients.[41] *B. burgdorferi* is one of several spirochetes that cause neurologic disease. As a group, these spirochetes show a peculiar feature compared to other bacterial neurologic infections: the organisms can be present in CSF without inducing inflammatory changes.[43,60] This is well-documented for neurosyphilis, leptospirosis, and relapsing fever, and appears to be occasionally true for Lyme disease as well. In Europe, *B. burgdorferi* has been cultured from otherwise normal CSF.[57-59] Preliminary antigen and PCR studies also suggest that *B. burgdorferi* components may be present in normal CSF.[14,36,41a] This is most likely to be true early in the infection, before an immune response has been mounted, and late in the infection, when organisms are particularly scarce and may be in sequestered parts of brain remote from CSF. In early Lyme disease, patients who have headache, stiff neck, and flulike symptoms but do not have CSF changes may well represent the earliest phase of meningitis. In late stages of the infection, it is conceivable that organisms are present in neurologic tissue without producing sufficient abnormalities to affect CSF parameters. *B. burgdorferi* seems capable of invading human tissue without causing a marked inflammatory response. Particularly in chronic infections, organisms are sparse and are not associated with much in the way of a host pathologic response. Normal CSF should not be used to exclude neurologic infection in a symptomatic seropositive patient. When there is a sufficiently strong clinical suspicion, such patients should be given a course of treatment to determine their therapeutic response. In the future, it is likely that some of the current experimental studies will become part of the routine CSF assessment for neurologic Lyme disease. They are likely to provide a much more definitive laboratory test for neurologic infection.

ACKNOWLEDGMENT

This article was supported in part by Grant AR 40470 from the National Institutes of Health.

REFERENCES

1. Baig S et al: Anti-*Borrelia burgdorferi* antibody response over the course of Lyme neuroborreliosis, *Infect Immun* 59:1050, 1991.
2. Baig S et al: Cells secreting antibodies to myelin basic protein in cerebrospinal fluid of patients with Lyme neuroborreliosis, *Neurology* 41:581, 1991.
3. Barbour AG: Isolation and cultivation of Lyme disease spirochetes, *Yale J Biol Med* 57:521, 1984.
4. Barbour AG, Hayes SF: Biology of *Borrelia* species, *Microbiol Rev* 50:381, 1986.
5. Benach JL, Coleman JL, Golightly MG: A murine IgM monoclonal antibody binds an antigenic determinant in outer surface protein A, an immunodominant basic protein of the Lyme disease spirochete, *J Immunol* 140:265, 1988.
6. Berlit P, Pohlmann-Eden B, Henningsen H: Brown-Sequard syndrome caused by *Borrelia burgdorferi, Eur Neurol* 31:18, 1991.
7. Bjerkhoel A, Carlsson M, Ohlsson J: Peripheral facial palsy caused by the *Borrelia* spirochete, *Acta Otolaryngol* 108:424, 1989.
8. Boeer A, Schipper HI, Prange HW: Local IgM production in meningoradiculitis Bannwarth and neurosyphilis, *J Neuroimmunol* 20:315, 1988.
9. Bourke SJ et al: Lyme disease with acute persistent meningitis, *Br Med J* 297:460, 1988.
10. Broderick JP, Sandok BA, Mertz LE: Focal encephalitis in a young woman 6 years after the onset of Lyme disease: tertiary Lyme disease? *Mayo Clin Proc* 62:313, 1987.
11. Clark RA et al: Spectrum of *Cryptococcus neoformans* infection in 68 patients infected with human immunodeficiency virus, *Rev Infect Dis* 12:768, 1990.
12. Cohen SR et al: A diagnostic index of active demyelination: myelin basic protein in cerebrospinal fluid, *Ann Neurol* 8:25, 1980.
13. Coyle PK et al: Cerebrospinal fluid immune complexes in patients exposed to *Borrelia burgdorferi:* detection of *Borrelia* specific and nonspecific complexes, *Ann Neurol* 28:739, 1990.
14. Coyle PK et al: Detection of *Borrelia burgdorferi* antigens in cerebrospinal fluid, *Neurology* 42:371, 1992.
15. Daffner KR, Saver JL, Biber MP: Lyme polyradiculoneuropathy presenting as increasing abnormal girth, *Neurology* 40:373, 1990.
16. Debue M et al: Detection of *Borrelia burgdorferi* in biological samples using the polymerase chain reaction assay, *Res Microbiol* 142:565, 1991.
17. Dorward DW, Schwan TG, Garon CF: Immune capture and detection of *Borrelia burgdorferi* antigens in urine, blood, or tissues from infected ticks, mice, dogs, and humans, *J Clin Microbiol* 29:1162, 1991.
18. Epstein LG et al: HIV expression in CSF of children with progressive encephalopathy, *Ann Neurol* 21:297, 1987.
19. Feder HM, Zalneraitis EL, Reik L: Lyme disease: acute focal meningoencephalitis in a child, *Pediatrics* 82:931, 1988.
20. Fishman RA: *Cerebrospinal fluid in diseases of the nervous system,* Philadelphia, 1980, WB Saunders.
21. Garcia-Monco JC, Benach JL: The pathogenesis of Lyme disease, *Rheum Dis Clin North Am* 15:711, 1989.
22. Garcia-Monco JC, Coleman JL, Benach JL: Antibodies to myelin basic protein in Lyme disease, *J Infect Dis* 158:667, 1988.
23. Garcia-Monco JC et al: *Borrelia burgdorferi* in the central nervous system: experimental and clinical evidence for early invasion, *J Infect Dis* 161:1187, 1990.
24. Garon CF, Dorward DW, Corwin MD: Structural features of *Borrelia burgdorferi*—the Lyme disease spirochete: silver staining for nucleic acids, *Scanning Microsc* 3:109, 1989.
25. Goodman JL et al: Persistent cardiac and urinary tract infections with *B. burgdorferi* in experimentally infected Syrian hamsters, *J Clin Microbiol* 29:894, 1991.
26. Goodman JS, Kaufman L, Koenig MG: Diagnosis of cryptococcal meningitis. Value of immunologic detection of cryptococcal antigen, *N Engl J Med* 285:434, 1971.
27. Greenlee JE: Approach to diagnosis of meningitis: cerebrospinal fluid evaluation, *Infect Dis Clin North Am* 4:583, 1990.
28. Halperin JJ, Volkman DJ, Wu P: Central nervous system abnormalities in Lyme neuroborreliosis, *Neurology* 41:1571, 1991.
29. Halperin JJ et al: Lyme neuroborreliosis: central nervous system manifestations, *Neurology* 39:753, 1989.
30. Hansen K, Cruz M, Link H: Oligoclonal *Borrelia burgdorferi*-specific IgG antibodies in cerebrospinal fluid in Lyme neuroborreliosis, *J Infect Dis* 161:1194, 1990.

31. Hansen K, Lebech A-M: Lyme neuroborreliosis: a new sensitive diagnostic assay for intrathecal synthesis of *Borrelia burgdorferi*-specific immunoglobulin G, A, and M, *Ann Neurol* 30:197, 1991.

32. Hedberg CW et al: An interlaboratory study of antibody to *Borrelia burgdorferi, J Infect Dis* 155:1325, 1987.

33. Henriksson A et al: Immunoglobulin abnormalities in cerebrospinal fluid and blood over the course of lymphocytic meningoradiculitis (Bannwarth's syndrome), *Ann Neurol* 20:337, 1986.

34. Hyde FW et al: Detection of antigens in urine of mice and humans infected with *Borrelia burgdorferi,* etiologic agent of Lyme disease, *J Clin Microbiol* 27:58, 1989.

35. Jacobson DM, Marx JJ, Dlesk A: Frequency and clinical significance of Lyme seropositivity in patients with isolated optic neuritis, *Neurology* 41:706, 1991.

36. Jaulhac B et al: Detection of *Borrelia burgdorferi* in cerebrospinal fluid of patients with Lyme borreliosis, *N Engl J Med* 324:1440, 1991.

37. Kaplan SL: Antigen detection in CSF-pros and cons, *Am J Med* 75(1B):109-118, 1983.

38. Kohlhepp W, Kuhn W, Kruger H: Extrapyramidal features in central Lyme borreliosis, *Eur Neurol* 29:150, 1989.

39. Leland DS, Kohler RB: Evaluation of the L-clone *Legionella pneumophila* serogroup 1 urine antigen latex test, *J Clin Microbiol* 29:2220, 1991.

40. Logigian EL, Kaplan RF, Steere AC: Chronic neurologic manifestations of Lyme disease, *N Engl J Med* 323:1438, 1990.

41. Logigian EL, Steere AC: *Lyme borreliosis*. In Lambert HP, editor: *Infections of the central nervous system*, Philadelphia, 1991, BC Decker.

41a. Luft BJ et al: Invasion of the central nervous system by *Borrelia burgdorferi* in acute disseminated infection, *JAMA* 267:1364, 1992.

42. Luger SW, Krauss E: Serologic tests for Lyme disease, *Arch Intern Med* 150:761, 1990.

43. Lukehart SA et al: Invasion of the central nervous system by *Treponema pallidum:* implications for diagnosis and treatment, *Ann Intern Med* 109:855, 1988.

44. Magnarelli LA et al: Cross-reactivity of nonspecific treponemal antibody in serologic tests for Lyme disease, *J Clin Microbiol* 28:1276, 1991.

45. Martin R et al: *Borrelia burgdorferi*-specific and autoreactive T cell lines from cerebrospinal fluid in Lyme radiculomyelitis, *Ann Neurol* 24:509, 1988.

46. Martin R et al: Persistent intrathecal secretion of oligoclonal, *Borrelia burgdorferi*-specific IgG in chronic meningoradiculomyelitis, *J Neurol* 235:229, 1988.

47. Martin R et al: *Borrelia burgdorferi* myelitis presenting as a partial stiff man syndrome, *J Neurol* 237:51, 1990.

48. Midgard R, Hofstad H: Unusual manifestations of nervous system *Borrelia burgdorferi* infection, *Arch Neurol* 44:781, 1987.

49. Mokry M et al: Chronic Lyme disease with an expansive granulomatous lesion in the cerebellopontine angle, *Neurosurgery* 27:446, 1990.

50. Nadelman RB et al: Isolation of *Borrelia burgdorferi* from the blood of seven patients with Lyme disease, *Am J Med* 88:21, 1990.

51. Olsson I et al: Tick-borne borreliosis and facial palsy, *Acta Otolaryngol* 105:100, 1988.

52. Pachner AR, Duray P, Steere AC: Central nervous system manifestations of Lyme disease, *Arch Neurol* 46:790, 1989.

53. Pachner AR, Itano A: *B. burgdorferi* infection of the brain: characterization of the organism and response to antibiotics and immune sera in the mouse model, *Neurology* 40:1535, 1990.

54. Pachner AR, Steere AC: The triad of neurologic manifestations of Lyme disease: meningitis, cranial neuritis, and radiculoneuritis, *Neurology* 35:47, 1985.

55. Pachner AR et al: Antigen-specific proliferation of CSF lymphocytes in Lyme disease, *Neurology* 35:1642, 1985.

56. Persing DH: PCR: trenches to benches, *J Clin Microbiol* 29:1, 1991.

57. Pfister H-W et al: Latent Lyme neuroborreliosis: presence of *Borrelia burgdorferi* in the cerebrospinal fluid without concurrent inflammatory signs, *Neurology* 39:1118, 1989.

58. Pfister H-W et al: Randomized comparison of ceftriaxone and cefotaxime in Lyme neuroborreliosis, *J Infect Dis* 163:311, 1991.

59. Preac-Mursic V et al: Survival of *Borrelia burgdorferi* in antibiotically treated patients with Lyme borreliosis, *Infection* 17:355, 1989.

60. Reik L: *Spirochetal infections of the nervous system.* In Kennedy PGE, Johnson RT, editors: *Infections of the nervous system,* London, 1987, Butterworths.

61. Reik L, Burgdorfer W, Donaldson JO: Neurologic abnormalities in Lyme disease without erythema chronicum migrans, *Am J Med* 81:73, 1986.

62. Reik L et al: Neurologic abnormalities of Lyme disease, *Medicine* 58:281, 1979.

63. Reik L et al: Demyelinating encephalopathy in Lyme disease, *Neurology* 35:267, 1985.

64. Roberg M et al: Acute peripheral facial palsy: CSF findings and etiology, *Acta Neurol Scand* 83:55, 1991.

65. Rodriquez-del Valle M et al: Detection of antigens and antibodies in the urine of humans with *Plasmodium falciparum* malaria, *J Clin Microbiol* 29:1236, 1991.

66. Ryberg B: Bannwarth's syndrome (lymphocytic meningoradiculitis) in Sweden, *Yale J Biol Med* 57:499, 1984.

67. Schwan TG, Burgdorfer W, Schrumpf ME: The urinary bladder, a consistent source of *B. burgdorferi* in experimentally infected white-footed mice *(Peromipcus leucopus), J Clin Microbiol* 26:893, 1988.

68. Schwartz BS et al: Antibody testing in Lyme disease, *JAMA* 262:3431, 1989.

69. Sellors J et al: Rapid, on-site diagnosis of chlamydial urethritis in men by detection of antigens in urethral swabs and urine, *J Clin Microbiol* 29:407, 1991.

70. Sindic CJM et al: Lymphocytic meningoradiculitis and encephalomyelitis due to *Borrelia burgdorferi:* a clinical and serological study of 18 cases, *J Neur Neurosurg Psych* 50:1565, 1987.

71. Stanek G et al: Isolation of *B. burgdorferi* from the myocardium of a patient with longstanding cardiomyopathy, *N Engl J Med* 322:249, 1990.

72. Steere AC: Lyme disease, *N Engl J Med* 321:586, 1989.

73. Steere AC, Pachner AR, Malawista SE: Neurologic abnormalities of Lyme disease: successful treatment with high-dose intravenous penicillin, *Ann Intern Med* 99:767, 1983.

74. Steere AC et al: The spirochetal etiology of Lyme disease, *N Engl J Med* 308:733, 1983.

75. Steere AC et al: Evaluation of the intrathecal antibody response to *Borrelia burgdorferi* as a diagnostic test for Lyme neuroborreliosis, *J Infect Dis* 161:1203, 1990.

76. Stiernstedt GT et al: Diagnosis of spirochetal meningitis by enzyme-linked immunosorbent assay and indirect immunofluorescence assay in serum and cerebrospinal fluid, *J Clin Microbiol* 21:819, 1985.

77. Szer IS, Taylor E, Steere AC: The long-term course of Lyme arthritis in children, *N Engl J Med* 325:159, 1991.

78. Veenendaal-Hilbers JA et al: Basal meningovasculitis and occlusion of the basilar artery in two cases of *Borrelia burgdorferi* infection, *Neurology* 38:1317, 1988.

79. Von Stedingk L-V et al: Intrathecally produced antibodies to *Borrelia burgdorferi* measured by IgG-capture ELISA, *Serodiagn Immunother Infect Dis* 4:387, 1990.

80. Weder B et al: Chronic progressive neurological involvement in *Borrelia burgdorferi* infection, *J Neurol* 234:40, 1987.

81. Wheat LJ et al: Significance of *Histoplasma* antigen in the cerebrospinal fluid of patients with meningitis, *Arch Intern Med* 149:302, 1989.

82. Wilske B et al: Intrathecal production of specific antibodies against *Borrelia burgdorferi* in patients with lymphocytic meningoradiculitis (Bannwarth's syndrome), *J Infect Dis* 153:304, 1986.

83. Wokke JHJ et al: Chronic forms of *Borrelia burgdorferi* infection of the nervous system, *Neurology* 37:1031, 1987.

84. Wright PA, Wynford-Thomas D: The PCR: miracle or mirage? A critical review of its uses and limitations in diagnosis and research, *J Pathol* 162:99, 1990.

85. Zimmerman SE et al: Comparison of sandwich solid-phase radioimmunoassay and two enzyme-linked immunosorbent assays for detection of *Histoplasma capsulatum* polysaccharide antigen, *J Infect Dis* 160:678, 1989.

Therapy

John Nowakowski and Gary P. Wormser

Lyme disease is the most common vectorborne disease in the United States.[24] In a discussion of the treatment of early disease, it is important to indicate at the outset that "early" versus other stages of Lyme disease cannot always be easily differentiated. Because the route of infection is inoculation of the organism into the skin by a tick bite, it seems reasonable to consider, as others have done,[4,16,61,105] that the resulting local cutaneous infection, known as erythema migrans (EM), is a manifestation of early Lyme disease. The typical appearance of EM is an expanding circular or oval erythematous lesion with or without central clearing. The antecedent tick bite occurred several days to more than a month earlier and is usually painless and unnoticed.[112] Less than one third of patients presenting with EM recall having been bitten.[5,105] EM is associated with fever, malaise, and other nonspecific symptoms such as headache, myalgia, and arthralgia in up to 80% of cases.[105] Such early disease, however, does not imply lack of dissemination of the etiologic spirochete, *Borrelia burgdorferi,* because blood cultures may grow the organism in up to 21% of EM cases,[72] and there may be other clinical evidence of dissemination, such as secondary EM lesions or objective neurologic, rheumatologic, or cardiologic findings.

Patients without EM typically present with manifestations such as intermittent monoarticular arthritis,[102] facial nerve palsy or other evidence of neurologic involvement,[85] and heart block.[66,104] Although these abnormalities may be the first and only recognized manifestation of Lyme disease for perhaps 20% to 40% of patients and may have been present for only a brief period when the diagnosis of Lyme disease is made, they are generally not considered to represent "primary" stage Lyme disease. It is also known that some nonspecific febrile illnesses (flu-like illnesses) are actually Lyme disease based on either the development of an EM lesion within a few days of onset, seroconversion for anti-*B. burgdorferi* antibodies, or recovery of *B. burgdorferi* from the blood of such individuals.[72]

Lyme disease should be considered in the differential diagnosis of such illnesses for patients who have been in endemic regions during the peak season for transmission, May through July.[100] Patients presenting with flulike manifestations but without EM can be very difficult to diagnose because the symptoms are nonspecific, blood cultures may be negative or may take weeks to months to show growth and are generally not available, and serum antibodies may not be detectable at this stage.[95] The literature is sparse concerning the diagnosis and treatment of early Lyme disease without EM. Thus, for purposes of this chapter, early Lyme disease implies the presence of EM, with or without other symptoms or signs.

The goals of therapy in early infection are to resolve the EM lesion and associated constitutional symptoms; to prevent the development of more serious later manifestations involving the musculoskeletal system, the central and peripheral nervous system, and the cardiovascular system; to prevent the occurrence (or recurrence) of less severe symptoms such as fatigue, arthralgias, myalgias, brief arthritis; and to minimize adverse effects of therapy including high cost. In this chapter, we review the history of therapeutic intervention for patients with early Lyme disease associated with EM; examine in vitro and in vivo susceptibility data of chemotherapeutic agents against *B. burgdorferi;* make suggestions for the management of EM and other manifestations of early infection; and offer guidelines for prevention of disease including an approach to patients presenting with bites from ticks that may transmit *B. burgdorferi* to humans.

HISTORICAL PERSPECTIVES OF THERAPY FOR ERYTHEMA MIGRANS

In 1909, Afzelius made the initial clinical description of erythema chronicum migrans Afzelius before a meeting of the Dermatological Society of Stockholm. He thought the disease may be transmitted to humans by ticks.[1] Over the next half century, it became clear that this dermatologic condition could be associated with nervous system involvement,[6,7,39,42] including meningitis, radiculopathy, and peripheral and cranial neuritis. Involvement of the seventh cranial nerve with facial paralysis was particularly common. The neurologic entity was variously called the Bannwarth syndrome, Garin-Bujadoux syndrome, or chronic lymphocytic meningoradiculitis. By the mid 1940s, it was well-established that EM and its neurologic consequences usually followed a tick bite; however, the causal factor remained obscure.

In 1948, Lennhoff presented his findings of spirochetelike elements, visualized with a mercury stain, in skin biopsy preparations from patients with erythema chronicum migrans.[54] Over the next few years, under Lennhoff's direction, various spirocheticidal agents including bismuth salts, arsenicals, and penicillin were tested for therapeutic efficacy in groups of patients diagnosed with EM. Sixteen treated patients from Sweden were reported by Hollström in 1951.[43] He noted that 8 of the 16 patients reported prior tick bites at the site of the EM rash and 3 had multiple EM lesions. Although all of the therapies resulted in fading or disappearance of the lesions, penicillin gave the most dramatic results. This was consistent with the observation that penicillin was also the most effective spirocheticide available at the time to treat early syphilis. Hollström noted that the rash could recur if inadequate amounts of therapy were used. In this report, several patients presented with neurologic symptoms including meningitis and focal weakness that reversed after therapy with penicillin.

From 1948 to 1957, Hollström treated 77 patients presenting with EM using penicillin and reported his results in 1958.[44] The total dose used in most cases was between 600,000 and 2,400,000 units given intramuscularly, although some patients received both oral and intramuscular preparations of penicillin. Of the 65 patients available for follow-up, 89% had resolution of EM within 2 weeks after finishing therapy; an additional 7.7% were cured within 3 weeks. Two pediatric cases had recurrences after total doses of 300,000 units. These reports provided strongly suggestive evidence that EM was an infectious disease. In 1955, Binder successfully transferred the lesion to others by inoculating tissue obtained from the leading edge of the rash.[19] In 1962, several authors reported improvement in EM after therapy with tetracycline.[35,40] The impetus for such therapy was the apparent coincidental finding of a positive microagglutination titer against *Rickettsia* in a patient with EM.[35]

In 1970, the first reported case of EM in the United States was described.[94] Transmission occurred after a tick bite in Wisconsin. The rash and associated radicular pain cleared within 48 hours of a single intramuscular dose of 1.2 million units of benzathine penicillin G. In 1975, four cases of EM occurring within a 1-month period were seen in southeastern Connecticut.[65] Three were treated with oral penicillin V and one with erythromycin stearate. This was the first reported use of erythromycin to treat this condition. All resolved within several days of beginning therapy. Interestingly, this was the same year investigations began surrounding a cluster of cases of arthritis in children and adults in the same geographic area of southeastern Connecticut.[102] Epidemiologic studies led by Steere found that many of these cases were preceded by an enlarging circular rash consistent with EM. In the summer of 1976, Steere began the prospective investigation that defined the clinical entity now known as Lyme disease[101] (also called Lyme borreliosis). The above reports provided the basis for the choice of antibiotics used in the first controlled trials of therapy for EM discussed below.

IN VITRO AND IN VIVO SUSCEPTIBILITY OF *B. BURGDORFERI* TO ANTIBIOTICS

The choice of therapy for most bacterial infections is guided by isolation of the causative organism from infectious material and subsequent in vitro susceptibility testing. This type of information gathered over the years has allowed certain generalizations regarding appropriate initial therapy in a given clinical setting. Once the organism and its antimicrobial susceptibility pattern are identified, therapy can be specifically tailored to the offending pathogen. The success of this model in spirochetal infections is limited by the fastidious nature of these organisms making growth in culture difficult, the relatively low number of spirochetes in many clinical specimens reducing the likelihood of isolating the organism, and the unexplained discordance of in vitro data with clinical results for certain antibiotics. Isolation techniques and antibiotic sensitivity testing for spirochetes are the subject of a recent review by Johnson.[46]

Suggestive evidence that Lyme disease was caused by a tickborne spirochete came in 1982 when a previously unrecognized spirochete was grown from *Ixodes dammini* ticks,[23] thought to be the primary insect vector for human transmission in the northeastern United States.[112] In 1983, the same spirochete, subsequently named *Borrelia burgdorferi,* was isolated from blood, skin lesions, and cerebrospinal fluid (CSF) of patients with Lyme disease,[13,106] using Barbour-Stoenner-Kelly (BSK) media.[9] The clinical utility of culture as a diagnostic tool is limited by low recovery rates from blood, generally less than 10%[9,108] (although higher in some series [21%][72]), and the weeks to months it may take for cultures to become positive. Cultures obtained from the leading edge of the EM lesion, however, can yield the organism in up to 70% of cases[18,83] (also Wormser GP, unpublished data). The isolation and propagation of *B. burgdorferi* in the laboratory have led to numerous studies of in vitro susceptibility to various antibiotics* and to the development of a variety of animal models and test systems involving rabbits,[14,22,52,53] guinea pigs,[53] hamsters,[48,91] rats,[11] mice,[12,89] and gerbils.[56] Experimental infections in several animal species have been used for evaluating the activity of antimicrobials against the organism in vivo.[47,49,67,69,70] A qualitative comparison of antimicrobial efficacy based on studies done in vitro, and in vivo using laboratory animals, is shown in Table 18–1.[118]

Results of in vitro testing of antimicrobial agents against *B. burgdorferi* should be viewed cautiously due to lack of standardization in the methodologies used and no proven correlation with clinical effectiveness. The clinical utility of antimicrobial susceptibility testing depends on the development of standardized procedures that are widely accepted. The National Committee for Clinical Laboratory Standards (NCCLS) publishes standards for in vitro susceptibility testing,[75,76] which are updated periodically. These standards are useful for most bacteria that have a relatively short generation time. They may not apply to organisms such as *B. burgdorferi* that typically have generation times ranging from 11 to 20 hours.[9,46] Inconsistencies among published studies in the reported minimum inhibitory concentration (MIC) and minimum bactericidal concentrations (MBC) for various antibiotics against *B. burgdorferi* may be related more to differences in assay technique than to true strain variations. Table 18–2 reviews the various methodologies that have been published for in vitro susceptibility testing of *B. burgdorferi*. The most obvious methodologic difference is the amount of time in which spirochetes were exposed to the antibiotics tested, which ranged from 2 days to 6 weeks. This has practical significance because many antibiotics, especially the beta-lactams, may degrade at temperatures above $-20°$ C,[51] particularly when in solution. There are also major differences in the endpoint assessed ranging from inhibition of motility to lack of growth in subculture.

In addition, the MIC may also be strain dependent. This is especially evident for penicillin to which *B. burgdorferi* is often labeled as moderately susceptible. It is not known if the range in penicillin susceptibility among isolates is clinically signifi-

*References 17, 18, 47, 49, 50, 56, 67-70, 97.

Table 18–1 Antimicrobial activity in vitro and in laboratory animal test systems from reported studies*

	Activity	
Antimicrobial	**In vitro**	**Animal test systems**
Amikacin	0	NA
Amoxicillin	+ +	+ +
Amoxicillin-clavulanic acid	+ +	+ +
Ampicillin	+ +	NA
Azithromycin	+ + +	+ +
Cefotaxime	+ + +	+ +
Ceftriaxone	+ + +	+ +
Cefuroxime	+ +	+ +
Chloramphenicol	+	NA
Ciprofloxacin	+	NA
Clarithromycin	+ + +	+
Doxycycline	+ +	+ +
Erythromycin	+ + +	+
Gentamicin	0	NA
Imipenem	+ +	+ +
Lincomycin	+ +	NA
Mezlocillin	+ +	+
Minocycline	+ +	NA
Ofloxacin	+	NA
Oxacillin	+ +	NA
Penicillin	+	+
Rifampin	0	NA
Roxithromycin	+ + +	0
Tetracycline	+ +	+ +
Trimethoprim-sulfamethoxazole	0	NA

Modified from Wormser GP: Treatment of *Borrellia burgdorferi* infection. *Lab Med* 21:316, 1990.
*NA indicates not available; 0, not active, and +, + +, + + + indicate degrees of activity, from least to most.

cant. Consistently, the most favorable MICs have been reported for erythromycin and derivatives, ceftriaxone, and cefotaxime. Acceptable MICs are usually reported for tetracycline and its derivatives, and for extended spectrum beta-lactam derivatives such as ampicillin and amoxicillin.

Most interesting is the large variability in the MBCs of antibiotics against *B. burgdorferi,* particularly the beta-lactam derivatives. In one study, Luft et al[56] reported MBCs for penicillin and ceftriaxone ranging from 2 to 50 μg/ml and from 1 to 50 μg/ml, respectively. Others[18,47,50] have generally found the MBC for penicillin to be less than 10 μg/ml and for ceftriaxone less than 1 μg/ml. Luft postulated that the higher MBCs they observed may be due to the short time of incubation with antibiotic (2 days) employed.

Regardless of technique, the MBCs for penicillin against *B. burgdorferi* are consistently higher than

Table 18–2 Methodologies used for in vitro susceptibility testing of *Borrelia burgdorferi*

First author and reference	Isolates used	*B. burgdorferi* concentration	Incubation time with antibiotics	Endpoint used*
Johnson SE[50]	3 tick 2 human	10^5/ml	5 days	MIC: Least concentration of antibiotic with $\leq 10^5$ motile spirochetes/ml detected on darkfield
Berger BW[18]	6 human	0.5×10^6/ml	3 days	MIC: Least concentration of antibiotic with > 90% motile spirochetes on darkfield and total not greater than inoculum MBC: Least concentration of antibiotic with no growth by darkfield from < 1% (vol/vol) transfer by 11 days
Mursic VP[68]	5 human 2 tick	10^5/ml	4 days	MIC: Least concentration of antibiotic with no growth by darkfield in subculture by 5 days (amount subcultured not specified)
Mursic VP[70]	10 human	10^5/ml	4 days	MIC: Least concentration of antibiotic with no growth by darkfield in subculture by 4 days (amount subcultured not specified)
Johnson RC[47]	1 human	10^5/ml	42 days	MBC: Least concentration of antibiotic "in which spirochetes could not be detected" by darkfield and no growth in 10% (vol/vol) transfer (duration of subculture incubation not specified)
Luft BJ[56]	3 human 2 tick	2×10^6/ml	2 days	MIC: Least concentration of antibiotic with number of motile organisms not greater than inoculum MBC: Least concentration of antibiotic with no growth by darkfield from transfer of MIC pellet (duration of subculture incubation not specified)
Berger BW[17]	6 human	10^5/ml	21 days	MBC: Least concentration of antibiotic with no growth by darkfield in 10% (vol/vol) transfer by 21 days
Mursic VP[69]	10 human	10^5/ml	8 days	MIC: Least concentration of antibiotic with no growth by darkfield in subculture by 8 days (amount subcultured not specified)
Johnson RC[49]	8 human	10^5/ml	21 days	MBC: Least concentration of antibiotic with no growth by darkfield in 10% (vol/vol) subculture by 21 days

*MIC = minimum inhibitory concentration; MBC = minimum bactericidal concentration.

those reported for tetracyclines, amoxicillin, and most cephalosporins. Indeed, the MBCs for penicillin in some studies exceed the average peak serum concentration (4 μg/ml) achievable with oral administration of 500 mg of phenoxymethyl penicillin in the fasting state. Steady-state serum levels of tetracycline 500 mg PO qid during fasting are similar[117] to those of an equivalent dose of phenoxymethyl penicillin; however, tetracycline levels usually exceed its reported MICs and MBCs. Doxycycline, having much better absorption, reaches a peak serum level of over 2 μg/ml with a dose of only 100 mg,[117] which is close to the reported MICs for this agent. Despite the temptation to develop treatment strategies based on the comparison of MICs or MBCs with measurable serum levels of antibiotics, and thus avoid oral penicillin preparations, the fact remains that for the vast majority of patients with EM, treatment with oral penicillin is successful.[5,15,114] Thus, the clinical significance of in vitro susceptibility testing for penicillin is unclear.

The validity of in vitro susceptibility data for certain macrolide antibiotics is also dubious. Erythromycin is consistently among the most active drugs in vitro with MICs and MBCs frequently below 0.2 μg/ml. However, studies in laboratory animals and clinical trials in humans[45,107] suggest a relatively lower degree of activity compared to tetracycline or penicillin preparations. In a recent report comparing the antiborrelial activity of newer macrolides,[70] the authors noted the inability of these agents to clear experimental infection in gerbils, with the exception of azithromycin, despite MICs below 0.2 μg/ml for the four agents studied. The reasons for the differences between in vitro and in vivo activity for this class of antibiotics are unknown. In general, studies comparing antibiotic efficacy in infected laboratory animals are limited by the failure to demonstrate comparability of dosing regimens on the basis of antibiotic blood levels. An underappreciated but important piece of information learned from in vivo susceptibility testing, however, is that 5[47,49] to 7[69] days of appropriate antibiotic therapy can completely clear all organ systems, including the central nervous system, of *B. burgdorferi*, based on histologic examination and culture.

There have been few attempts to correlate the outcome of therapy in human infection with in vitro or in vivo (animal) susceptibility results using the patient's own isolate. In one study, Berger and Johnson[17] could not demonstrate resistance of the organism in vitro despite a poor clinical response in two patients. More such studies are indicated to determine if relative antibiotic resistance may explain why some patients develop progressive manifestations of infection despite apparently appropriate therapy for erythema migrans.[32,33,55,109]

WHICH ANTIMICROBIAL AGENTS ARE USEFUL?

After their initial description of Lyme arthritis,[102] Steere and colleagues subsequently documented its association with EM and constitutional symptoms,[101,105] carditis,[101,104] and neurologic manifestations,[86] which led to an appreciation of the systemic nature of the infection. Early in the course of these investigations, the authors were skeptical of the value of antibiotics based on the inherent variability in the natural history of the illness and the occasional development of late manifestations despite antibiotic therapy.[101] In 1980, Steere et al[103] published a report describing the clinical course of patients with and without antibiotic therapy. During a 4-year interval, patients presenting with EM were treated with penicillin G (42 patients) or followed without antibiotic intervention (55 patients). Tetracycline (7 patients) or erythromycin (9 patients) was used for penicillin-allergic patients. The decision to treat or not was based primarily on which year the patients presented with the rash. The authors found that treatment with penicillin or tetracycline but not erythromycin significantly reduced the duration of EM. Penicillin therapy also significantly reduced the subsequent development and severity of arthritis. The development of neurologic symptoms and the clinical outcome of cardiac conduction abnormalities did not seem affected by therapy, but these complications were, in general, very uncommon.

These encouraging results led to a prospective, randomized trial[107] comparing phenoxymethyl penicillin (40 patients), tetracycline (39 patients), and erythromycin (29 patients). Equal efficacy in time to resolution of EM and associated symptoms was observed for penicillin and tetracycline. The EM lesion resolved significantly more slowly in the group receiving erythromycin, and these patients required retreatment for persistence of symptoms or immediate relapse more frequently. Major late complications described as myocarditis, recurrent arthritis, or meningoencephalitis did not occur in any of 39 patients treated with tetracycline, compared to 3 of 40 treated with penicillin and 4 of 29 treated with erythromycin (p = .07 by chi square). Minor late complications including facial palsy, supraventricular tachycardia, arthritis lasting less than 2 weeks, and musculoskeletal pain occurred in all treatment groups frequently (50% with penicillin, 44% with tetracycline, and 38% with erythromycin). It should be pointed out that tetracycline therapy has not been uniformly successful in preventing serious late complications of Lyme disease in other studies.[32,33,55]

It is noteworthy that very few therapeutic trials for EM have been conducted in a prospective randomized fashion and none has been double-blinded. It was not until 1990 that a second randomized prospective trial was published.[34] Nevertheless, several retrospective studies deserve mention. Åsbrink[5] published results on 161 Swedish patients with EM. In this group, 145 were treated with antibiotics (132 with phenoxymethyl penicillin, 9 with erythromycin, 4 with tetracycline) and 16 patients primarily with fading rashes refused therapy. As expected, neurologic and musculoskeletal complaints occurred with much greater frequency in those untreated (6 of 16 [37.5%] untreated versus 12 of 145 [8.3%] treated), although, in general, late musculoskeletal manifestations were observed much less frequently than in the U.S. experience. Such clinical differences may be related to molecular or antigenic variations between European and North American *B. burgdorferi* isolates[8,10] or possibly to differences in genetic susceptibility of the indigenous human populations.

A retrospective analysis by Berger[15] of his experience treating patients with EM in Long Island, New York, led to several provocative observations. He confirmed the earlier findings by Steere[107] that the greater the severity of the initial symptoms, the worse the outcome. Virtually all 80 patients with mild symptoms at onset responded to initial therapy, usually phenoxymethyl penicillin 500 mg PO qid for 15 days, whereas 17 of the 81 patients more severely ill required retreatment. The author suggested that the addition of probenecid to the initial oral penicillin regimen resulted in fewer treatment failures in the more severely ill group. However, patients were not randomized prospectively to receive additional therapy with probenecid, and it is not noted if the treatment groups were comparable. Also, the precise reasons for retreatment were not explicitly stated. Because it was known whether probenecid had been given, it is possible that this information may have affected patient assessment or the decision to retreat. A prospective, controlled, and blinded study is needed to substantiate whether probenecid enhances the efficacy of oral penicillin therapy.

A nonrandomized, prospective evaluation by Weber[114] in Germany found no significant difference in outcome among 65 patients treated with oral penicillin, 36 with tetracycline derivatives, or 20 with amoxicillin/clavulanate. In all, 33 patients (27%) developed late manifestations but only 6 required retreatment. The precise reasons for retreatment were not stated. This is an important omission because the decision to retreat patients is often based solely on the presence of subjective complaints, which may or may not reflect persistent infection. Weber's study, like others,[34,36,73,96,107] found that a certain proportion of patients have persistence of such subjective symptoms as fatigue and arthralgias after initial therapy, which rarely, if ever, respond to repeat courses of antibiotics and usually resolve spontaneously within 6 months, but may persist for up to 2 years.

Many of the more recent antibiotic studies, as well as physician preference among practitioners in the community, demonstrate a trend toward the use of oral antibiotics that are newer, given in higher doses, or administered for longer durations than in older published studies. However, there is no evidence of enhanced benefit of these regimens based on controlled trials. For example, amoxicillin and doxycycline have replaced penicillin and tetracycline, respectively, based on improved pharmacokinetic parameters such as increased bioavailability, wider tissue distribution, and longer dosing interval. These factors may help to increase patient compliance by allowing, for example, less frequent dosing, or the consumption of dairy products. Nevertheless, the less severe manifestations are still frequently seen after therapy, although the incidence may not be as high as previously reported by Steere.[107] Unfortunately, there are no controlled prospective randomized trials comparing the effectiveness of penicillin versus either amoxicillin alone, amoxicillin/probenecid, or even penicillin/probenecid. No trial has ever compared tetracycline to doxycycline. Most recent studies have compared the newer agents against one another based on suppositions that improved pharmacokinetic parameters would enhance clinical outcome, and thus justify the higher cost of these agents (Table 18–3).

Dattwyler et al[34] in 1990 reported results of a randomized, prospective trial comparing amoxicillin/probenecid (37 patients) versus doxycycline (35 patients) given for 21 days to patients with EM at the University of Stony Brook, New York. No significant advantage was observed for either therapy. No patient in either group developed major late complications using the criteria developed by Steere et al.[107] A total of 13.5% in the amoxicillin/probenecid group and 6% in the doxycycline group developed mild fatigue or arthralgias. These symptoms resolved within the 6-month follow-up period. Although the frequency of minor complications was less than observed by Steere,[107] these results should not be interpreted to mean that the antibiotic regimens are superior to those used in the Steere study. The two clinical trials are not comparable for several reasons. In the Steere trial,

Table 18–3 Cost comparison of various antibiotic regimens for early Lyme disease from least to most expensive*

Antibiotic regimen	10 to 14 day duration	21 day duration
Tetracycline 500 mg PO qid	$3.24-$4.54	$6.80
Phenoxymethyl penicillin 500 mg PO qid	$3.36-$4.70	$7.05
Phenoxymethyl penicillin 500 mg PO qid and probenecid 500 mg PO qid	$7.28-$10.19	$15.28
Doxycycline 100 mg PO bid (generic formulation)	$7.60-$10.64	$15.96
Doxycycline 100 mg PO tid (generic formulation)	$11.40-$15.96	$23.94
Amoxicillin 500 mg PO tid	$13.80-$19.32	$28.98
Amoxicillin 500 mg PO tid and probenecid 500 mg PO tid	$16.74-$23.44	$36.15
Doxycycline 100 mg PO bid (brand name, e.g., Vibramycin)	$55.00-$77.00	$115.50
Cefuroxime axetil 500 mg PO bid	$80.00-$112.00	$168.00

*Based on prices listed in the 1991 Red Book. Oradell, NJ, 1991, Medical Economics.

EM was present in the majority of patients for over 10 days before beginning therapy. Although not specifically stated in the Dattwyler study, it is likely that these patients were more promptly diagnosed and treated as is the present community standard. The follow-up period in the Dattwyler trial was only 6 months compared to several years in the Steere trial. Those with only mild fatigue after therapy were not considered to have minor late complications in the Stony Brook study. Finally, patients were excluded from the Stony Brook study if they presented with acute objective neurologic or cardiac abnormalities. It is not stated how vigorously these abnormalities were sought, but such exclusion criteria may have removed patients complaining of severe headache and neck stiffness, whether or not cerebrospinal fluid analysis was performed. Excluding such patients who may be at greater risk for developing late manifestations[107] even in the absence of "objective" CSF abnormalities, would tend to bias study results toward a more salutary outcome.

Results of a relatively small, randomized, multicenter, prospective trial comparing doxycycline, amoxicillin/probenecid, and azithromycin (an azalide antibiotic recently released in the United States) in 57 patients from Massachusetts, Connecticut, or Minnesota with EM showed no significant differences.[64] Major late neurologic manifestations developed in 3 (one in each group) of the 25 patients who presented with "symptoms suggestive of dissemination of the spirochete to the nervous system," whereas the 14 patients with uncomplicated EM and the 18 with other systemic symptoms remained well during 5 months of follow-up. This study suggests that azithromycin, despite other evidence gathered against the use of macrolide agents, may have clinical utility equivalent to doxycycline and amoxicillin/probenecid, even when used for only 5 days. Larger comparative studies are needed to confirm these findings.

We participated in a multicenter, investigator-blinded, randomized comparison of cefuroxime axetil 500 mg PO bid versus doxycycline 100 mg PO tid, both for 20 days, in patients with EM.[73] One month after treatment, clinical success (*cure* or *improvement*) was noted in 93% of those treated with cefuroxime axetil compared to 88% in the doxycycline group. At 1 year follow-up, clinically successful outcomes were maintained in 43 (90%) of 48 evaluable patients who received cefuroxime and 35 (92%) of 38 evaluable patients with doxycycline (Nadelman R et al, unpublished data).

In summary, the results of treatment trials for patients with early Lyme disease using agents such as doxycycline and amoxicillin/probenecid cannot be compared accurately to earlier trials using oral penicillin preparations and tetracycline. Despite earlier diagnosis and therapy of EM, major and minor post-treatment complications are still observed in all recent trials. New oral agents tested, azithromycin and cefuroxime axetil, also appear efficacious and may be advantageous for patients intolerant of tetracyclines and certain penicillins.

DURATION OF THERAPY

In an introduction to a session regarding therapy for Lyme disease at an international conference in 1987, Dr. Harold Neu concluded that there are no data supporting whether therapy should be continued for "7, 10, 14, or 21 days."[77] It is still difficult to find an answer to this question. A surprisingly short duration of therapy, one dose of oral doxycycline or tetracycline, is curative in louseborne relapsing fever caused by *B. recurrentis*,[78] and 5 to 10 days of tetracycline or erythromycin is considered effective in tickborne relapsing fever due to various species of *Borrelia*.[88]

Only one randomized, controlled trial to date has addressed the issue of duration of therapy for EM. Steere[107] found that 10 days of low-dose tetracycline therapy (25 patients) was equivalent to the same regimen given for 20 days (24 patients) in regard to resolution of EM and to prevention of major late complications of infection. Despite these results, many authoritative sources recommend that antibiotics be administered up to 21[57,82,92,111] or 30[28,100] days to all[57] or at least certain patients[13,28,82,92,100,111] with EM.

In animal test systems, infection with *B. burgdorferi* can be completely eradicated with as few as 5 days of therapy[47,49] provided a sufficient dose of an appropriate antibiotic is given. These studies did not evaluate whether shorter courses of therapy might do just as well. In a controlled randomized trial of patients in Germany with EM, 5 days of intramuscular ceftriaxone (40 patients) was equally as effective, or better, than 12 days of oral phenoxymethyl penicillin (33 patients).[116] A total of 24% in the penicillin group versus 15% in the ceftriaxone group developed minor late manifestations. *B. burgdorferi* could be cultured from the site of resolved EM 3 months after therapy with penicillin in one patient. Also, one patient had recurrence of EM and arthralgias 8 weeks after ceftriaxone therapy. It is not clear if this represented reinfection.

To investigate further the effect of duration of therapy, we compared the outcome of patients enrolled in the cefuroxime axetil versus doxycycline study discussed above in which patients were treated for 20 days,[73] with the outcome of patients who refused or were ineligible for the study. The group not entered included 20 patients treated with doxycycline 100 mg bid or tid for 14 days and 25 patients treated with tetracycline 500 mg PO qid for 14 days. The percentage of patients with associated systemic complaints at the beginning of therapy and the duration of EM before therapy were similar between those enrolled in the formal study and those who were not. The *cure* rate as defined by resolution of both EM and symptoms immedi-

ately after completion of therapy was similar in all four groups (71.4% for 20 day cefuroxime, 64.7% for 20 day doxycycline, 65% for 14 day doxycycline, and 84% for 14 day tetracycline). We also found that the percentage of patients maintaining successful outcomes at 1 year was similar in all four groups (unpublished data).

In summary, there is no evidence supporting increased benefit of treating patients with EM for longer than 10 to 14 days. Extending therapy brings additional cost and possibly added toxicity. Comparative costs for various treatment regimens used for 10 to 14 versus 21 days are presented in Table 18–3.[84]

THERAPEUTIC RECOMMENDATIONS
Preventive strategies

The primary vectors for transmission of *B. burgdorferi* to humans are hard-bodied ticks of the genus *Ixodes*. An excellent review of the *Ixodes* tick vectors and reservoir hosts of *B. burgdorferi* has recently been published.[2] Three North American (*I. dammini* in northeastern and midwestern United States, *I. scapularis* in southeastern United States, *I. pacificus* in western United States) and two European (*I. ricinus* from Europe to western Asia, *I. persulcatus* from eastern Europe through Asia) spe-

Table 18–4 Recommendations for preventing Lyme disease*

Avoid known heavily tick-infested areas especially from May through July when *I. dammini* nymphs are abundant.

Wear light-colored clothing for easier detection of ticks.

Keep shirt tucked into pants. Wear long pants and tape trouser cuffs and/or place trousers in socks.

Avoid open-toed shoes especially without socks or stockings.

Inspect yourself and other family members carefully when returning from a potentially infested area.

Use an insect skin repellant containing N,N-diethyl-m-toluamide (DEET) or other agent of proven effectiveness especially when exposure to heavily infested areas is unavoidable.

Use a clothing pesticide such as permethrin especially on trouser legs and socks.

Inspect outdoor pets for ticks frequently.

Promptly remove ticks using forceps with steady upward pressure. Do not burn the tick or attempt to suffocate it before removal. Cleanse the area with soap and water afterwards.

*Adapted from References 3 and 71 with emphasis on endemic areas of the northeastern and midwestern United States.

cies of *Ixodes* are considered to be vectors of *B. burgdorferi* to humans. The geographic distribution of competent *Ixodes* vectors parallels the observed epidemiologic distribution of Lyme disease cases.[26,27,99] Other insects including deer flies, horse flies, mosquitoes, and soft-bodied ticks are capable of carrying *B. burgdorferi*[60,93] but have been implicated only rarely in transmission to humans.[41,58] The duration of tick attachment is an important factor in transmitting infection with most effective transmission occurring after prolonged (more than 2 days) feeding.[80,81] Therefore, prompt removal of ticks may prevent infection with *B. burgdorferi*. Although nymphal ticks are relatively small, they are not undetectable. The importance of close inspection after returning indoors especially from late spring through midsummer in endemic regions cannot be overemphasized. Recommended strategies to prevent infection are summarized in Table 18–4.[3,71]

It is not always possible to avoid exposure to tick-infested areas. Relatively large numbers of ticks can be found on residential landscapes in suburban regions in endemic areas.[37] The use of tick repellents is not without risk, and routine application of these agents to the skin each time a person ventures outdoors cannot be recommended. N,N-diethyl-m-toluamide (DEET) is partially absorbed from the skin into the systemic circulation; its use has been associated with dermatitis, anaphylaxis, and neurotoxicity including grand mal seizures.[25] Short-term use of these agents for exposure to highly infested areas is reasonable and can be recommended.

Therapy for erythema migrans with and without systemic manifestations

Our treatment approach in early Lyme disease is summarized in Table 18–5. Any of the choices listed under regimen A are acceptable therapy for patients with EM with or without associated systemic manifestations. The use of erythromycin is discouraged except if unable to use the other agents because of intolerance or allergy. Doxycycline is

Table 18–5 Therapy of early Lyme disease

Manifestation	Recommended therapy*	Duration
Erythema migrans with or without systemic symptoms	Regimen A	10-14 days
Erythema migrans with cranial nerve palsy	Regimen A	10-14 days
Erythema migrans with meningitis	Regimen B	10-14 days
Erythema migrans with arthritis	Regimen A	30 days
Erythema migrans with heart block (PR interval < 0.30 sec)	Regimen A	10-14 days
(PR interval ≥ 0.30 sec)†	Regimen B	10-14 days
Miscellaneous situations		
Viral-like illness presumed to be Lyme disease	Regimen A	10-14 days
Asymptomatic seropositive (never treated)	Regimen A (or observation)	10-14 days
Lymphocytoma	Regimen A	30 days
Ixodes tick bite in endemic area (asymptomatic)	Observation	
Ixodes tick bite in pregnant woman (asymptomatic)	Regimen A (not tetracyclines)	10-14 days
Lyme disease during pregnancy (any clinical manifestation)	Regimen B	10-14 days

Modified from Wormser GP: Treatment of *Borrelia burgdorferi* infection, *Lab Med* 21:316, 1990.

*The recommended treatments are as follows:

Regimen A for adults includes tetracycline 500 mg PO qid, doxycyline 100 mg PO bid, phenoxymethyl penicillin 500 mg PO qid, amoxicillin 500 mg PO tid, or cefuroxime axetil 500 mg PO bid. For patients unable to take either penicillin or tetracycline and their derivatives, use 500 mg erythromycin PO qid.

For children 9 years old and over, tetracycline 12.5 mg/kg PO qid (up to 2 g/day), doxycycline 100 mg PO bid, phenoxymethyl penicillin 12.5 mg/kg PO qid (up to 2 g/day), or amoxicillin 12.5 mg/kg PO tid (up to 1.5 g/day), or cefuroxime axetil 250 mg PO bid. For children younger than 9 years of age, phenoxymethyl penicillin 12.5 mg/kg PO qid (up to 2 g/day) or amoxicillin 12.5 mg/kg PO tid (up to 1.5 g/day), or cefuroxime axetil 250 mg PO bid (125 mg PO bid for children less than 2 years of age). Alternative regimen is erythromycin 12.5 mg/kg PO qid (up to 2 g/day).

Regimen B for adults includes 3 to 4 million U of penicillin intravenously every 4 hours or ceftriaxone 2 g intravenously daily. For children, ceftriaxone 75 to 100 mg/kg intravenously daily (up to 2 g/day) or penicillin G 50,000 U/kg intravenously every 4 hours (up to 24 million U/day).

†A temporary pacemaker may be indicated for certain patients with advanced heart block.

preferable to tetracycline for people over 60 years of age because of the possibility of occult kidney disease. The convenience of twice daily dosing argues for doxycycline over tetracycline generally.

Occasionally, a patient presents with a rash that is somewhat similar to EM but atypical based, for example, on smaller size or other characteristics of its general appearance. Such lesions may be due to poison ivy, ringworm, cellulitis, contact dermatitis, granuloma annulare, and insect bite reactions. If the patient is otherwise well, we usually ask the patient to return for reevaluation of the lesion in 1 to 2 days. Typically, the rash of Lyme disease continues to expand over this relatively short time period. In contrast, the sometimes intense local reactions to the bite of an *Ixodes* tick or other insects tend to disappear rather than expand during this interval.

For patients whose rash is indistinguishable from bacterial cellulitis based on its appearance or the presence of toxic symptoms, we recommend oral amoxicillin/clavulanate 500 mg PO tid for 10 to 14 days, which should be adequate therapy for both *B. burgdorferi* infection and *Staphylococcus aureus,* streptococcal, or *Hemophilus influenzae* cellulitis. Patients presenting with EM accompanied by cranial nerve palsy may be treated with one of the choices in regimen A. Those presenting with clinical evidence of meningeal irritation should have a lumbar puncture performed and, if abnormal, should be treated with one of the choices from regimen B.

Approximately 15% of patients treated for EM, especially those presenting with systemic complaints or other evidence of dissemination, such as multiple EM, will develop a Jarisch-Herxheimer–like response.[34,107,114] This is described as an intensification of symptoms after the first several doses of antibiotics. Its occurrence in syphilis and relapsing fever may be linked to release of pyrogenic material from spirochetes after exposure to appropriate antibiotics, and a similar mechanism is likely in Lyme disease.[21,119] Patients should be alerted to the possibility of this reaction.

Therapy for miscellaneous situations involving early *B. burgdorferi* infection

Patients presenting with flulike symptoms after an *Ixodes* tick bite or those with such symptoms found to be seropositive and residing in an endemic area may be treated with one of the choices presented in regimen A. One must be careful to establish that these symptoms began during the peak transmission period for *B. burgdorferi*. We have evaluated numerous individuals with vague complaints and low positive or equivocal antibody levels against *B. burgdorferi* referred to us because of failure to respond to antimicrobial regimens used for Lyme disease. Frequently, these patients have fairly long-standing complaints, and subsequent serologic evaluation typically fails to demonstrate significant or specific antibody responses. We refrain from treating such people with prolonged, potentially harmful courses of antibiotics and instead search for alternative diagnoses.

Asymptomatic seropositive patients are occasionally encountered in clinical practice. Such people are tested because a family member, neighbor, or pet is diagnosed with Lyme disease. Some are tested as part of a routine health examination or epidemiologic survey. The prevalence of such asymptomatic seropositives is highest in populations at greatest risk for exposure and can approach 10%.[98,110] There is little guidance on how to handle such patients in the available literature. We recommend clinical observation or therapy with an oral agent for 10 to 14 days. It is important to test these patients for latent syphilis because serologic cross-reactivity of the two spirochetes is well documented.[87] Of note, the rapid plasma reagin, VDRL, and microhemagglutination assay for *Treponema pallidum* are usually negative in Lyme disease.[30]

The approach to the patient sustaining an *Ixodes* tick bite in an endemic area remains controversial. Some physicians routinely treat such patients with oral antibiotics for several days to several weeks. This approach cannot be recommended based on the limited information available. As previously mentioned, there is evidence from animal studies[80,81] that ticks must feed more than 24 hours before effectively transmitting infection. In one small trial conducted in Connecticut,[29] 56 patients with witnessed or reported *Ixodes* tick bites were randomized to receive oral penicillin for 10 days or placebo. No patient in either group had either symptomatic or asymptomatic seroconversion. One patient (3%) in the placebo group developed EM 14 days after the bite, and one patient (4%) in the antibiotic group developed a drug rash. We have an ongoing, blinded, placebo-controlled study[74] evaluating the efficacy of a single dose of doxycycline (200 mg) in preventing Lyme disease within 72 hours of a proven *Ixodes* tick bite. Over 265 patients have been enrolled to date, and the study has not been decoded. However, of 230 patients who have completed the full follow-up period to date, only 3 have developed EM at the site of the original tick bite. These studies indicate that the incidence of clinical infection after a documented *Ixodes dammini* tick bite is less than 3%. In clinical practice when we encounter such patients, we do not give prophylactic therapy and only treat those patients who develop EM or systemic symptoms.

Lymphadenosis benigna cutica (*Borrelia* lymphocytoma) can occur at the site of a tick bite and frequently appears on the earlobe or nipple. It manifests as a firm reddish nodule or plaque, frequently surrounded by an EM lesion or it may follow the *Ixodes* tick bite by 6 to 10 months.[4] Histologically, a benign lymphocytic infiltration is observed. This manifestation has not been reported in the United States. Treatment with regimen A is appropriate; however, it is recommended by some that therapy be extended to 30 days.[61] Rarely, patients may present with cutaneous manifestations distinct from EM such as granuloma annulare, malar erythema, papular urticaria, erythema nodosum, or Henoch-Schönlein–like purpura. Spirochetes have not been cultured from these lesions. The choice of therapy should be guided by the associated manifestations consistent with *B. burgdorferi* infection.

Management of early infection during pregnancy

The precise risk to the developing fetus of maternal Lyme disease during pregnancy is unknown, but appears to be small.[20] However, it is well-documented that fetal infection can occur and can have deleterious outcomes, including malformations and death.[59,90,115] Maternal-fetal transmission has occurred when EM developed during the first trimester of pregnancy in a mother who was untreated and, in one instance, in a mother who received an oral penicillin preparation (propicillin 1 million U tid) for 7 days.[115] Another study demonstrated the occurrence of diverse fetal abnormalities among children born to mothers with onset of Lyme disease during pregnancy, most of whom were treated with appropriate oral antibiotics; the defects, all of which were different, however, could not be clearly linked to infection with *B. burgdorferi*.[63] Despite the likely low incidence of transmission of *B. burgdorferi* to the fetus, pending definitive studies, we routinely recommend intravenous therapy (regimen B) to all pregnant women with active Lyme disease. In our experience, all pregnant women with EM who have received such antibiotic therapy have delivered healthy babies.

Assessment of response to therapy

Judging the adequacy of treatment for Lyme disease poses special problems due to the organism's latency and the intermittent pattern of exacerbations and remissions in the natural history of untreated infection. Antibody titers tend to fall after treatment but may persist in asymptomatic individuals for years. Conversely, some patients with objective late Lyme disease are consistently seronegative.[33] Therefore, unlike syphilis, there is no simple laboratory test to gauge the adequacy of treatment for Lyme disease.

To complicate matters further, reinfection with *B. burgdorferi*, leading to recurrence of clinical disease, is well reported.[79,113] Recurrent infection in a recently treated patient could easily be misinterpreted as a treatment failure. In addition, the *Ixodes* group of ticks may simultaneously transmit other infectious agents such as *Babesia* in the United States,[38,62] or tickborne encephalitis virus in Europe.[31] Clinical symptoms from these disorders may overlap those of Lyme disease but would not respond to therapeutic interventions designed to treat *B. burgdorferi* infection.

Careful monitoring is essential in all patients treated for Lyme disease. Patients should be informed of the various manifestations of late infection. Those manifesting subjective symptoms of fatigue, arthralgias, and so forth ("post-Lyme syndrome") should be reassured and treated symptomatically. If residual symptoms are consistent with fibromyalgia, these individuals may benefit from interventions geared toward this condition, such as exercise and low-dose amitriptyline.[96]

Important questions still remain regarding therapy for early Lyme disease such as optimal duration and choice of therapy; which patients, if any, may benefit from very aggressive interventions; and are treatment failures or slow responders due to antimicrobial resistance, other properties of the organism, or host factors. Hopefully, future trials will provide the necessary answers.

ACKNOWLEDGMENTS

We thank Drs. Robert Nadelman and Durland Fish for their assistance and critical review of this manuscript. We also extend our thanks to Gilda Forseter, R.N., Donna McKenna, R.N., Diane Holmgren, R.N., Ulrich Jorde, M.D., Susan Bittker, BS, Denise Cooper, BS, and Charles Pavia, Ph.D. for their technical assistance.

REFERENCES

1. Afzelius A: Erythema chronicum migrans, *Acta Derm Venereol (Stockh)* 2:120, 1921.
2. Anderson JF: Epizootiology of *Borrelia* in *Ixodes* tick vectors and reservoir hosts, *Rev Infect Dis* 11(suppl 6):1451, 1989.
3. Anderson JF: Preventing Lyme disease, *Rheum Clin North Am* 15:757, 1989.
4. Åsbrink E, Hovmark A: Early and late cutaneous manifestations in *Ixodes*-borne borreliosis, *Ann NY Acad Sci* 539:4, 1988.
5. Åsbrink E, Olsson I: Clinical manifestations of erythema chronicum migrans Afzelius in 161 patients, *Acta Derm Venereol (Stockh)* 65:43, 1985.
6. Bannwarth A: Chronische lymphocytäre meningitis, enzüdliche polyneuritis und "rheumatismus," *Arch Psychiatr Nervenkr* 113:284, 1941.
7. Bannwarth A: Zur klinik und pathogenese der "chronischen lymphocytären meningitis," *Arch Psychiatr Nervenkr* 117:161, 1944.
8. Barbour AG: Immunochemical analysis of Lyme disease spirochetes, *Yale J Biol Med* 57:581, 1984.

9. Barbour AG: Isolation and cultivation of Lyme disease spirochetes, *Yale J Biol Med* 57:521, 1984.

10. Barbour AG, Heiland RA, Howe TR: Heterogeneity of major proteins in Lyme disease borreliae: A molecular analysis of North American and European isolates, *J Infect Dis* 152:478, 1985.

11. Barthold SW et al: An animal model for Lyme arthritis, *Ann NY Acad Sci* 539:264, 1988.

12. Barthold SW et al: Lyme borreliosis in selected strains and ages of laboratory mice, *J Infect Dis* 162:133, 1990.

13. Benach JL et al: Spirochetes isolated from the blood of two patients with Lyme disease, *N Engl J Med* 308:740, 1983.

14. Benach JL et al: Experimental transmission of the Lyme disease spirochete to rabbits (letter), *J Infect Dis* 150:786, 1984.

15. Berger BW: Treatment of erythema chronicum migrans of Lyme disease, *Ann NY Acad Sci* 539:346, 1988.

16. Berger BW: Dermatologic manifestations of Lyme disease, *Rev Infect Dis* 11(suppl 6):1475, 1989.

17. Berger BW, Johnson RC: Clinical and microbiologic findings in six patients with erythema migrans of Lyme disease, *J Am Acad Dermatol* 21:1188, 1989.

18. Berger BW et al: Isolation and characterization of the Lyme disease spirochete from the skin of patients with erythema chronicum migrans, *Am Acad Dermatol* 13:444, 1985.

19. Binder E, Doepfmer R, Horstein O: Übertragung des erythema chronicum migrans von mensch zu mensch in zwel passagen, *Klin Wochenschr* 33:727, 1955.

20. Bracero LA et al: Prevalence of seropositivity to the Lyme disease spirochete during pregnancy in an endemic area, Manuscript submitted for publication.

21. Bryceson ADM et al: Studies on the mechanism of the Jarisch-Herxheimer reaction in louse-borne relapsing fever: evidence for the presence of circulating *Borrelia* endotoxin, *Clin Sci* 43:343, 1972.

22. Burgdorfer W: The New Zealand white rabbit: an experimental host for infecting ticks with Lyme disease spirochete, *Yale J Biol Med* 57:609, 1984.

23. Burgdorfer W et al: Lyme disease—a tick-borne spirochetosis? *Science* 216:1317, 1982.

24. Centers for Disease Control: Lyme disease—United States, 1987 and 1988, *MMWR* 38:668, 1989.

25. Centers for Disease Control: Seizures temporally associated with use of DEET insect repellent, *MMWR* 38:678, 1989.

26. Chengxu A et al: Clinical manifestations and epidemiological characteristics of Lyme disease in Hailin County, Heilongjiang province, China, *Ann NY Acad Sci* 539:302, 1988.

27. Ciesielski CA et al: The geographic distribution of Lyme disease in the United States, *Ann NY Acad Sci* 539:283, 1988.

28. Committee on Infectious Diseases: Treatment of Lyme borreliosis, *Pediatrics* 88:176, 1991.

29. Costello CM et al: A prospective study of tick bites in an endemic area for Lyme disease, *J Infect Dis* 159:136, 1989.

30. Craft JE, Grodzicki RL, Steere AC: Antibody response in Lyme disease: evaluation of diagnostic tests, *J Infect Dis* 149:789, 1984.

31. Craven RB: *Toga viruses.* In Belshe RB, editor: *Textbook of human virology,* p 617, Littleton, MA, 1984, PSG Publishing.

32. Dattwyler RJ, Halperin JJ: Failure of tetracycline therapy in early Lyme disease, *Arthritis Rheum* 30:448, 1987.

33. Dattwyler R et al: Seronegative Lyme disease, *N Engl J Med* 319:1441, 1988.

34. Dattwyler RJ et al: Amoxicillin plus probenecid versus doxycycline for treatment of erythema migrans borreliosis, *Lancet* 2:1404, 1990.

35. Degos R, Touraine R, Arouete J: Erythema chronicum migrans: discussion of rickettsial origin, *Ann Dermatol Syphiligr* 89:247, 1962.

36. Dinerman H, Steere AC: Fibromyalgia following Lyme disease: association with neurologic involvement and lack of response to antibiotic therapy, *Arthritis Rheum* 33(suppl):S136, 1990 (abstract).

37. Falco RC, Fish D: Prevalence of *Ixodes dammini* near the homes of Lyme disease patients in Westchester County, New York, *Am J Epidemiol* 127:826, 1988.

38. Gadbaw JJ et al: Babesiosis—Connecticut, *MMWR* 38:649, 1989.

39. Garin et Bujadoux C: Paralysie par les Tiques, *J Med Lyon* 71:765, 1922.

40. Giroud P, Capponi M, Dumas N: Rickettsioses et lésions cutanées en dehors de syndromes fébriles, *Bull Soc Pathol Exot* 55:958, 1962.

41. Hård S: Erythema chronicum migrans (Afzelii) associated with mosquito bite, *Acta Derm Venereol (Stockh)* 46:473, 1966.

42. Hellerström S: Erythema chronicum migrans Afzelii, *Acta Derm Venereol (Stockh)* 11:315, 1930.

43. Hollström E: Successful treatment of erythema migrans Afzelius, *Acta Derm Venereol (Stockh)* 31:235, 1951.

44. Hollström E: Penicillin treatment of erythema chronicum migrans Afzelius, *Acta Derm Venereol (Stockh)* 38:285, 1958.

45. Hovmark A et al: A comparative study of efficacy of roxithromycin and phenoxymethyl penicillin in the treatment of erythema migrans. IV International Conference on Lyme Borreliosis, Stockholm, 1990 (abs P117).

46. Johnson RC: Isolation techniques for spirochetes and their sensitivity to antibiotics in vitro and in vivo, *Rev Infect Dis* 11(suppl 6):1505, 1989.

47. Johnson RC, Kodner C, Russell M: In vitro and in vivo susceptibility of the Lyme disease spirochete, *Borrelia burgdorferi,* to four antimicrobial agents. *Antimicrob Agents Chemother* 31:164, 1987.

48. Johnson RC, Marek N, Kodner C: Infection of Syrian hamsters with Lyme disease spirochetes, *J Clin Microbiol* 20:1099, 1984.

49. Johnson RC et al: Comparative in vitro and in vivo susceptibilities of the Lyme disease spirochete to cefuroxime and other antimicrobial agents, *Antimicrob Agents Chemother* 34:2133, 1990.

50. Johnson SE et al: Susceptibility of the Lyme disease spirochete to seven antimicrobial agents, *Yale J Biol Med* 57:549, 1984.

51. Koneman EW et al: *Antimicrobial susceptibility testing.* In *Color atlas and textbook of diagnostic microbiology,* ed 3, p 473, Philadelphia, 1988, JB Lippincott.

52. Kornblatt AN, Steere AC, Brownstein DG: Experimental Lyme disease in rabbits: spirochetes found in erythema migrans and blood, *Infect Immun* 46:220, 1984.

53. Krinsky WL, Brown SJ, Askenase PW: *Ixodes dammini* induced skin lesions in guinea pigs and rabbits compared to erythema chronicum migrans in patients with Lyme arthritis, *Exp Parasitol* 53:318, 1982.

54. Lennhoff C: Spirochaetes in aetiologically obscure diseases, *Acta Derm Venereol (Stockh)* 28:295, 1948.

55. Logigian EL, Kaplan RF, Steere AC: Chronic neurologic manifestations of Lyme disease, *N Engl J Med* 323:1438, 1990.

56. Luft BJ et al: New chemotherapeutic approaches in the treatment of Lyme borreliosis, *Ann NY Acad Sci* 539:352, 1988.

57. Luft BJ et al: A perspective on the treatment of Lyme borreliosis, *Rev Infect Dis* 11(suppl 6):1518, 1989.

58. Luger SW: Lyme disease transmitted by a biting fly, *N Engl J Med* 322:1752, 1990.

59. MacDonald AB: Gestational Lyme borreliosis—implications for the fetus, *Rheum Dis Clin North Am* 15:657, 1989.

60. Magnarelli LA, Anderson JF, Barbour AG: The etiologic agent of Lyme disease in deer flies, horse flies, and mosquitoes, *J Infect Dis* 154:355, 1986.

61. Malane MS et al: Diagnosis of Lyme disease based on dermatologic manifestations, *Ann Intern Med* 114:490, 1991.

62. Marcus LC et al: Fatal pancarditis in a patient with coexistent Lyme disease and babesiosis, *Ann Intern Med* 103:374, 1985.

63. Markowitz LE et al: Lyme disease during pregnancy, *JAMA* 255:3394, 1986.

64. Massarotti EM et al: Treatment of early Lyme disease, *Am J Med* 92:396, 1992.

65. Mast WE, Burrows WM: Erythema chronicum migrans in the United States, *JAMA* 236:859, 1976.

66. McAlister HF et al: Lyme carditis: an important cause of reversible heart block, *Ann Intern Med* 110:339, 1989.

67. Mursic VP, Wilske B: Comparison of in vitro and in vivo activity of various antibiotics against *Borrelia burgdorferi*, IV International Conference on Lyme Borreliosis 1990 Stockholm (abs P112).

68. Mursic VP, Wilske B, Schierz G: European *Borrelia burgdorferi* isolated from humans and ticks: culture conditions and antibiotic susceptibility, *Zentralbl Bakteriol Mikrobiol Hyg* 263:112, 1986.

69. Mursic VP et al: In vitro and in vivo susceptibility of *Borrelia burgdorferi*, *Eur J Clin Microbiol Infect Dis* 6:424, 1987.

70. Mursic VP et al: Comparative antimicrobial activity of the new macrolides against *Borrelia burgdorferi*, *Eur J Clin Microbiol Infect Dis* 8:651, 1989.

71. Nadelman RB, Wormser GP: A clinical approach to Lyme disease, *Mount Sinai J Med* 57:144, 1990.

72. Nadelman RB et al: Isolation of *Borrelia burgdorferi* from the blood of seven patients with Lyme disease, *Am J Med* 88:21, 1990.

73. Nadelman RB et al: A multicenter, investigator-blinded, randomized comparison of the efficacy and safety of cefuroxime axetil and doxycycline in the treatment of patients with early Lyme disease. 30th Interscience Conference on Antimicrobial Agents and Chemotherapy 1990, Atlanta (abs 655).

74. Nadelman RB et al: Single dose doxycycline as prophylaxis for Lyme borreliosis after *I. dammini* bites in a Lyme endemic area, IV International Conference on Lyme Borreliosis, Stockholm, 1990 (abs L12).

75. National Committee for Clinical Laboratory Standards: *Performance standards for antimicrobial disk susceptibility tests*, ed 3, Publication M2-A3. Villanova, PA, 1984, NCCLS.

76. National Committee for Clinical Laboratory Standards: *Methods for dilution antimicrobial susceptibility tests for bacteria that grow aerobically*, Publication M7-A. Villanova, PA, 1985, NCCLS.

77. Neu HC: A perspective on therapy of Lyme infection, *Ann NY Acad Sci* 539:314, 1988.

78. Perine PL, Teklu B: Antibiotic treatment of louse-borne relapsing fever in Ethiopia: a report of 377 cases, *Am J Trop Med Hyg* 32:1096, 1983.

79. Pfister NW et al: Reinfection with *Borrelia burgdorferi*, *Lancet* 2:984, 1986.

80. Piesman J et al: Duration of tick attachment and *Borrelia burgdorferi* transmission, *J Clin Microbiol* 25:557, 1987.

81. Piesman J et al: Duration of adult female *Ixodes dammini* attachment and transmission of *B. burgdorferi*, with description of a needle aspiration isolation method, *J Infect Dis* 163:895, 1991.

82. Rahn DW, Malawista SE: Lyme disease: recommendations for diagnosis and treatment, *Ann Intern Med* 114:472, 1991.

83. Rawlings JA, Fournier PV, Teltow GJ: Isolation of *Borrelia* spirochetes from patients in Texas, *J Clin Microbiol* 25:1148, 1987.

84. 1991 Red Book, Oradell, NJ, 1991, Medical Economics.

85. Reik Jr L, Burgdorfer W, Donaldson JO: Neurologic abnormalities in Lyme disease without erythema chronicum migrans, *Am J Med* 81:73, 1986.

86. Reik L et al: Neurologic manifestations of Lyme disease, *Medicine (Baltimore)* 58:281, 1979.

87. Russell H et al: Enzyme-linked immunosorbent assay and indirect immunofluorescence assay for Lyme disease, *J Infect Dis* 149:465, 1984.

88. Sanford JP: *Relapsing fever—treatment and control.* In Johnson RC, editor: *The biology of parasitic spirochetes*, p 389, New York, 1976, Academic Press.

89. Schaible UE et al: Demonstration of antigen-specific T cells and histopathological alterations in mice experimentally inoculated with *Borrelia burgdorferi*, *Infect Immun* 57:41, 1989.

90. Schlesinger PA et al: Maternal-fetal transmission of the Lyme disease spirochete, *Borrelia burgdorferi*, *Ann Intern Med* 103:67, 1985.

91. Schmitz JL et al: Induction of Lyme arthritis in LSH hamsters, *Infect Immun* 56:2336, 1988.

92. Schoen RT: Treatment of Lyme disease, *Conn Med* 53:335, 1989.

93. Schulze TL et al: *Amblyomma americanum:* a potential vector of Lyme disease in New Jersey, *Science* 224:601, 1984.

94. Scrimenti RJ: Erythema chronicum migrans, *Arch Dermatol* 102:104, 1970.

95. Shrestha M, Grodzicki RL, Steere AC: Diagnosing early Lyme disease, *Am J Med* 78:235, 1985.

96. Sigal LH: Summary of the first 100 patients seen at a Lyme disease referral center, *Am J Med* 88:577, 1990.

97. Sköldenberg B et al: Treatment of Lyme borreliosis with emphasis on neurological disease, *Ann NY Acad Sci* 539:317, 1988.

98. Smith PF et al: Occupational risk of Lyme disease in endemic areas of New York state, *Ann NY Acad Sci* 539:289, 1988.

99. Stanek G et al: European Lyme borreliosis, *Ann NY Acad Sci* 539:274, 1988.

100. Steere AC: Lyme disease, *N Engl J Med* 321:586, 1989.

101. Steere AC et al: Erythema chronicum migrans and Lyme arthritis: the enlarging clinical spectrum, *Ann Intern Med* 86:685, 1977.

102. Steere AC et al: Lyme arthritis: an epidemic of oligoarticular arthritis in children and adults in three Connecticut communities, *Arthritis Rheum* 20:7, 1977.

103. Steere AC et al: Antibiotic therapy in Lyme disease, *Ann Intern Med* 93:1, 1980.

104. Steere AC et al: Lyme carditis: cardiac abnormalities of Lyme disease, *Ann Intern Med* 93:8, 1980.

105. Steere AC et al: The early clinical manifestations of Lyme disease, *Ann Intern Med* 99:76, 1983.

106. Steere AC et al: The spirochetal etiology of Lyme disease, *N Engl J Med* 308:733, 1983.

107. Steere AC, et al: Treatment of the early manifestations of Lyme disease, *Ann Intern Med* 99:22, 1983.

108. Steere AC et al: Recovery of Lyme disease spirochetes from patients, *Yale J Biol Med* 57:557, 1984.
109. Steere AC et al: Unilateral blindness caused by infection with the Lyme disease spirochete, *Borrelia burgdorferi*, *Ann Intern Med* 103:382, 1985.
110. Steere AC et al: Longitudinal assessment of the clinical and epidemiological features of Lyme disease in a defined population, *J Infect Dis* 154:295, 1986.
111. Treatment of Lyme disease, *Med Letter* 31:57, 1989.
112. Wallis RC et al: Erythema chronicum migrans and Lyme arthritis: field study of ticks, *Am J Epidemiol* 108:322, 1978.
113. Weber K et al: Reinfection with erythema migrans disease, *Infection* 14:32, 1986.
114. Weber K et al: Antibiotic therapy of early European Lyme borreliosis and acrodermatitis chronica atrophicans, *Ann NY Acad Sci* 539:324, 1988.
115. Weber K et al: *Borrelia burgdorferi* in a newborn despite oral therapy for Lyme borreliosis during pregnancy, *Pediatr Infect Dis J* 7:286, 1988.
116. Weber K et al: A randomized trial of ceftriaxone versus oral penicillin for the treatment of early European Lyme borreliosis, *Infection* 18:91, 1990.
117. Welling PG et al: Bioavailability of tetracycline and doxycycline in fasted and nonfasted subjects, *Antimicrob Agents Chemother* 11:462, 1977.
118. Wormser GP: Treatment of *Borrelia burgdorferi* infection, *Lab Med* 21:316, 1990.
119. Young EF et al: Studies on the pathogenesis of the Jarisch-Herxheimer reaction, *J Infect Dis* 146:606, 1982.

Treatment of *Borrelia burgdorferi* Infection: Acute and Chronic Disease

Raymond J. Dattwyler

In any discussion of the treatment of Lyme disease, one must bear in mind the fact that Lyme disease is an infection caused by the spirochete *Borrelia burgdorferi*. Basic infectious disease principles should be considered in the therapy of this disease. A clear concept of this disease is extremely important in interpreting treatment studies and rationally approaching therapy. There is no gold standard laboratory test for Lyme disease. Because serologic tests have a poor predictive value and markedly overpredict the disease, there is confusion on the part of many clinicians as to the scope of its clinical manifestations. In the past, Lyme disease was divided into three discrete stages: stage 1, erythema migrans; stage 2, acute neurologic or cardiac involvement; stage 3, arthritis, giving the impression that the clinical expression of this infectious disease proceeds in an orderly fashion from one stage to the next.[26] It is now generally recognized that this staging scheme is obsolete and that *B. burgdorferi* infection is better conceptualized as a progressive infectious disease.[2,12,21] Infection begins locally in the skin at the site of a tick bite with about two thirds of infected people developing erythema migrans (EM), a characteristic skin lesion at the site of the tick bite. Heralded by the onset of constitutional signs and symptoms, hematogenous dissemination of *B. burgdorferi* with seeding of multiple organs occurs early in the course of infection in a large number of patients. The most obvious evidence of dissemination is the development of additional EM lesions or major organ system involvement: meningitis, cranial neuropathy, arthritis, hepatitis or carditis. As the immune response develops, the disease can enter a chronic phase. Yet, not unlike people with syphilis, many people with *B. burgdorferi* infection never develop progressive disease. Consequently, rather than classifying the disease by which organ system is involved, in judging appropriate treatment it is better to consider if the infection is localized or disseminated, and acute or chronic. Unfortunately, few studies have approached treatment in this manner.

In the past, studies lumped together patients with both simple local infection and disseminated infection.[24] Only recently have investigators begun to address this disease more as an infectious disease. If one simply approaches it as any other bacterial disease, Lyme disease can be demystified. As in any infectious disease, one would ideally like to culture the causative organism, determine its sensitivity, and, based on that information, treat with the antibiotic that seems most appropriate for that cultured organism. Unfortunately, in Lyme disease, *B. burgdorferi* has generally been difficult to culture from the infected host.[1,23] However, that does not mean that there is no information on the sensitivity of this spirochete. *B. burgdorferi* has been cultured from infected individuals and isolated from ticks; a number of studies of the in vitro antibiotic sensitivity of this organism have been carried out on these isolates.[9,13] This information can be used to help decide which antimicrobials should be used to treat this infectious process. Although there was no standardization of the methods used in these studies, it is clear from these reports that *B. burgdorferi* is sensitive in vitro to penicillins, tetracyclines, third-generation cephalosporins, and macrolides.[9,13,17]

Agents that are not active in vitro can be eliminated from consideration, but the mere demonstration that an antibiotic is effective in vitro does not mean that it will be effective in vivo. The macrolides, erythromycin[24] and roxithromycin (Asbrink, personal communication), are highly active in vitro, yet are relatively ineffective in vivo. Thus, in addition to in vitro sensitivity, absorption, tissue penetration, and pharmacokinetics all must be considered in the choice of an antibiotic. Experiments have demonstrated that an antimicrobial must be kept together with *B. burgdorferi* for a prolonged period (72 to 96 hours) for the antibiotic to effect a kill.[13] In addition, it is clear that *B. burgdorferi* can enter the central nervous system (CNS) early in the course of infection. Thus, when designing a treatment regimen, one must pay attention not only to the sensitivity of the organism but also to the ability of the regimen to provide adequate CNS levels and to the pharmacokinetics of the particular antibiotics used.

In reviewing the literature on the treatment of this disease, one finds that there is a limited number of well-designed randomized prospective trials. The largest studies have been carried out in EM patients and are reviewed in Chapter 18. Oral agents that were evaluated in the early studies included penicillin, erythromycin, and tetracycline.[24] In retrospect, the poor response to these antimicrobial agents can be explained in part by the fact that none of the dosage regimens provided adequate antimicrobial concentrations in important systems like the CNS.

A more recent treatment study of EM compared amoxicillin 500 mg plus 500 mg of probenecid three times a day for 21 days to doxycycline 100 mg twice a day for 21 days.[5] The pharmacokinetics, in vitro sensitivity, and the CNS penetrations of these regimens were considered in the study design. In contrast to earlier studies, there were no major late complications, and minor complications were limited to arthralgias and fatigue, which was self-limited in all cases. None of the patients in that trial needed further treatment. Both regimens were highly effective. Further analysis of the results of that study revealed that people who presented with constitutional signs or symptoms such as fever, arthralgias, myalgias (complicated EM) were more likely to have posttreatment fatigue or arthralgias than those without constitutional signs or symptoms. This raises the possibility that in some patients with EM and constitutional signs and symptoms, alternative regimens that provide even better CNS levels may be required.

Other oral agents are currently under study for the treatment of EM, but there are no clear-cut data that either oral cephalosporins or new macrolides like azithromycin should be used in place of either amoxicillin plus probenecid or doxycycline for the treatment of patients with EM. Azithromycin may prove to be an excellent drug in people who cannot or should not receive these other agents. A significant drawback of many oral regimens, especially the oral cephalosporins, is the failure to provide adequate antimicrobial levels in the CNS. Inadequate treatment of the CNS is quite a worrisome possibility and, until more definitive studies are published, oral therapy with alternatives to doxycycline, minocycline, and amoxicillin plus probenecid cannot be recommended in patients with signs or symptoms suggestive of acute disseminated infection. This is especially true of the oral cephalosporins, because none of those currently in use in the United States have been shown to provide adequate CNS levels.

The treatment of acute and chronic disseminated disease is somewhat more controversial because case definitions have varied and most of the trials are small and limited in scope. It is clear, with more recent studies reporting a high success rate, that this is an eminently treatable disease. In acute disseminated infection, constitutional signs and symptoms are associated with acute neurologic, cardiac, and musculoskeletal manifestations. As the infection enters a chronic phase, constitutional signs and symptoms are absent or mild and the disease is characterized by focal inflammation in the affected organ system, usually the nervous system, joints, or skin. Intravenous penicillin and ceftriaxone have been the most widely used antibiotics for the treatment of disseminated infection with major organ system manifestations.[3,4,15,16,27]

Patients with acute meningitis or meningoencephalitis normally respond quite well to intravenous penicillin.[11,14,20] However, there are reports of progressive disease despite penicillin therapy.[6] Third-generation parenteral cephalosporins, ceftriaxone and cefotaxime, appear to be highly effective in patients with acute CNS infection and can be used as primary therapy or in cases where penicillin has been ineffective.[15,18] Lipid-soluble tetracyclines, like doxycycline and minocycline, with the ability to cross the blood-brain barrier, may be attractive agents to treat disseminated infection. Doxycycline has been shown to have efficacy in acute neuroborreliosis, but more experience is needed before a clear role for these agents can be delineated.[7,10] In Bannwarth's syndrome, meningopolyradiculitis, penicillin usually halts progression, but as many as 50% of patients with this syndrome continue to have serious neurologic signs such as spastic paraparesis after treatment.[11,14] The treatment response of peripheral neuropathy in Lyme disease has not been specifically studied. However, anecdotally, the response to ceftriaxone is quite good.[8] One must realize when treating patients with neurologic involvement that the nervous system heals slowly and that significant insults to the CNS may be associated with permanent deficits. Also, it is extremely important to define objectively the clinical manifestations so that the response to therapy can be clearly assessed. A lumbar puncture and analysis of the cerebrospinal fluid (CSF) is virtually mandatory in patients suspected of having CNS infection.

The treatment of Lyme arthritis has to be considered in light of the natural course of this disease. Steere described the outcome of 55 patients who initially presented with EM who were not treated.[22] Of these 55 patients, 34 developed arthritis, but the arthritis was self-limited in 28 and only became chronic in 6. In a study of the treatment of Lyme arthritis, Steere compared benzathine penicillin to placebo (saline). He reported that 7 of 16 patients given benzathine penicillin had resolution of their arthritis as compared to 0 of 20 given saline.[25] In a nonrandomized extension of that study, he found that 11 of 20 patients given 20 million U of intravenous penicillin a day for 10 days had remission of their arthritis.[25] Thus, approximately 50% of patients with arthritis secondary to *B. burgdorferi* continued to have episodes of arthritis after parenteral penicillin. In recent experiments using polymerase chain reaction, we were able to demonstrate the presence of bacterial DNA in the CSF of patients with recurrent Lyme arthritis. This finding raises the possibility that the CNS may be a reservoir for *B. burgdorferi*, suggesting that any regimen that does not adequately treat the neural compartment may not provide a cure. Penicillin, even when give intravenously, may not reach adequate levels in the CSF in the absence of meningeal inflammation and disruption of the blood-brain barrier. It also raises questions as to the treatment of chronic disease with oral antibiotics.

In a prospective, randomized study comparing penicillin to ceftriaxone in patients with chronic disseminated disease (arthritis or neurologic manifestations), ceftriaxone was shown to be superior to penicillin.[4] Ceftriaxone provides adequate levels in the CNS, even in the absence of meningeal inflammation. Questions still remain as to the optimal treatment of disseminated infection. Pfister et al reported that 10 days of cefotaxime was equal to 10 days of ceftriaxone in the treatment of neuroborreliosis but that 10 of the 27 patients in the study remained symptomatic.[16] Ten days of treatment may be too short.

Third-generation cephalosporins like ceftriaxone appear to be the treatment of choice for disseminated infection with a high probability of CNS involvement. Unlike penicillin, with an approximate 50% failure rate, ceftriaxone has a failure rate of only 15% or less. However, larger long-term studies are required to determine the optimal treatment of this disease and the precise role ceftriaxone and other third-generation cephalosporins should play in the treatment of this infection. Questions remain as to the optimal duration of therapy and if parenteral therapy should be used for patients with early disseminated infection. A multicenter trial is being carried out to try to answer these questions.

In refractory patients, long-term antibiotic therapy has not been studied in a systematic way. Anecdotal reports would suggest that this is not an effective means of therapy. Questions have been raised as to the cause of continued objective disease in patients who have been adequately treated with antibiotics. Although there is no clear scientific proof, many investigators hypothesize that immune mechanisms play an important role in those patients to antibiotics. Schoen reported that in 20 patients who underwent arthroscopic synovectomy for refractory chronic Lyme arthritis of the knee, 16 had resolution of joint inflammation.[19] Other modalities aimed at reducing inflammation may be effective but further clinical trials are required.

REFERENCES

1. Benach JL et al: Spirochetes isolated from the blood of two patients with Lyme disease, *N Engl J Med* 308:740, 1983.
2. Berger BW: Treatment of erythema chronicum migrans of Lyme disease, *Ann NY Acad Sci* 539(346):346, 1988.
3. Dattwyler RJ, Luft BJ: Antibiotic treatment of Lyme borreliosis, *Biomed Pharmacother* 43(6):421, 1989.
4. Dattwyler RJ et al: Treatment of late Lyme borreliosis—randomised comparison of ceftriaxone and penicillin, *Lancet* 1(8596):1191, 1988.
5. Dattwyler RJ et al: Amoxicillin plus probenecid versus doxycycline for treatment of erythema migrans borreliosis, 336:1404, 1990.
6. Diringer MN, Halperin JJ, Dattwyler RJ: Lyme meningoencephalitis: report of a severe, penicillin-resistant case, *Arthritis Rheum* 30(6):705, 1987.
7. Dotevall L, Hagberg L: Penetration of doxycycline into cerebrospinal fluid in patients treated for suspected Lyme neuroborreliosis, *Antimicrob Agents Chemother* 33:1078, 1989.
8. Halperin JJ et al: Lyme disease: cause of a treatable peripheral neuropathy, *Neurology* 37(11):1700, 1987.
9. Johnson RC, Kodner C, Russell M: In vitro and in vivo susceptibility of the Lyme disease spirochete, *Borrelia burgdorferi*, to four antimicrobial agents, *Antimicrob Agents Chemother* 31(2):164, 1987.
10. Kohlhepp W, Oschmann P, Mertens HG: Treatment of Lyme borreliosis. Randomized comparison of doxycycline and penicillin G, *J Neurol* 236:464, 1989.
11. Kristoferitsch W et al: High-dose penicillin therapy in meningopolyneuritis Garin-Bujadoux-Bannwarth. Clinical and cerebrospinal fluid data, *Zentralbl Bakteriol Mikrobiol Hyg [A]* 263(3):357, 1987.
12. Luft BJ, Dattwyler RJ: *Lyme borreliosis: problems in diagnosis and treatment.* In Remington JS, Swartz MV, editors: *Current clinical topics in infectious diseases*, vol II, p 56. New York, 1989, McGraw-Hill.
13. Luft BJ et al: New chemotherapeutic approaches in the treatment of Lyme borreliosis, *Ann NY Acad Sci* 539(352):352, 1988.
14. Pfister HW et al: Bannwarth's syndrome and the enlarged neurological spectrum of arthropod-borne borreliosis, *Zentralbl Bakteriol Mikrobiol Hyg [A]* 263(3):343, 1987.
15. Pfister HW et al: Cefotaxime vs penicillin G for acute neurologic manifestations in Lyme borreliosis. A prospective randomized study, *Arch Neurol* 46(11):1190, 1989.
16. Pfister HW et al: Randomized comparison of ceftriaxone and cefotaxime in Lyme neuroborreliosis, *J Infect Dis* 163(2):311, 1991.
17. Preac MV, Wilske B, Schierz G: European *Borrelia burgdorferi* isolated from humans and ticks culture conditions and antibiotic susceptibility, *Zentralbl Bakteriol Mikrobiol Hyg [A]* 263(1-2):112, 1986.

18. Rahn DW, Malawista SE: Lyme disease: recommendations for diagnosis and treatment, *Ann Intern Med* 114(6):472, 1991.
19. Schoen RT et al: Treatment of refractory chronic Lyme arthritis with arthroscopic synovectomy, *Arthritis Rheum* 34:1056, 1991.
20. Skoldenberg B et al: Treatment of Lyme borreliosis with emphasis on neurological disease, *Ann NY Acad Sci* 539(317):317, 1988.
21. Steere AC: Lyme disease, *N Engl J Med* 321:586, 1989.
22. Steere AC, Schoen RT, Taylor E: The clinical evolution of Lyme arthritis, *Ann Intern Med* 107:725, 1987.
23. Steere AC et al: The spirochetal etiology of Lyme disease, *N Engl J Med* 308:733, 1983.
24. Steere A et al: Treatment of the early manifestations of Lyme disease, *Ann Intern Med* 99:22, 1983.
25. Steere AC et al: Successful parenteral penicillin therapy of established Lyme arthritis, *N Engl J Med* 312(14):869, 1985.
26. Steere AC et al: Clinical manifestations of Lyme disease, *Zentralbl Bakteriol Mikrobiol Hyg [A]* 263(1-2):201, 1986.
27. Steere AC et al: Treatment of Lyme disease, *Zentralbl Bakteriol Mikrobiol Hyg [A]* 263(3):352, 1987.

20 New Antibiotic Agents

Carl Urban and Benjamin J. Luft

Antibiotics have played a pivotal role in the reduction or eradication of many different pathogens. Lyme borreliosis caused by the bacterium *Borrelia burgdorferi* is no exception. Numerous classes of antibiotics have been tested on this organism including the penicillins,[11,24,27,46,52] cephalosporins,[11,24,37,52,54] tetracyclines,[12,14,24,27] and macrolides,[24,26,38,52] but the exact role these compounds play in the eradication of symptoms or disease remains controversial.[13,30] No new antibiotics have shown any equal or better efficacy over the older ones with the exception of some of the newer macrolides[16,26,38] and cefuroxime.[25,32] What has been evolving over the past few years are newer chemotherapeutic strategies for the treatment of Lyme borreliosis[28,30] and investigations into the ultrastructure,[53] physiology,[2,47] and macromolecular structures[50-52] of this bacterium. Hopefully, these newer approaches will give us a better understanding of the pathogenesis of the organism and identify those sites that are amenable to abating, altering, or eradicating the disease. This chapter reviews some of the more recent in vitro and in vivo *Borrelia burgdorferi* studies performed with the newer macrolides and cefuroxime, mentions some of the newer chemotherapeutic modalities in the treatment of Lyme borreliosis, and discusses investigations undertaken to discern those proteins or glycoproteins that are involved in beta-lactam binding.

IN VITRO AND IN VIVO SUSCEPTIBILITY STUDIES

Considering the worldwide distribution and increasing frequency of Lyme disease, only a few laboratories have published information on the susceptibility of *Borrelia burgdorferi* to antibiotics.[24-27,28,38,52] This is due to a number of reasons, including the specialized media and techniques involved in cultivating the organism and strain variation.[2,52] More importantly, there is no standardized methodology employed in the testing of the organisms.[30] However, important information can be gleaned from in vitro and animal studies as pointed out by Luft et al[30] and others.[55]

Preac-Mursic et al[38] have recently published interesting in vitro and in vivo data from studies with gerbils showing the antibacterial activity of the new macrolides, azithromycin, clarithromycin, and roxithromycin, compared with erythromycin. All of the newer compounds had better minimal inhibitory concentration (MIC) values—MIC 50 and MIC 90—than erythromycin, but in the animal model studies only azithromycin demonstrated both high in vitro and in vivo activity. Although the in vivo studies involved only three gerbils for each of the new macrolides tested, the results are quite promising considering their long half-lives, high blood and tissue concentrations, high oral bioavailability, and low protein binding.

A similar study by Johnson et al[26] also compared the in vitro and in vivo susceptibilities of *Borrelia burgdorferi* to tetracycline, erythromycin, and azithromycin. Their data also supported the earlier results of Preac-Mursic et al[38] that azithromycin had superior in vitro values (Preac-Mursic et al, MIC 90, 0.015 μg/ml; Johnson et al, minimal bactericidal concentration (MBC), 0.04 μg/ml). In addition, azithromycin also demonstrated excellent results when used in a Syrian hamster animal model testing system. These investigators as well as others all agree that although erythromycin does well when tested in vitro, it does not perform as well in animal studies.

A letter in the *Lancet*[16] reported on the treatment of a 30-year-old man infected with *Borrelia burgdorferi* with the administration of co-trimoxazole and roxithromycin. Although the relative contribution of co-trimoxazole is questionable, as pointed out by Bowman,[6] both authors agree that the ability of roxithromycin to penetrate the blood-brain barrier may be the reason for its remarkable activity against the organisms. Results of clinical trials with these newer macrolide antibiotics are eagerly awaited.

Johnson et al[25] have recently compared the in vitro and in vivo susceptibilities of *Borrelia burgdorferi* to cefuroxime and several other agents. Their in vitro data demonstrated an MBC of 1 μg/ml for cefuroxime, which was comparable to amoxicillin, more than tenfold greater than ceftriaxone, and threefold higher than erythromycin. Their 50% curative dose data using golden Syrian hamsters showed a 60% protection rate (three of five animals) with cefuroxime. These data taken together with cefuroxime's oral bioavailability suggest a utility for this compound in humans.

A recent abstract by Nadelman et al[32] reported on a randomized clinical comparison of cefuroxime axetil and doxycycline in the treatment of early Lyme disease. Of the 123 patients enrolled, 93% or 52 out of 56 patients in the cefuroxime group and 88% or 45 out of 51 patients in the doxycycline group showed a cure or improvement. As with other cephalosporins, there was a high incidence of diarrhea in the cefuroxime group and a greater incidence of skin photosensitivity reactions in the doxycycline cohort. They concluded that a 500-mg dose of cefuroxime twice a day is as effective as a 100-mg dose of doxycycline three times a day. Because it is easier to take a drug twice a day and most humans acquire Lyme borreliosis symptoms during the spring or summer months when the sun is most prevalent, cefuroxime may be the better oral drug for early Lyme borreliosis.

The superiority of ceftriaxone and cefotaxime in the treatment of the later stages of Lyme borreliosis is unequivocal. The results of in vitro and in vivo MIC and MBC studies demonstrate the efficacy of these cephalosporins.* Although ceftriaxone has been shown by many authors to be the treatment of choice for the later stages of Lyme disease,[9,30,45,49] it is only recently that a randomized study has been published comparing ceftriaxone and cefotaxime in Lyme neuroborreliosis.[36] This randomized study gave patients who presented with Lyme neuroborreliosis either ceftriaxone (2 g IV every 24 hours, 17 patients) or cefotaxime (2 g IV every 8 hours, 16 patients) for 10 days. The authors concluded that patients with Lyme neuroborreliosis may benefit from a 10-day course of either antibiotic and suggest that a longer period of administration may be required because 10 of these patients still presented with symptoms.

Although excellent antibiotics are available for the treatment of Lyme disease, clinical failures still occur.[11,49] This is probably due to a number of reasons including our lack of understanding of the pathogenesis of the disease.[47] However, there is general agreement that early Lyme disease is more treatable than the later stages.[49]

OUTER MEMBRANE STRUCTURE OF *BORRELIA BURGDORFERI*

Information on the molecular architecture of *Borrelia burgdorferi* is just beginning to surface. The

---

*References 11, 21, 25, 26, 27, 37, 52.

recent analysis of the outer membrane ultrastructure of several spirochetes using freeze-fracture election microscopy methods by Walker et al[53] indicates that, unlike *Treponema pallidum, Borrelia burgdorferi* contains concentrated populations of intramembranous particles on the concave outer membrane fracture surface, which is a typical feature of gram-negative organisms. However, unlike gram-negative bacteria, all of the spirochetes tested fractured within the outer membrane and not the inner membrane. A lipopolysaccharide (LPS) moiety has also been described in this organism with properties similar to typical gram-negative LPS.[4] Whether this is LPS or some other component of the organism is controversial.[48] The outer membrane serves as an excellent barrier to many compounds including the hydrophobic beta-lactam and macrolide antibiotics.[35] These compounds do not penetrate the outer membrane because of the charges imparted mostly by the LPS. In addition, porins, which are also present in the outer membranes of typical gram-negative organisms, are rather selective and specific in allowing molecules to enter and exit.[35] Because porin proteins have never been described in *Borrelia burgdorferi*, it is not known whether these structures play a role in antibiotic resistance in Lyme borreliosis.

PENICILLIN-BINDING PROTEINS IN *BORRELIA BURGDORFERI*

Investigations into the molecular targets of beta-lactam antibiotics have recently been reported.[50-52] These proteins, termed penicillin-binding proteins (PBPs) as first described by Spratt,[42,43] are enzymes involved in the synthesis of the bacterial cell wall, and ultimately they define the relative shape of any particular bacterium. Urban et al[51] have demonstrated at least 10 proteins that routinely bind radiolabeled penicillin in *Borrelia burgdorferi* (ATCC B31) using a penicillin-binding assay as first described by Spratt. These investigators determined the relative affinity of the proteins using several methods, including adding increasing concentrations of radiolabeled penicillin to equal amounts of sonicated or freeze-thawed *Borrelia burgdorferi* membranes and then subjecting these membranes to polyacrylamide gel electrophoresis. The results of autoradiographic analysis indicated that, of the 10 PBPs, a 94-kD and a 57-kD protein were the first proteins to be labeled at the lowest concentration of radiolabeled penicillin. The 94-kD PBP was also the first protein to be eliminated when increasing amounts of cold penicillin were incubated with membranes of *Borrelia burgdorferi* using a classic competition binding assay. These investigators compared the PBP profiles before and after boiling aliquots of membranes to determine if the enzymatic activity of any PBPs could be destroyed. While the 94-kD high-affinity PBP disappeared, small amounts of bound radiolabeled penicillin could be observed with some of the other proteins, suggesting two types of PBPs. The large number of PBPs observed was somewhat surprising, although an argument could be made for an increased number of these proteins in spirochetes because of their unusual shape. The demonstration of the 94-kD and 57-kD high-affinity PBPs was in general agreement with the report by Radolf et al,[40] who also demonstrated 94-kD and 58-kD PBPs in *T. pallidum*. At increasing concentrations of penicillin, they also observed several other proteins labeled with penicillin. Radolf et al[40] and Cunningham et al[8] questioned whether the labeled proteins were true PBPs.

Several papers have put these observations into perspective. Luft et al[29] used biotin and labeled iodine to characterize the surface topology of *Borrelia burgdorferi*. They were able to identify 13 distinct proteins or glycoproteins, presumably on the surface of the organism. Many of these surface antigens had molecular weights similar to some of the PBPs shown by Urban et al,[51] especially the 31-kD OspA (outer surface protein A) and 34-kD OspB proteins. Several of these major surface proteins possessed cross-reacting epitopes with many other proteins in *Borrelia burgdorferi*.[23] This information, coupled with the observation that the OspA protein also contained sequence homology to a beta-lactamase from *Staphylococcus aureus*,[5] suggests a family of proteins sharing similar structure and function with conserved regions. A report by Brandt et al[7] indicated that the two major outer surface proteins, OspA and OspB, as well as several other proteins, are also lipoproteins that were selectively extracted with the detergent Triton X-114. This provided additional information supporting the contention that a family of proteins sharing similar structure and function is present in *Borrelia burgdorferi*, some of which are positioned on the outer surface of *Borrelia burgdorferi* and others more integrally associated with the spirochete.

Further investigation into the PBPs of *Borrelia burgdorferi* was undertaken by Urban et al[50] using the beta-lactamase inhibitor tazobactam. In vivo experiments with this compound demonstrated a decrease in the growth rate of *Borrelia burgdorferi* (ATCC B31) at a concentration of 31 μg/ml as compared with 7.8 μg/ml of penicillin at 24 hours. When tazobactam was used in competition binding experiments, preincubation with 9.6 μg/ml of tazobactam resulted in a 34% reduction in binding to the 57-kD protein and a 59% reduction in binding to the 94-kD protein at the same concentration.

After preincubation with 96 μg/ml of tazobactam, virtually all of the 57-kD band disappeared, whereas a further reduction in binding down to 29% was observed with the 94-kD band. These data also support previous suggestions that the 94-kD and 57-kD PBPs represent lethal targets in *Borrelia burgdorferi*. Interestingly, many of the other previously reported PBPs present in these organisms were not as affected by tazobactam when scanning densitometry tracings were compared, suggesting the existence of a rather selective affinity for this beta-lactamase inhibitor by the 94-kD and 57-kD PBPs.

These authors were not the first to use beta-lactamase inhibitors in the study of PBPs. Spratt et al[44] demonstrated earlier that clavulanic acid also competed with many PBPs in *Escherichia coli* with low affinity. More importantly, they suggested a utility for this class of compounds in studying structure-function relationships. The observation by Urban et al[50] that tazobactam is able to discriminate between high-affinity PBPs and other proteins capable of binding penicillin with lower affinities may stimulate investigators to probe similar proteins with antibiotics that have MICs and MBCs in therapeutic ranges. We recently performed competition binding assays comparing ceftriaxone and penicillin on *Borrelia burgdorferi* (unpublished data). The 94-kD and 57-kD PBPs were removed with a tenfold lower concentration of penicillin. Such results indicated that these proteins have a higher affinity for penicillin despite the in vitro and in vivo data suggesting that ceftriaxone is a superior drug especially for the later stages of Lyme borreliosis. These results are not surprising because most PBP experiments are performed on bacterial membranes rather than whole cells and are not influenced by the ability of an antibiotic to penetrate the organisms. The unusual pharmacologic characteristics of ceftriaxone are well known, including its long serum half-life.[31] It is tempting to speculate that ceftriaxone also has a lower affinity for nonessential proteins that bind penicillin or that it penetrates the spirochete more rapidly, leading to enhanced triggering of endogenous autolysins that eventually kill the cells.

FUTURE EXPERIMENTS

Now that many of the proteins in *Borrelia burgdorferi* have been cloned and sequenced, more definitive work can be performed on those proteins that have been found to possess penicillin-binding activity. Our preliminary experiments have demonstrated that a recombinant form of OspA is a protein that binds penicillin (unpublished data). Sequence analysis indicates that at least two sites on the protein contain the necessary conserved tetrapeptide sequence consisting of Ser-Xaa-Xaa-Lys. The tertiary structure of OspA also changes dramatically in the presence of penicillin (unpublished data). Another interesting feature of the OspA protein is the reported lipoprotein nature, as mentioned earlier. This protein, as well as all other proteins, contains a consensus site consisting of Leu-Xaa-Yaa-Cys, which is a requirement for protein processing.[39] Many proteins that possess this site are processed[20] and exported.[19] One well-characterized lipoprotein is the *Bacillus licheniformis* penicillinase, which exists in a membrane-bound form and a secreted form.[22,34] Unpublished observations by Luft et al have demonstrated the presence of large amounts of OspA protein in media that can be precipitated with anti-*Borrelia burgdorferi* antisera. Whether these proteins are secreted or are present as a result of the intrinsic fragility of the organisms, as suggested by Brandt et al,[7] remains to be determined. Again, it would be interesting if these proteins are hyperproduced or shed normally in response to a beta-lactam signal. Zhu et al[56] have reported such a molecule (designated Bla R) that binds penicillin and acts as a signal transducer for beta-lactamase production in *Bacillus licheniformis*. The Bla R protein does not contain any beta-lactamase activity although it contains sequence homology to another beta-lactamase. Amanuma and Strominger[1] have previously demonstrated that PBP 5 in *E. coli* possesses weak beta-lactamase activity, and many investigators have described various relationships between beta-lactamases and PBPs.[17,33] Urban et al[52] have postulated that similar events could be taking place in *Borrelia burgdorferi*. Because PBPs are essential for the survival of all bacteria, different subsets of this protein could be tailored according to their final destination. Some of the proteins would perform as classic PBPs, others would remain on the surface of the organism acting as attractants for beta-lactam compounds, and some of the proteins could be secreted into the external milieu. Although many of these suggestions are speculative, in vitro labeling experiments should be performed to verify these exciting possibilities.

X-ray protein crystallography allows very high resolution, and it is conceivable that many of the PBPs in *Borrelia burgdorferi* are amenable to such analysis. One should be able to design an antibiotic to "fit" any particular PBP as has been done with synthetic peptides and mimetics.[41]

Investigators and clinicians have contributed significantly to the study of Lyme borreliosis. Because it is a difficult disease to diagnose clinically[3] and serologically,[10] much of their effort has been spent characterizing those proteins to which the host responds.[15,18] As mentioned previously, earlier diagnosis results in a greater chance for clinical cure with antibiotics. Only within the last 3 to 4 years have significant clinical trials indicated which antibiotics are useful for short- and long-term treatment. Newer chemotherapeutic modalities have been employed using higher doses of more potent drugs for longer periods of time. Investigators have been probing the antimicrobial molecular targets in *Borrelia burgdorferi*. When these targets are more fully characterized using a wider variety of borrelial isolates and antibiotics, clinicians may be able to treat this disease with even greater success rates.

REFERENCES

1. Amanuma H, Strominger JL: Purification and properties of penicillin binding proteins 5 and 6 from *Escherichia coli, J Biol Chem* 255:1173, 1980.
2. Barbour AG: Laboratory aspects of Lyme borreliosis, *Clin Microbiol Rev* 1:399, 1988.
3. Barbour AG: The diagnosis of Lyme disease: rewards and perils, *Ann Intern Med* 110:501, 1989.
4. Beck G et al: Chemical and biologic characterization of a lipopolysaccharide from Lyme disease spirochete (*Borrelia burgdorferi*), *J Infect Dis* 152:108, 1985.
5. Bergstrom SV, Bundoc G, Barbour AG: Molecular analysis of linear plasmid encoded major surface proteins (OSP A and OSP B) of the Lyme disease spirochete, *Borrelia burgdorferi, Mol Microbiol* 3:479, 1989.
6. Bowman CA: Oral treatment of late borreliosis with roxithromycin plus cotrimoxazole, *Lancet* 336:1514, 1990.
7. Brandt ME et al: Immunogenic integral membrane proteins of *Borrelia burgdorferi* are lipoproteins, *Infect Immun* 58:983, 1990.
8. Cunningham TM, Miller JN, Lovett MA: Identification of *Treponema pallidum* penicillin-binding proteins, *J Bacteriol* 169:5298, 1987.
9. Dattwyler RJ et al: Ceftriaxone as effective therapy in refractory Lyme disease, *J Infect Dis* 155:1322, 1987.
10. Dattwyler RJ et al: Seronegative Lyme disease dissociation of specific T- and B-lymphocyte responses to *Borrelia burgdorferi, N Engl J Med* 319:1441, 1988.
11. Dattwyler RJ et al: Treatment of late Lyme borreliosis— randomized comparison of ceftriaxone and penicillin, *Lancet* 1:1191, 1988.
12. Dattwyler RJ et al: Amoxicillin plus probenecid versus doxycycline for treatment of erythema migrans borreliosis, *Lancet* 336:1404, 1990.
13. Diringer MN, Halpern JJ, Dattwyler RJ: Lyme meningoencephalitis: report of a severe, penicillin resistant case, *Arthritis Rheum* 30:705, 1987.
14. Dotevall L, Hagberg L: Penetration of doxycycline into cerebrospinal fluid in patients treated for suspected Lyme neuroborreliosis, *Antimicrob Agents Chemother* 33:1078, 1989.
15. Finn AF, Dattwyler RJ: The immunology of Lyme borreliosis, *Lab Med* 21:305, 1990.
16. Gasser R, Durslag J: Oral treatment of late borreliosis with roxithromycin plus co-trimoxazole, *Lancet* 336:1189, 1990.
17. Ghuysen JM: Bacterial active-site serine penicillin-interactive proteins and domains: mechanism, structure and evolution, *Rev Infect Dis* 10:726, 1988.
18. Golightly MG, Thomas JA, Viciana AL: The laboratory diagnosis of Lyme borreliosis, *Lab Med* 21:299, 1990.

19. Guzzo J et al: *Pseudomonas aeruginosa* alkaline protease: evidence for secretion genes and study of secretion mechanisms, *J Bacteriol* 173:5290, 1991.
20. Hara H et al: Genetic analyses of processing involving C-terminal cleavage in penicillin-binding protein 3 of *Escherischia coli, J Bacteriol* 171:5882, 1990.
21. Hassler D et al: Cefotaxime versus penicillin in the late stage of Lyme disease—prospective, randomized therapeutic study, *Infection (Munich)* 18:24, 1990.
22. Hayashi S, Wu H: Biosynthesis of *Bacillus licheniformis* penicillinase in *Escherichia coli* and in *Bacillus subtilis, J Bacteriol* 156:773, 1983.
23. Jiang W et al: Cross antigenicity between the major surface proteins (OSP A and OSP B) and other proteins of *Borrelia burgdorferi, J Immunol* 144:284, 1990.
24. Johnson RC, Kodner C, Russell M: *In vitro* and *in vivo* susceptibility of Lyme disease spirochete, *Borrelia burgdorferi*, to four antimicrobial agents, *Antimicrob Agents Chemother* 31:164, 1987.
25. Johnson RC et al: Comparative *in vitro* and *in vivo* susceptibilities of the Lyme disease spirochete *Borrelia burgdorferi* to cefuroxime and other antimicrobial agents, *Antimicrob Agents Chemother* 34:2133, 1990.
26. Johnson RC et al: *In vitro* and *in vivo* susceptibility of *Borrelia burgdorferi* to azithromycin, *Antimicrob Agents Chemother* 25(suppl A):33, 1990.
27. Johnson SE et al: Susceptibility of Lyme disease spirochete to seven antimicrobial agents, *Yale J Biol Med* 57:549, 1984.
28. Luft BJ et al: New chemotherapeutic approaches in the treatment of Lyme disease, *Ann NY Acad Sci* 539:93, 1988.
29. Luft BJ et al: Biochemical and immunochemical characterization of the surface proteins of *Borrelia burgdorferi, Infect Immun* 57:3637, 1989.
30. Luft BJ et al: A perspective on the treatment of Lyme borreliosis, *Rev Infect Dis* 11(suppl 6):1518, 1989.
31. Moellering RC, editor: Ceftriaxone: a long acting cephalosporin, *Am J Med* 77(4c):1, 1984.
32. Nadelman R et al: Clinical comparison of cefuroxime axetil (CAE) and doxycycline (DOC) in the treatment of patients with early Lyme disease (LD) (Abstract # 1369) 17th International Congress of Chemotherapy, Berlin, Germany, June 23-28, 1991.
33. Nicholas RA, Strominger JL: Relations between beta-lactamases and penicillin-binding proteins: beta-lactamase activity of penicillin-binding protein 5 from *Escherichia coli, Rev Infect Dis* 10:733, 1988.
34. Nielsen JB, Caulfield MP, Lampen JO: Lipoprotein nature of *Bacillus licheniformis* membrane penicillinase, *Proc Natl Acad Sci USA* 78:3511, 1981.
35. Nikaido H: Outer membrane barrier as a mechanism of antimicrobial resistance, *Antimicrob Agents Chemother* 33:1831, 1989.
36. Pfister HW et al: Cefotaxime vs penicillin G for acute neurologic manifestations in Lyme neuroborreliosis. A prospective randomized study, *Arch Neurol* 46:1190, 1989.
37. Pfister HW et al: Randomized comparison of ceftriaxone and cefotaxime in Lyme neuroborreliosis, *J Infect Dis* 163:311, 1991.
38. Preac-Mursic V et al: Comparative antimicrobial activity of the new macrolides against *Borrelia burgdorferi, Eur J Clin Microbiol Infect Dis* 8:651, 1989.
39. Pugsley AB, Schwartz M: Export and secretions of proteins by bacteria, *FEMS Microbiol Rev* 32:3, 1985.
40. Radolf JD et al: Penicillin-binding proteins and peptidoglycan of *Treponema pallidum* subsp. *pallidum, Infect Immun* 57:1248, 1989.
41. Saragoui MU et al: Design and synthesis of a mimetic from an antibody complementary determining region, *Science* 253:792, 1991.
42. Spratt BG: Distinct penicillin binding proteins in the division, elongation, and shape of *Escherichia coli* K12, *Proc Natl Acad Sci USA* 72:2999, 1975.
43. Spratt BG: Properties of the penicillin-binding proteins of *Escherichia coli* K12, *Eur J Biochem* 72:341, 1977.
44. Spratt BG, Jobanputra V, Zimmerman W: Binding of thienamycin and clavulanic acid to the penicillin binding proteins of *Escherichia coli* K12, *Antimicrob Agents Chemother* 12:406, 1977.
45. Steere AC: Lyme disease, *N Engl J Med* 321:586, 1989.
46. Steere AC et al: Successful parenteral penicillin therapy of established Lyme arthritis, *N Engl J Med* 312:869, 1985.
47. Szczepanski A, Benach JL: Lyme borreliosis: host response to *Borrelia burgdorferi, Microbiol Rev* 55:21, 1991.
48. Takayama K, Rothenberg RJ, Barbour AG: Absence of lipopolysaccharide in the Lyme disease spirochete, *Borrelia burgdorferi, Infect Immun* 55:2311, 1987.
49. Treatment of Lyme disease, *Medical Letter* 31:57, 1989.
50. Urban C, Rahal JJ, Luft B: Effect of a beta-lactamase inhibitor, tazobactam on growth and penicillin-binding proteins of *Borrelia burgdorferi, FEMS Microbiol Lett* 82:113, 1991.
51. Urban C et al: Penicillin-binding proteins in *Borrelia burgdorferi, J Bacteriol* 172:6139, 1990.
52. Urban C et al: The *in vitro* response of *Borrelia burgdorferi* to antibiotics. In Einhäupl KM et al, eds: Lyme borreliose, Symposium EIBSEE, September 6-7, 1989, Basel/Grenzach-Wymlen, 1990, Editiones Rocme.
53. Walker EM et al: Analysis of outer membrane ultrastructure of pathogenic treponema and borrelia species by freeze fracture electron microscopy, *J Bacteriol* 173:5585, 1991.
54. Weber K et al: A randomized trial of ceftriaxone versus oral penicillin for the treatment of early European lyme borreliosis, *Infection (Munich)* 18:91, 1990.
55. Zak O, O'Reilly T: Animal models in the evaluation of antimicrobial agents, *Antimicrob Agents Chemother* 35:1527, 1991.
56. Zhu YF et al: Identification of beta-lactamase production in *Bacillus licheniformis*, as a penicillin-binding protein with strong homology to the oxa-2 beta-lactamase (class d) of *Salmonella typhimurium, J Bacteriol* 172:1137, 1990.

21 Vaccine Development

P. K. Coyle

Immunization involves the artificial induction of immunity to protect a person from disease. Immunization can be active (where the person is made to form their own natural protective immune responses) or passive (where the person is given exogenous antibodies to provide temporary protection).[12] Natural protective responses are induced by means of vaccination. Vaccines may consist of suspensions of attenuated or killed microorganisms, or subunit fractions of the organisms. The ultimate goal of all such vaccines, however, is to induce active immunity and prevent an infectious disease. Development of an effective specific vaccine provides prophylactic treatment for a human infection. Such preventive therapy is always more desirable than symptomatic treatment provided after disease has occurred. Active immunization has already led to the eradication of one deadly disease (smallpox) and the control of a number of other major infections (including diphtheria, measles, mumps, pertussis, polio, rubella, tetanus, and yellow fever).[19] The ideal vaccine needs to be safe, effective, and inexpensive. Although modern vaccines approach this ideal, they do not fully achieve it. They all have potential adverse side-effects, and they do not provide 100% protection. Therefore, the decision to use a vaccine must first weigh the risks of the natural disease against the risks of the vaccination. A vaccine needs to activate not only antibody-producing B cells, but also T cells.[1] It needs to generate in the vaccinated person both humoral and cellular immune responses, to produce high numbers of memory B and T cells. The way in which a person's immune system responds to a given vaccine depends on a number of factors, including the route of administration, the chemical and physical properties of the vaccine antigen, its metabolic fate, and a number of host-related factors, which include genetic factors.[12] Generally, vaccination with live, attenuated organisms best mimics the natural infection. It triggers a host immune response to provide lifelong immunity. However, there are obvious risks to deliberately inoculating live infectious agent. Vaccination with killed organisms generally does not provide permanent immunity, so repeated vaccinations become necessary. Subunit preparations often give a poor immune response. They typically require multiple vaccinations in combination with an adjuvant. The addition of adjuvant (such as aluminum salts) to a vaccine enhances the vaccine's immunogenicity. The adjuvant helps keep antigen at the injection site and activates antigen-presenting cells to enhance processing of the vaccine antigen.[1] One area of current vaccine research involves the search for improved adjuvants, as well as the optimal antigen preparation (such as a lipopeptide combination). Finally, once an effective vaccine is developed, decisions need to be made about the optimal population who should receive the vaccine.

POTENTIAL PROBLEMS

A number of problems need to be addressed in the development of a vaccine for Lyme disease (Table 21–1). The first involves the choice of immunogen. Inoculation of live spirochetes carries the risk of producing an infection that might not be controllable. *Borrelia burgdorferi* is known to cause a persistent chronic infection.[24] Viable organisms have been found in sequestered tissues of infected hosts years after the original exposure. The idea of deliberately injecting live *B. burgdorferi* into a person is particularly troublesome because the mechanisms involved in controlling dissemination and persistence of these organisms in the host are, for the most part, unknown. Unless extensive studies were carried out to document its safety, it is unlikely that a live vaccine will be used in Lyme disease.

The use of inactivated spirochetes requires a manufacturing process that will ensure killing of all viable organisms without structurally destroying their immunogenicity. This technique also requires cultivating large supplies of *B. burgdorferi* in vitro, which is not an easy task. Inoculation of either attenuated or inactivated organisms involves injection of impurities from their culture process, which is another potential problem.

A more modern approach to vaccine production involves the use of synthetic proteins or peptides.[4]

Table 21–1 Potential problems associated with a Lyme disease vaccine

Choice of immunogen	Live attenuated *B. burgdorferi*
	Inactivated *B. burgdorferi*
	Synthetic peptides/proteins/ lipopeptides/lipoproteins
	OspA, other antigens
	Single versus multiple antigens
Vaccine safety	Induction of autoimmune reaction
	Immune enhancement
	Jarisch-Herxheimer reaction
Vaccine efficacy	Protective immune mechanisms not delineated
	Role of antigenic variation and strain differences
	Duration of immunity

Identification of genes that code for immunogenic proteins can be used to clone DNA. Such DNA can be inserted into an expression vector such as *Escherichia coli* to produce large amounts of purified protein or protein epitope sites (peptides). Large amounts of very pure antigens can be generated in this manner. These antigens can be used as a vaccine, along with an adjuvant to improve their immunogenicity. Of course, creation of such a vaccine presupposes that the antigens chosen are critical for protective immunity. Such antigens have not yet been identified for human Lyme disease. The best candidate antigen to date is the lipoprotein OspA, although this is based solely on animal models.

Several concerns have been raised about the safety of a Lyme disease vaccine. *B. burgdorferi* infection can trigger autoimmune responses that are both humoral and cellular, presumably on the basis of molecular mimicry between spirochetal antigens and host antigens.[24] The spirochete proteins that appear to be involved in autoimmune reactions include the 41-kD flagellin and several stress (heat shock) proteins. Certain antibodies directed against *B. burgdorferi* cross-react with peripheral nerves and nerve axons, neurons, hepatocytes, synovial joint cells, and cardiac muscle cells. Patients with Lyme disease can develop autoantibodies, including anticardiolipin antibodies, rheumatoid factor, and antineuronal and antimyelin antibodies. Lyme disease can also trigger T cells which react to autoantigens such as cardiolipin, myelin basic protein, and galactocerebroside. Such reports raise the possibility that vaccination with *B. burgdorferi* antigens might trigger an autoimmune process, particularly in a genetically susceptible person. An-

other potential concern about vaccination relates to the suggestion that some of the pathologic damage in Lyme disease is actually bystander damage due to immune reactions triggered by the infection. In such a case, the immune enhancement induced by vaccination might actually lead to tissue damage. In fact, certain vaccines developed for measles and respiratory syncytial virus infections have produced hypersensitivity reactions in vaccinated persons.[1,12] It has also been speculated that vaccination of a recently infected person might lead to a Jarisch-Herxheimer reaction, identical to that seen with initiation of antibiotic therapy.[8] This reaction might occur if sufficient accessible spirochetes were destroyed by the generated immune response and induced a secondary inflammatory cascade.

Finally, some basic questions need to be addressed to ensure vaccine efficacy. Although neutralizing antibodies are presumed to be important in controlling *B. burgdorferi* infection, the crucial protective immune mechanisms that control disease spread in humans are unknown.[24] Cellular mechanisms are likely to be as important as humoral mechanisms in this disease. The precise role of the phagocyte, complement, antibody, T cell, natural killer cell, and so forth have not been delineated for acute and chronic Lyme disease. Such an understanding becomes critical to develop and test an optimal vaccine. It is also unclear whether a single vaccine will be able to offer immunity to different strains of *B. burgdorferi*. In vitro, *B. burgdorferi* can change antigens and lose plasmids.[10] Although systematic antigenic variation has not been documented to occur in vivo with *B. burgdorferi*, it certainly does occur in the related borreliae which produce relapsing fever.[17] A programmed antigenic variation might allow *B. burgdorferi* to evade the host immune response and set up a persistent infection. The role of antigenic variation and spirochetal strain differences in human Lyme disease needs to be addressed to optimize vaccine therapy. The duration of immunity after vaccination also needs to be examined to determine the optimal immunization protocol.

Vaccination has been used to control infection with spirochetes other than *B. burgdorferi*. A successful animal vaccine has been developed for the spirochete that causes leptospirosis.[11] This vaccine uses whole inactivated organisms. In syphilis, however, a vaccine using a synthetic surface antigen has only been able to provide partial immunity in rabbits, despite multiple inoculations in combination with a powerful adjuvant.[3]

ANIMAL STUDIES

Animal models provide the opportunity to test vaccine efficacy and safety before initiating any human trials. In addition, there is animal Lyme disease. Dogs, cats, horses, and cows can become ill when infected by *B. burgdorferi*. Therefore, there is a need for a veterinary as well as a human vaccine for Lyme disease. A series of reports have shown that both passive and active immunization in hamster and mouse models can protect against infection or pathologic tissue damage by *B. burgdorferi* (Table 21–2).[9,13–16,22,23] These animal studies have indicated that antibodies, particularly those directed against the OspA outer surface lipoprotein, can be protective if they are given in sufficient quantity before or at the time of spirochete exposure. Antibodies to the major flagellin protein do not appear to be protective.[22] There is evidence that complement fixing antibodies and Fc receptor binding antibodies are especially important.[9,22] Recent data also suggest that the protective antibodies have borreliacidal activity. In a hamster model, this borreliacidal activity due to IgG peaked at 3 weeks after infection and then gradually declined.[18] The authors speculated that this might make the animal susceptible to reinfection. Rats have been shown to develop borreliacidal activity after infection.[20] Humans with Lyme disease also show this activity in their serum, and preliminary studies suggested that this activity might to detectable even in seronegative patients.[5] This implies that antibodies that kill *B. burgdorferi* may not be measured by current antibody assays. The successful use of a synthetic OspA protein vaccine in animals is particularly exciting, because OspA shows a high degree of conservation among different *B. burgdorferi* isolates. It took a very large quantity of OspA to protect the animals however, suggesting that OspA is a poor immunogen and should probably be combined with an adjuvant. A truncated OspA has recently been cloned. This shorter protein is much more soluble and easily purified than the whole protein. The truncated OspA is currently being tested as a vaccine in a hamster model. OspB has also been shown to be protective recently in a mouse model.[9a]

Table 21–2 Animal models used to test Lyme vaccines

Animal model	Disease manifestations	Immunization protocol	Results
Syrian hamster[15,16]	Subclinical infection	Passive immunization with hamster, rabbit immune sera	1. Protection from infection 2. Some strain specificity 3. Immune sera must be given before infection
Syrian hamster[13,14,16]	Subclinical infection	Active immunization with inactivated *B. burgdorferi*	1. Protection from infection 2. Dose-dependent 3. Protection decreases over time
Irradiated LSH hamster[23]	Arthritis	Passive immunization with hamster immune sera	1. Protection from infection and disease
Immunodeficient (scid) mouse[22]	Arthritis, carditis	Passive immunization with mouse immune sera; monoclonal antibodies to OspA, flagellin	1. Immune sera and OspA antibodies protect or mitigate infection and disease 2. Must be given at the time of infection
Immunocompetent (C3H/HeJ) mouse[9]	Arthritis, carditis	Passive immunization with mouse, rabbit immune sera; monoclonal antibodies to OspA. Active immunization with *E. coli* expressing OspA; purified recombinant OspA fusion protein	1. Immune sera and OspA antibodies protect from infection and disease 2. *E. coli* expressing OspA protect from infection and mitigates disease 3. OspA fusion protein protects from infection and disease
Immunocompetent (C3H/HeJ) mouse[9a]	Arthritis, carditis	Passive immunization with rabbit immune sera lacking anti-OspA; or anti-OspA and OspB antibodies Active immunization with recombinant OspA; OspB; flagellin	1. Immune sera lacking anti-OspA antibodies protect; sera lacking anti-OspA and OspB antibodies do not protect 2. OspA or OspB protect from spirochete challenge; protection is dose-dependent

A veterinary Lyme vaccine is already in active use.[8] It has been conditionally licensed while safety and efficacy trials are in progress. This is a dog vaccine that consists of inactivated whole spirochetes. The vaccine is designed for healthy dogs aged 3 months and older. It is administered intramuscularly twice (several weeks apart), with an annual booster dose. Lyme vaccines for cats, cows, and horses are under development.

HUMAN VACCINES

The apparent success of Lyme vaccines in animals has led to the hope that a human vaccine can be developed. However, these animal models do not completely mimic human Lyme disease. There is an emphasis on OspA as the key *B. burgdorferi* antigen to promote protective immune responses. Antibodies to OspA appear very early in animal infections. In humans, however, the antibody response to OspA appears late and is variable.[2,6,7] It is unclear whether a subunit OspA vaccine is sufficiently immunogenic in humans to trigger a protective response. It is also unclear whether a vaccine with this single antigen will work. The precise mechanisms for protection in the human infection, including the role of OspA, are unknown. This hampers human vaccine development. It is not known whether antibodies are truly protective in the human infection. However, in the few cases of reinfection in the literature in which this question was addressed, it appears as though reinfected subjects lacked antibodies.[21,25] This implies antibodies are indeed protective. Once a vaccine is developed, it is likely to be used only for people at high risk for Lyme disease: those who live in very endemic areas or those who have job exposures that put them at particular risk. Because *B. burgdorferi* infection may never result in clinical disease, any human vaccine will have to be quite safe to justify its prophylactic use. It is also likely that periodic booster vaccinations should be required to maintain protection. Even if vaccine therapy for human Lyme disease never comes to fruition however, the studies being carried out in this area are likely to result in a much better understanding of the disease. Ultimately, such knowledge will lead to optimal management and therapy for Lyme disease.

ACKNOWLEDGMENT

This article was supported in part by Grant AR 40470 from the National Institutes of Health.

REFERENCES

1. Ada GL: The immunological principles of vaccination, *Lancet* 335:523, 1990.
2. Barbour AG et al: Antibodies of patients with Lyme disease to components of the *Ixodes dammini* spirochete, *J Clin Invest* 72:504, 1983.
3. Borenstein LA et al: Immunization of rabbits with recombinant *Treponema pallidum* surface antigen 4D alters the course of experimental syphilis, *J Immunol* 140:2415, 1988.
4. Brown F: From Jenner to genes—the new vaccines, *Lancet* 335:587, 1990.
5. Callister SM, Schell RF, Lovrich SD: Lyme disease assay which detects killed *Borrelia burgdorferi, J Clin Microbiol* 29:1773, 1991.
6. Coleman JL, Benach JL: Isolation of antigenic components from the Lyme disease spirochete: their role in early diagnosis, *J Infect Dis* 155:756, 1987.
7. Craft JE et al: Antigens of *Borrelia burgdorferi* recognized during Lyme disease. Appearance of a new immunoglobulin M response and expansion of the immunoglobulin G response late in the illness, *J Clin Invest* 78:934, 1986.
8. Edelman R: Perspective in the development of vaccines against Lyme disease, *Vaccine* 9:531, 1991.
9. Fikrig E et al: Protection of mice against the Lyme disease agent by immunizing with recombinant OspA, *Science* 250:553, 1990.
9a. Fikrig E et al: Roles of OspA, OspB, and flagellin in protective immunity to Lyme borreliosis in laboratory mice, *Infect Immun* 60:657, 1992.
10. Georgilis K, Steere AC, Klempner MS: Infectivity of *Borrelia burgdorferi* correlates with resistance to elimination by phagocytic cells, *J Infect Dis* 163:150, 1991.
11. Gyles CL, Thoen CO: *Pathogenesis of bacterial infections in animals.* Ames, 1986, Iowa State University Press.
12. Hinman AR et al: *Immunization.* In Mandell GL, Douglas RG Jr, Bennett JE, editors: *Principles and practice of infectious disease,* ed 3. New York, 1990, Churchill Livingstone.
13. Johnson RC, Kodner CL, Russell ME: Active immunization of hamsters against experimental infection with *Borrelia burgdorferi, Infect Immun* 54:897, 1986.
14. Johnson RC, Kodner CL, Russell ME: Passive immunization of hamsters against experimental infection with the Lyme disease spirochete, *Infect Immun* 53:713, 1986.
15. Johnson RC, Kodner CL, Russell ME: Vaccination of hamsters against experimental infection with *Borrelia burgdorferi, Zentralbl Bakteriol Mikrobiol Hyg [A]* 263:45, 1986.
16. Johnson RC et al: Experimental infection of the hamster with *Borrelia burgdorferi, Ann NY Acad Sci* 539:258, 1988.
17. Kehl KSC et al: Antigenic variation among *Borrelia* spp. in relapsing fever, *Infect Immun* 54:899, 1986.
18. Lovrich SD et al: Borreliacidal activity of sera from hamsters infected with the Lyme disease spirochete, *Infect Immun* 59:2522, 1991.
19. Moxon ER: The scope of immunization, *Lancet* 335:448, 1990.
20. Pavia CS et al: Antiborrelial activity of serum from rats injected with the Lyme disease spirochete, *J Infect Dis* 163:656, 1991.
21. Pfister H-W et al: Reinfection with *Borrelia burgdorferi, Lancet* 2:984, 1986.
22. Schaible UE et al: Monoclonal antibodies specific for the outer surface protein A (OspA) of *Borrelia burgdorferi* prevent Lyme borreliosis in severe combined immunodeficiency (scid) mice, *Proc Natl Acad Sci USA* 87:3768, 1990.
23. Schmitz JL et al: Passive immunization prevents induction of Lyme arthritis in LSH hamsters, *Infect Immun* 58:144, 1990.
24. Szczepanski A, Benach JL: Lyme borreliosis: host responses to *Borrelia burgdorferi, Microbiol Rev* 55:21, 1991.
25. Weber K et al: Reinfection in erythema migrans disease, *Infection* 14:32, 1986.

Special Topics

 Pathogenesis of Lyme Disease

James L. Coleman and *Jorge L. Benach*

An overview of the pathogenesis of Lyme disease can include factors of virulence (none are known for *Borrelia burgdorferi*); host-pathogen relationships at the molecular and cellular levels; immune, inflammatory, and autoreactive responses; and host-associated factors. In this book, many of these topics are covered separately so this overview is confined to areas of pathogenesis that are not represented elsewhere. The topic of pathogenesis of Lyme borreliosis has been covered in two recent reviews.[33,64]

PATHOGENESIS

After leaving the skin, *B. burgdorferi* enters the bloodstream, enabling it to disseminate throughout the body and invade various organ systems. The extreme difficulty encountered in isolating the spirochete from the blood[11,62] suggests that the spirochetemia is transient, and isolations are probably the result of fortunate timing. Isolation of spirochetes from skin lesions,[15] myocardium,[47] synoviae[42] and synovial fluid[53,58] has been successful only infrequently. This is a point of difference between Lyme disease and syphilis, in which *Treponema pallidum* is found in large numbers in the primary chancre and also in infected tissues and organs. By what mechanisms can such a small number of organisms enter the body through a tick bite and subsequently affect, either directly or indirectly, distant organs and tissues? This question has led investigators to search for host-associated factors that could amplify the pathogenicity of a small number of organisms. There is evidence to support the idea that *B. burgdorferi* is a potent inducer of interleukin-1 (IL-1) production.[39]

Production of interleukin-1

IL-1 is a powerful immune mediator secreted by mononuclear phagocytes and is known for its wide range of effects on host cells.[29,30] Murine macrophages and cultured human monocytes produce IL-1 when stimulated by *B. burgdorferi*.[39] Several cell types associated with the joint capsule are known to be capable of secreting IL-1, including macrophages[29] and synoviocytes.[70] IL-1 has also

been shown to be present in the synovial fluid of Lyme disease patients.[8] As a result of this evidence, investigations have focused on spirochete-associated factors capable of eliciting host cell IL-1 production. A lipopolysaccharide (LPS)-like molecule was extracted from *B. burgdorferi* by both a modified hot phenol-water method and a phenol-chloroform-petroleum ether method. The extract in either case demonstrated LPS-like properties in that it was pyrogenic in rabbits, mitogenic for mononuclear cells and murine splenocytes, and cytotoxic for murine macrophages. The extract was also positive in the *Limulus* amebocyte lysate assay for endotoxin.[9] Sodium dodecyl sulfate polyacrylamide gel electrophoresis (SDS-PAGE) and silver staining of the extract showed it to have properties characteristic of rough-form LPS.[9] Although the extract demonstrated a number of biologic activities similar to classic LPS, another study has reported the absence of lipid-A,[67] the lipid portion of the molecule, which is known to be associated with its toxicity.

Autoimmunity

Another possible mechanism by which *B. burgdorferi* could indirectly cause damage to organ systems is by the development of an immune response to self antigens that contain similarities to spirochetal antigens. Such a phenomenon has been documented for viral and other bacterial infections.[49] Monoclonal antibodies generated against a number of viruses show reactivity to normal tissues from noninfected mice.[59] There is evidence to suggest that autoimmunity also occurs in Lyme disease.[1,56] Patients with neurologic symptoms have serum IgM antibodies that cross-react with normal, human axons.[56] This antiaxonal binding is removable by preabsorption of the sera with *B. burgdorferi*. In this study, a murine monoclonal antibody directed against the spirochete endoflagellae was also shown to bind to normal human axons.[56] Similar results were obtained in another study using monoclonal antibodies in which antigenic determinants were found to be shared by *B. burgdorferi* flagellin and myelin, and Schwann cells from the peripheral nervous system as well as hepatocytes, synovial cells, and cardiac muscle.[1] However, in this case, the possibility of direct immune-mediated tissue damage is in doubt because the monoclonal antibody reactivity is limited to the cytoplasm of the cells, not to the cell surface.[1] Antibodies to myelin and myelin basic protein have been found in the sera and cerebrospinal fluid (CSF) of Lyme disease patients.[34,63] In addition, anticardiolipin antibodies[46] and rheumatoid factor[43] have been found in Lyme disease patients. Genetic susceptibility, which is an important component for the development of autoreactivity, is the subject of chapter 5 in this book. It is important to mention that associations with HLA phenotypes were made for Lyme disease before the organism was discovered.[61]

A special class of proteins called heat shock proteins has been identified in *B. burgdorferi*.[19,20,45,60] Heat shock proteins are among the most conserved of all proteins in procaryotic and eucaryotic cells[71] and thus are extremely likely to act as autoantigens. Significant amino acid identity has been shown to exist between a 58-kD spirochetal protein and proteins of the *Escherichia coli* GroEL family.[48]

Spirochete attachment

Direct injury to cells as a result of spirochetal attachment is another means by which *B. burgdorferi* can inflict damage. Spirochete attachment presumably would also be the requisite first step in transendothelial migration out of the bloodstream before invasion of various organ tissues. *B. burgdorferi* is capable of infecting a wide range of organ systems in humans[31] and has also been isolated from organs of experimentally infected rodents.[7,41] Cultured tick cells showed cytopathic effects when exposed to *B. burgdorferi*.[44] In another study, neuronal cells coincubated with *B. burgdorferi* also showed evidence of damage as measured by ^{51}Cr release and electron microscopy.[37] In addition, *B. burgdorferi* has been shown to adhere to rat primary brain cells,[35] endothelial monolayers,[66,68] and human epithelial cells.[14,40] The adherence phenomenon appears to be strain-specific. B31, a high-passage strain[18] showed a reduced capacity to bind to cultured cells compared to lower passage isolates.[66,68] Assays designed to demonstrate the ability of *B. burgdorferi* to penetrate human umbilical vein endothelial cells (HUVEC) have also shown strain differences. Experiments have also suggested that spirochete viability is important for *B. burgdorferi*/cell adherence. Heat or formalin fixation of *B. burgdorferi* was associated with reduced adherence for primary rat brain cells[35] and HUVEC.[66] It is also important to point out that epitopes on adhesion molecules may have been altered or destroyed in the process.

Studies on the nature of *B. burgdorferi* adhesions have been incomplete. Exposure of *B. burgdorferi* to human antisera significantly reduced spirochetal adherence to HUVEC,[66] however, pretreatment of *B. burgdorferi* with immune rat serum had no effect on its adherence to rat primary brain cells.[35] Pretreatment of *B. burgdorferi* with monoclonal antibodies specific for outer surface protein A (OspA) have shown mixed results, with one report showing an inhibitory effect with HEp-2 cells[14] whereas other reports failed to demonstrate any effect with HUVEC[66] or primary rat brain cultures.[35] A monoclonal antibody specific for *B. burgdorferi* outer surface protein B (OspB) has been shown to be effective in reducing adherence to HUVEC.[66] Monoclonal antibodies directed against the 41-kD endoflagellar protein have been shown to be only slightly effective in reducing cytoadherence.[14,66]

Studies have also been conducted to elucidate the nature of the cell surface receptor involved in the adhesion process. In HEp-2 cells, pretreatment of the cells with neuraminidase to eliminate sialic acid residues reduced spirochete adherence by 43%.[14] Culturing the cells in the presence of tunicamycin, a glycosylation inhibitor, and sialidase also reduced the binding of *B. burgdorferi*.[14]

Evidence has also been provided for the adherence of *B. burgdorferi* to glycolipids found in neuronal cells, specifically oligodendroglia and Schwann cells in which the spirochete was found to have a greater capacity for adherence to galactocerebroside than other structurally related molecules such as glucocerebroside, ceramide, and sphingosine.

The ability of *B. burgdorferi* to adhere to and subsequently penetrate endothelium, either through the cytoplasm[25] or through intracellular spaces[66] is shown by damage caused to the blood-brain barrier after intravenous injection of spirochetes and subsequent detection of spirochetes in the CSF of rats.[36] In addition, IL-1 has been shown to increase vascular permeability and elicit blood vessel damage.[30] In this regard, cells of neural origin can contribute to the process of pathogenesis as *B. burgdorferi* induces synthesis of interleukin-6 (IL-6) in these cells.[38]

IMMUNE RESPONSE

Evidence suggests that professional phagocytes such as polymorphonuclear leukocytes (PMN), monocytes, and macrophages play an important role in the host's initial defense against *B. burgdorferi*. Macrophages have been consistently found to be present at the site of the erythema migrans (EM) lesion in close proximity with spirochetes.[31] When the spirochetes reach the bloodstream and begin the process of dissemination to other sites, they come into contact with circulating PMN and monocytes. In the chronic stage of the disease, PMN are found in the synovial fluid and spirochetes in both synovium and synovial fluid.[42,53,58] Studies have been carried out to determine the nature of the interaction between *B. burgdorferi* and phagocytes in vitro. *B. burgdorferi* have been shown to be internalized by human PMN and peripheral blood monocytes, murine macrophages, and rabbit peritoneal exudate macrophages.[1,12,50,65] Phagocytosis of *B. burgdorferi* by PMN and mononuclear phagocytes occurred regardless of whether opsonized or unopsonized spirochetes were used in the assay,[12] however, the process was more efficient when the spirochetes were preincubated with immune serum or synovial fluid, even when low spirochete-to-phagocyte ratios were used.[2,12,50] Evidence suggests that the Fc receptors (FcR) play an important role in the process. When FcR were inactivated by prior incubation with monomeric IgG or a monoclonal antibody to FcγRIII, the uptake of radiolabeled spirochetes was reduced by 90%. When the assay was adjusted to simulate presumed conditions in vivo, in which a low spirochete-to-phagocyte ratio would be the norm, the process of phagocytosis was inefficient. This scenario may parallel conditions in vivo in which inefficient phagocytosis of unopsonized spirochetes as the first line of host defense allows the spirochetes to spread to secondary sites.

Previous studies have shown that *B. burgdorferi* lose their ability to infect rodent models after prolonged passage in culture.[41,54] In one report, there was no difference between phagocytosis of spirochetes routinely grown in culture and spirochetes freshly isolated from the spleens of Syrian hamsters.[50]

Analysis of the phagocytic process by transmission electron microscopy demonstrated further that *B. burgdorferi* were indeed internalized by PMN[12,50,65] and monocytes,[50] with pseudopodia clearly extending around the spirochete.[65] Evidence suggests that *B. burgdorferi* do not survive inside phagocytic cells after being internalized. Electron microscopic examination of PMN phagosomes revealed internalized spirochetes that were disrupted.[12,64] Similar results were obtained using FITC-labeled anti-*B. burgdorferi* antibodies and fluorescence microscopy with mononuclear phagocytes.[12] Acridine orange, a dye often used to demonstrate cell viability, was used to show that spirochetes internalized by PMN and monocytes were nonviable.[50]

The humoral response in Lyme disease is characterized by the initial recognition of a limited number of antigens, followed by a marked expansion in the number of antigens recognized later in the illness.[5,22,26] Specifically, the early antibody response is of the IgM class and is directed against a polypeptide of Mr 41-kD, which has been shown to be a major component of the spirochetal endoflagellum.[6] These IgM antibodies normally appear 3 to 6 weeks after infection and may persist in some cases.[5,22,26] The IgG response begins to develop after approximately 6 weeks and is also directed initially to the 41-kD endoflagellar protein. As the infection progresses, antibodies are produced to a number of other polypeptides, including the 31-kD OspA and the 34-kD OspB,[4,22,26] although in some cases immune recognition of one or both of these proteins may be lacking. IgE antibodies have also been reported in Lyme disease patients.[13]

The cellular immune response has been measured[27,28] and is the subject of chapter 15 in this book so it will not be dealt with further.

Of much recent interest are the investigations on the outer surface proteins, flagellin, and others as potential vaccine candidates and/or diagnostic markers. Two polypeptides, a 39-kD[57] and a 93-kD,[69] have been found to be specific and possibly useful in diagnostic serology. The variable nature of OspB has been known for some time and has been proposed as a possible source of strain typing.[3] The surface location of OspA and OspB was initially discovered by electron microscopy.[3,4] The basic nature of these proteins was established by two-dimensional gel electrophoresis of outer envelope[21] and whole cell preparations.[10] The sequence of OspA and OspB was elucidated, and the lipidated nature of these molecules was deduced.[16] The fact that both OspA and OspB are lipoproteins was confirmed by chemical means.[17] The function of other lipoproteins in gram-negative bacteria is thought to be as anchors of the outer envelope onto the cell wall; thus, these proteins are likely to have important structural functions. The fact that B-cell responses to OspA and OspB in patients develop late, and often not at all, is well known,[5,14,22,26] but when it does develop it is considered to be specific for *B. burgdorferi*. The opposite is true of the antibody response to the flagellin of this organism, which appears rapidly but has little specificity.[5,14,22-24] Despite this, OspA is being actively promoted as a potential immunogen. Rodents in experimental situations produce a strong antibody response to OspA.[14] Monoclonal antibodies to OspA can neutralize infectivity in mice,[52] and a recombinant OspA vaccine has been shown to protect mice from challenge.[32] Two studies have enhanced the possibilities that vaccination with OspA may be a promising endeavor. It has just been shown that the reacting epitopes for OspA are the same in mice as in humans.[55] In another study, it has been shown that both OspA and OspB are potent inducers of tumor necrosis factor.[51] The specific and nonspecific biologic activity of these proteins is becoming quite clear and may yet show that they can be used for prevention.

ACKNOWLEDGMENT

This article was supported in part by grants AI27044 and AR40445 from the National Institutes of Health and by a grant from the Mathers Charitable Foundation.

REFERENCES

1. Aberer E et al: Molecular mimicry and Lyme borreliosis: a shared antigenic determinant between *Borrelia burgdorferi* and human tissue, *Ann Neurol* 26:732, 1989.
2. Banfi E et al: Rapid flow cytometric studies of *Borrelia burgdorferi* phagocytosis by human polymorphonuclear leukocytes, *J Appl Bacteriol* 67:37, 1989.
3. Barbour AG, Tessier SL, Hayes SF: Variation in a major surface protein of Lyme disease spirochetes, *Infect Immun* 45:94, 1984.
4. Barbour AG, Tessier SL, Todd WJ: Lyme disease spirochetes and *Ixodid* tick spirochetes share a common surface antigenic determinant as defined by a monoclonal antibody, *Infect Immun* 41:795, 1983.
5. Barbour AG et al: Antibodies of patients with Lyme disease to components of the *Ixodes dammini* spirochete, *J Clin Invest* 72:504, 1983.
6. Barbour AG et al: A *Borrelia* specific monoclonal antibody binds to a flagellar epitope, *Infect Immun* 52:549, 1986.
7. Barthold SW et al: Experimental Lyme arthritis in rats infected with *Borrelia burgdorferi*, *J Infect Dis* 157:842, 1988.
8. Beck G, Benach JL, Habicht GS: Isolation of interleukin-1 from joint fluids of patients with Lyme disease, *J Rheumatol* 16:800, 1989.
9. Beck G et al: Chemical and biologic characterization of a lipopolysaccharide extracted from the Lyme disease spirochete (*Borrelia burgdorferi*), J Infect Dis 152:108, 1985.
10. Benach JL, Coleman JL, Golightly MG: A murine IgM monoclonal antibody binds an antigenic determinant in OSP-A, an immunodominant basic protein of the Lyme disease spirochete, *J Immun* 140:265, 1988.
11. Benach JL et al: Spirochetes isolated from the blood of two patients with Lyme disease, *N Engl J Med* 308:740, 1983.
12. Benach JL et al: Interactions of phagocytes with the Lyme disease spirochete: role of the Fc receptor, *J Infect Dis* 150:497, 1984.
13. Benach JL et al: An IgE response to spirochete antigen in patients with Lyme disease, *Zentralbl Bakteriol Mikrobiol Hyg [A]* 263:127, 1986.
14. Benach JL et al: Biological activity of *Borrelia burgdorferi* antigens, *Ann NY Acad Sci* 539:115, 1988.
15. Berger BW et al: Isolation and characterization of the Lyme disease spirochete from the skin of patients with eythema chronicum migrans, *J Am Acad Dermatol* 13:444, 1985.
16. Bergstrom S, Bundoc VG, Barbour AG: Molecular analysis of linear plasmid encoded major surface proteins OSP-A and OSP-B of the Lyme disease spirochete, *Borrelia burgdorferi*, *Mol Microbiol* 3:479, 1989.
17. Brandt ME et al: Immunogenic integral membrane proteins of *Borrelia burgdorferi* are lipoproteins, *Infect Immun* 58:983, 1990.
18. Burgdorfer W et al: Lyme disease—a tick borne spirochetosis? *Science* 216:1317, 1982.
19. Carriero MM, Laux DC, Nelson DR: Characterization of the heat shock response and identification of heat shock protein antigens of *Borrelia burgdorferi*, *Infect Immun* 58:2186, 1990.
20. Cluss RG, Boothby JT: Thermoregulation of protein synthesis in *Borrelia burgdorferi*, *Infect Immun* 58:1038, 1990.
21. Coleman JL, Benach JL: Isolation of the outer envelope from *Borrelia burgdorferi*, *Zentralbl Bakteriol Mikrobiol Hyg [A]* 263:123, 1986.
22. Coleman JL, Benach JL: Isolation of antigenic components from the Lyme disease spirochete: their role in early diagnosis, *J Infect Dis* 155:756, 1987.
23. Coleman JL, Benach JL: Identification and characterization of an endoflagellar antigen of *Borrelia burgdorferi*, *J Clin Invest* 84:322, 1988.
24. Collins C, Peltz G: Immunoreactive epitopes on an expressed recombinant flagellar protein of *Borrelia burgdorferi*, *Infect Immun* 59:514, 1991.
25. Comstock LE, Thomas DD: Penetration of endothelial cell monolayers by *Borrelia burgdorferi*, *Infect Immun* 57:1626, 1989.
26. Craft JE et al: Antigens of *Borrelia burgdorferi* recognized during Lyme disease. Appearance of a new immunoglobulin M response and expansion of the immunoglobulin G response late in the illness, *J Clin Invest* 78:934, 1986.
27. Dattwyler RJ et al: Cellular immune response in Lyme disease: the response to mitogens, live *Borrelia burgdorferi*, NK cell function, and lymphocyte subsets, *Zentralbl Bakteriol Mikrobiol Hyg [A]* 263:151, 1986.
28. Dattwyler RJ et al: Specific immune responses in Lyme borreliosis, *Ann NY Acad Sci* 539:93, 1988.
29. Dinarello CA: Interluekin-1, *Rev Infect Dis* 6:51, 1984.
30. Dinarello CA: Interleukin-1 and its biologically related cytokines, *Adv Immunol* 44:153, 1989.
31. Duray PH, Steere AC: Clinical pathologic correlations of Lyme disease by stage, *Ann NY Acad Sci* 539:65, 1988.
32. Fikrig E et al: Protection of mice against the Lyme disease agent by immunizing with recombinant OSP-A, *Science* 250:553, 1990.
33. Garcia-Monco JC, Benach JL: The pathogenesis of Lyme disease, *Rheum Dis Clin North Am* 15:711, 1989.
34. Garcia-Monco JC, Coleman JL, Benach JL: Antibodies to myelin basic protein in Lyme disease, *J Infect Dis* 158:667, 1988.
35. Garcia-Monco JC, Fernandez Villar B, Benach JL: Adherence of Lyme disease spirochetes to glial cells and cells of glial origin, *J Infect Dis* 160:497, 1989.
36. Garcia-Monco JC et al: *Borrelia burgdorferi* in the central nervous system: experimental and clinical evidence for early invasion, *J Infect Dis* 161:1187, 1990.
37. Garcia-Monco JC et al: Cytotoxicity of *Borrelia burgdorferi* for cultured rat glial cells, *J Infect Dis* 163:1362, 1991.
38. Habicht GS, Katona LI, Benach JL: Cytokines and the pathogenesis of neuroborreliosis: *Borrelia burgdorferi* induces glioma cells to secrete interleukin 6, *J Infect Dis* 164:568, 1991.
39. Habicht GS et al: Lyme disease spirochetes induce human and murine interleukin-1 production, *J Immunol* 134:3147, 1985.
40. Hechemy KE et al: *Borrelia burgdorferi* attachment to mammalian cells, *J Infect Dis* 159:805, 1989.
41. Johnson RC, Marek N, Kodner C: Infection of Syrian hamsters with Lyme disease spirochetes, *J Clin Microbiol* 20:1099, 1984.
42. Johnston YE et al: Lyme arthritis. Spirochetes found in synovial microangiopathic lesions, *Am J Pathol* 118:26, 1985.

43. Kujala GA, Steere AC, Davis JS: IgM rheumatoid factor in Lyme disease: correlation with disease activity, total serum IgM, and IgM antibody to *Borrelia burgdorferi, J Rheumatol* 14:772, 1987.

44. Kurtti TJ et al: *Borrelia burgdorferi* in tick cell culture: growth and cellular adherence, *J Med Entomol* 25:256, 1988.

45. Luft BJ et al: Immunologic and structural characterization of the dominant 66- to 73-kDa antigens of *Borrelia burgdorferi, J Immunol* 146:2776, 1991.

46. Mackworth-Young CG et al: Anticardiolipin antibodies in Lyme disease, *Arthritis Rheum* 31:1052, 1988.

47. Marcus LC et al: Fatal pancarditis in a patient with co-existent Lyme disease and babesiosis: demonstration of spirochetes in the myocardium, *Ann Intern Med* 103:374, 1985.

48. Mensi N et al: Characterization of *Borrelia burgdorferi* proteins reactive with antibodies in synovial fluid of a patient with Lyme arthritis, *Infect Immun* 58:2404, 1990.

49. Oldstone MBA: Molecular mimicry as a mechanism for the cause and as a probe uncovering etiologic agent(s) of autoimmune disease, *Curr Top Microbiol Immunol* 145:127, 1989.

50. Peterson PK et al: Human phagocyte interactions with the Lyme disease spirochete, *Infect Immun* 46:608, 1984.

51. Radolf JD et al: Lipoproteins of *Borrelia burgdorferi* and *Treponema pallidum* activate cachectic / tumor necrosis factor synthesis, *J Immunol* 147:1968, 1991.

52. Schaible VE et al: Monoclonal antibodies specific for the outer surface protein A (OSP-A) of *Borrelia burgdorferi* prevent Lyme borrelisis in severe combined immunodeficiency (scid) mice. *Proc Natl Acad Sci USA* 87:3768, 1990.

53. Schmidli J et al: Cultivation of *Borrelia burgdorferi* from joint fluid three months after treatment of facial palsy due to Lyme borreliosis, *J Infect Dis* 158:905, 1988.

54. Schwan T, Burgdorfer W, Garon CF: Changes in infectivity and plasmid profile of the Lyme disease spirochete, *Borrelia burgdorferi*, as a result of *in vitro* cultivation, *Infect Immun* 56:1831, 1988.

55. Sears JE et al: Molecular mapping of OSP-A mediated immunity against *Borrelia burgdorferi*, the agent of Lyme disease, *J Immunol* 147;1995, 1991.

56. Sigal LH, Tatum AH: Lyme disease patients' serum contains IgM antibodies to *Borrelia burgdorferi* that cross react with neuronal antigens, *Neurology* 38:1439, 1988.

57. Simpson WJ, Schrumpf ME, Schwan TG: Reactivity of human Lyme borreliosis sera with a 39-kilodalton antigen specific to *Borrelia burgdorferi, J Clin Microbiol* 28:1329, 1990.

58. Snydman DR et al: *Borrelia burgdorferi* in joint fluids in chronic Lyme arthritis, *Ann Intern Med* 104:798, 1986.

59. Srinivasappa J et al: Molecular mimicry: frequency of reactivity of monoclonal antiviral antibodies with normal tissues, *J Virol* 57:397, 1986.

60. Stamm LV et al: Heat shock response of spirochetes, *Infect Immun* 59:1572, 1991.

61. Steere AC et al: Chronic Lyme arthritis. Clinical and immunogenetic differentiation from rheumatoid arthritis, *Ann Intern Med* 90:896, 1979.

62. Steere AC et al: The spirochetal etiology of Lyme disease, *N Engl J Med* 308:733, 1983.

63. Suchanek G et al: Antimyelin antibodies in cerebrospinal fluid and serum of patients with meningopolyneuritis Garin-Bujadoux-Bannwarth and other neurological diseases, *Zentralbl Bakteriol Mikrobiol Hyg [A]* 263:160, 1986.

64. Szczepanski A, Benach JL: Lyme borreliosis: host responses to *Borrelia burgdorferi, Microbiol Rev* 55:21, 1991.

65. Szczepanski A, Fleit HB: Interaction between *Borrelia burgdorferi* and polymorphonuclear leukocytes. Phagocytosis and the induction of the respiratory burst, *Ann NY Acad Sci* 539:425, 1988.

66. Szczepanski A et al: Interaction between *Borrelia burgdorferi* and endothelium *in vitro, J Clin Invest* 85:1637, 1990.

67. Takayama K, Rothenberg RJ, Barbour AG: Absence of lipopolysaccharide in the Lyme disease spirochete, *Borrelia burgdorferi, Infect Immun* 55:2311, 1987.

68. Thomas DD, Comstock LE: Interaction of Lyme disease spirochetes with cultured eucaryotic cells, *Infect Immun* 57:1324, 1989.

69. Volkman DJ et al: Characterization of an immunoreactive 93 kDa core protein of *Borrelia burgdorferi* with a human IgG monoclonal antibody, *J Immunol* 146:3177, 1991.

70. Wood DD, Ihrie EJ, Hamerman D: Release of interleukin-1 from human synovial tissue *in vitro, Arthritis Rheum* 28:853, 1985.

71. Young RA, Elliot TJ: Stress proteins, infection, and immune surveillance, *Cell* 59:5, 1989.

23 Lyme Disease in Pregnancy

Genevieve Sicuranza and *David Allan Baker*

Lyme borreliosis became a reportable disease in the United States in 1982, and in 1991 a national surveillance case definition was established. The Centers for Disease Control in its June 1991 report indicated an eighteenfold increase in the number of cases from 1982 through 1989 (13,500).[1] Lyme disease was first described in 1977 in Old Lyme, Connecticut, as a juvenile-arthritis type syndrome associated with tick bites.[12] Although cases are concentrated in the northeastern, midwestern, and Pacific United States, Lyme disease has now been reported from most states. It is clearly an international problem, with a marked increase in infected and symptomatic people in Europe and Asia as well. Due to the rising numbers of cases each year, there has been increasing concern about the potential impact of Lyme disease on the pregnant woman and her fetus.

Lyme disease is caused by a spirochete, *Borrelia burgdorferi*, classically carried by the deer tick, *Ixodes dammini*.[10] Other vectors have been identified in New Jersey and Texas *(Amblyomma americanum)*.[11] Although the deer is the preferred host of the adult tick, almost any bird or domestic animal can act as an intermediate host. It is known that the fetus is quite vulnerable to the transplacental passage of the syphilis spirochete, *Treponema pallidum*. Because the causative agent of Lyme disease is also a spirochete, there is concern that *B. burgdorferi* might also affect the fetus. This chapter reviews the available information pertaining to Lyme disease in pregnancy and discusses the diagnosis and management in this selected population. (See Color Plate 8.)

PREGNANCY

Maternal infection may involve transmission of the invading microorganism to the fetus. This may have no adverse consequences or may produce a range of sequelae from minor transient problems to fetal death and abortion. Among the spirochetal bacterial infections, syphilis is known to cause abortion, stillbirth, and congenital abnormalities. Maternal relapsing fever and leptospirosis have also been associated with an increased risk of fetal loss.

Among animals, borreliae have been associated with bovine abortion. Whether Lyme disease affects the pregnancy or the fetus has been a subject of several studies. In 1985, Schlesinger[8] documented transplacental transmission of *B. burgdorferi* for the first time. The infant involved showed congenital heart anomalies. An autopsy revealed numerous spirochetes in the spleen, kidney, and bone marrow. The chorionic villi had histologic evidence of involvement with increased numbers of Hofbauer cells. The mother in question had been infected during the first trimester and had not received treatment. The Centers for Disease Control conducted a retrospective study on 19 women with Lyme disease.[5] There were five poor outcomes: prematurity, cortical blindness, fetal demise, syndactyly, and rash. No association was noted between a poor outcome and the trimester in which infection occurred, or whether treatment was given. A second study conducted by the Centers for Disease Control[5] involved a prospective analysis of 17 females infected during the first trimester. In this small prospective study, one infant was born with syndactyly, and there was one spontaneous loss at 13 weeks. All the other pregnancies resulted in normal infants.

From 1986 through 1987, Nadal et al[7] surveyed over 1000 mothers at deliveries where *anti-B. burgdorferi* antibody titers were obtained. Of these 1000 mothers, 12 had elevated titers, but only one mother was symptomatic with Lyme disease during her first trimester. Her child was born with a ventricular-septal cardiac defect (VSD). None of the children born to mothers with a positive titer had detectable antibodies. Of the 12 mothers with positive titers, 8 delivered at term, 2 were preterm, and 2 were postterm. Seven infants had problems in the newborn period: there were two cases of hyperbilirubinemia and one case each of hypotonia (attributed to medication), microcephaly, supraventricular extrasystoles, VSD, and small for gestational age when examined between 9 and 17 months of age; however, only the child with the VSD remained abnormal.

MacDonald published two papers regarding

Lyme disease in pregnancy. He described four cases of fetal borreliosis found while prospectively studying abortuses.[4] His findings included one term stillbirth and three second-trimester losses. One of the second-trimester losses was complicated by toxemia and another by systemic lupus erythematosus. *B. burgdorferi* was cultured from the fetal liver in each case. From the term stillbirth, spirochetes were found in the liver, heart, adrenal, brain, kidney, meninges, and subarachnoid. Three of the cases had identifiable cardiac malformations: atrial-septal defect, VSD, and coarctation of the aorta. He questioned whether or not *B. burgdorferi* could be a cause of fetal demise, congenital heart defect, or fetal loss after toxemia. In 1989,[3] MacDonald described several other cases. One was a 25-year-old black woman at term in labor who delivered a male fetus who was small for gestational age with multiple anomalies including VSD in addition to central nervous system (CNS) anomalies. *B. burgdorferi* was identified in the fetal autopsy. Another was a term intrauterine growth-retarded infant who succumbed to a large VSD and absence of the left hemidiaphragm. This autopsy also found spirochetes in tissue. MacDonald also reports several second-trimester losses, with and without anomalies, that at autopsy revealed *B. burgdorferi*. In the same article, MacDonald refers to a retrospective study of 10 sudden infant deaths; he reported that 2 had spirochetes consistent with *B. burgdorferi* in the brain. No other laboratory, however, has confirmed this high report of spirochetal invasion of the fetal and placental tissue.

In contrast to these reports of MacDonald,[3,4] the Fourth International Conference on Lyme Borreliosis held in Stockholm in June of 1990 concluded that there is little risk to the fetus.[9] The symposium examined a large retrospective study in which there was no increased rate of congenital malformations in infants with seropositive mothers. The symposium referred to a study in which there were six pregnant women with Lyme disease, all of whom had healthy infants. Another study, which surveyed pediatric neurologists in areas highly endemic for Lyme disease, failed to discover any records of neurologic cases that could be attributed to Lyme disease.

In a series of 143 pregnant women from Wisconsin, titers for *B. burgdorferi* exposure were examined and correlated with pregnancy outcome. In the group, the incidence of first-trimester spontaneous abortions was no greater for seropositive women than for seronegative women.[2]

DIAGNOSIS

According to the Centers for Disease Control,[5] a diagnosis of Lyme disease in pregnancy can be made with certainty if erythema migrans (EM) is present or if there is the new onset of typical neurologic, cardiac, or joint involvement in a pregnant woman accompanied by laboratory confirmation of infection (typically diagnostic antibody levels or a significant rise in acute versus convalescent antibody levels; isolation of spirochetes from a clinical sample is also acceptable). In reality, however, patients in whom there is a reasonable clinical suspicion for Lyme disease warrant treatment.

TREATMENT

According to the Centers for Disease Control, any pregnant woman with the diagnosis of Lyme disease, or the suspicion of it, should be treated.[5] The diagnosis should be a clinical one and not based on serology because serologic conversion may occur too late in the disease process. The problems with current antibody assays, and the problem of seronegativity, are addressed in Chapters 14 and 25. In the Centers for Disease Control study, 3 of 13 patients treated had abnormal fetal outcomes (23%), as did 2 of the 6 patients who were not treated (33%). According to their study, the time of the disease in relation to poor outcome and whether the patient was treated were not significant. The Centers for Disease Control admitted that none of these adverse outcomes was documented to be a direct sequela of Lyme disease. These adverse outcomes are only possible associations of *Borrelia burgdorferi* maternal infection (Table 23–1). According to Mikkelsen and Palli,[6] to avoid a potential adverse effect on the fetus, the mother should be treated aggressively. Treatment is guided by the clinical manifestations of the disease (Table 23–2). Lyme disease limited to the skin can probably be treated with amoxicillin or erythromycin (see Chapter 18 for a different approach). Probenecid should not be used, and the tetracyclines should be avoided. Disseminated disease, and infections in the first trimester, should be treated with parenteral antibiotics (ceftriaxone or penicillin G).

In 1987, Mikkelsen and Palle[6] reported the case of a 29-year-old woman who during her 24th week was bitten by a tick. She developed EM without any systemic manifestations, with a positive antibody titer. She was treated with penicillin for 10

Table 23–1 Adverse pregnancy outcomes with possible association to Lyme disease

---

Congenital anomalies (especially heart, great vessels)
Congenital cortical blindness
Miscarriage
Small for gestational age
Stillbirth
Toxemia

Table 23–2 Treatment of Lyme disease during pregnancy

Disease stage	Antibiotic regimen
Uncomplicated erythema migrans after first trimester	Amoxicillin 500 mg PO tid-qid × 21-30 days Erythromycin 250 mg PO qid × 21-30 days* Avoid tetracyclines, probenecid

Disseminated or late disease; first trimester infection	Intravenous antibiotics for 2-4 weeks
	  Ceftriaxone 2g
	  Penicillin G 20 million U qd

*Newer macrolides such as Azithromycin may prove to be superior to erythromycin.

days and subsequently delivered a term baby. Histologic study of the placenta was negative, and the antibody titer in cord and maternal blood was not elevated.

SUMMARY

A body of evidence[3,4] suggests that the causative agent of Lyme disease, *B. burgdorferi*, can cross the placenta and infect the fetus. There are also several reports that suggest that this may be associated with a poor fetal outcome. However, the majority of studies have not been able to identify *B. burgdorferi* as a cause of spontaneous abortions, congenital anomalies, or neurologic sequelae in infants.

It is essential to realize that in the pregnant woman Lyme disease is a clinical diagnosis regardless of her serologic status. Because the precise risk to the fetus from an infected pregnant female is not yet clear, it is important to be aggressive in the diagnosis and management of Lyme disease. This is important not only for the fetus, but also for the mother. The mother is certainly at risk for serious and potentially debilitating manifestations of Lyme disease including arthritis, carditis, and neurologic problems.

In conclusion, Lyme disease in pregnancy is a clinical diagnosis irrespective of serologic status.

The diagnosis must be made promptly, and treatment must be instituted in the interest of maternal, in addition to fetal, welfare.

REFERENCES

1. Centers for Disease Control, *MMWR* 40(25):417, 1991.
2. Dlesk A et al: Lyme seropositivity and pregnancy outcome in the absence of symptoms of Lyme disease, *Arthritis Rheum* 32(suppl):S46, 1989.
3. MacDonald AB: Human fetal borreliosis, toxemia of pregnancy, and fetal death, *Zentralbl Bakteriol Mikrobiol Hyg [A]* 263:189, 1986.
4. MacDonald AB: Gestational Lyme borreliosis, *Rheum Dis Clin North Am* 15(4):657, 1989.
5. Markowitz LE et al: Lyme disease during pregnancy, *JAMA* 255(24):3394, 1986.
6. Mikkelsen AL, Palle C: Lyme disease during pregnancy, *Acta Obstet Gynecol Scand* 66:477, 1987.
7. Nadal D et al: Infants born to mothers with antibodies against *Borellia burgdorferi* at delivery, *Eur J Pediatr* 148:426, 1989.
8. Schlessinger PA et al: Maternal-fetal transmission of Lyme disease spirochete *Borrelia burgdorferi*, *Ann Intern Med* 103:67, 1985.
9. Sigal LH: Summary of the Fourth International Symposium on Lyme Borreliosis, *Arthritis Rheum* 34(3):367, 1991.
10. Steere AG: Lyme disease, *N Engl J Med* 321:586, 1989.
11. Steere AC, Malawista SE: Cases of Lyme disease in the United States: locations correlated with distribution of *Ixodes dammini*, *Ann Intern Med* 91:730, 1979.
12. Steere AC et al: The clinical spectrum and treatment of Lyme disease, *Yale J Biol Med* 57:453, 1984.

Persisting Symptoms

Leonard H. Sigal

There is much mystery and speculation about the chronicity of symptoms in some patients with Lyme disease. Some physicians and patients state that *Borrelia burgdorferi* can cause "resistant" or "dormant" infection, which then might explain the lack of response to courses of antibiotic therapy otherwise usually deemed adequate. That symptoms may persist is undeniable; that the explantion lies in persisting infection, the priviledge location of the infectious agent, or its diminished antibiotic sensitivity, is by no means established.

After careful analysis of the patients referred to The Lyme Disease Center at Robert Wood Johnson Medical School, patients seen elsewhere, and the extensive clinical experience of others, we have found that the population of patients with "persistent Lyme disease" can be divided into five categories:

1. True persisting Lyme disease: inadequate therapy
2. Permanent tissue damage, not responsive to antibiotics: adequate therapy
3. Slowly resolving Lyme disease
4. Post-Lyme disease: possible reactive phenomena
5. Symptoms unrelated to Lyme disease: initial misdiagnosis

TRUE PERSISTING LYME DISEASE: INADEQUATE THERAPY

Many of these patients have true infection with *B. burgdorferi* as the cause of their complaints and may benefit from further antibiotic therapy. In the initial controlled antibiotic trials, using a lower dose and shorter duration of therapy than is being suggested now, some patients had resolution of their clinical problems during their initial course of therapy, only to experience a significant relapse after termination of the drug. Many of these patients were cured by a longer duration or higher dose of therapy.[29] The likely explanation for this phenomenon was that the regimen used represented inadequate therapy for Lyme disease. In current practice, some patients have recrudescence of previously resolving symptoms, which may be due to less than adequate duration or dose of therapy.[6] Likewise, some patients with articular or central nervous system (CNS) infection may seem to improve on oral regimens, only to worsen later. In these patients, the likely explanation is that an inappropriate regimen was used, with insufficient penetration of drug to the site of infection and inflammation.[5,9]

In addition, some patients experience relapse despite having been treated with what would seem to be an adequate therapeutic regimen. Explanations offered for this phenomenon include inadequate penetration of drug to privileged sites where the organism resides, "resistance" of the strain of organism,[9,10,14,18,29] and coincidence (i.e., the second course of antibiotic was given coincident with the natural course of resolution). This occasional lack of response to first treatments occurs in the practice of even the most experienced clinicians. In this circumstance, retreatment is indicated,[18] with detailed clinical follow-up.

PERMANENT TISSUE DAMAGE, NOT RESPONSIVE TO ANTIBIOTICS: ADEQUATE THERAPY

It is possible that tissue damage induced by the initial infection has been so extensive that permanent tissue dysfunction has been produced. In this circumstance, total resolution of the resulting symptoms may be impossible. The lack of total resolution of *B. burgdorferi*–induced damage to antibiotic therapy has been described and discussed previously for facial palsy,[5] central and peripheral nervous system disease,[2,13,14,19] cardiac disease,[23] and arthritis.[30] In some patients, therapy merely halts the progression of disease, rather than leading to resolution.[13] In North American Lyme disease, peripheral neuropathy and radiculoneuropathy seem to have a greater tendency to become chronic than does CNS disease.[18] The tendency to chronicity also correlates with a longer duration of disease before the institution of therapy[14,19] and with the severity of the initial manifestations of Lyme disease.[10,29] It seems likely that with longer or more severe disease, permanent tissue damage may result that is refractory to further antibiotic therapy.

Not infrequently, such patients are subjected to repeated courses of ineffective theapy because the clinician has obtained serologic testing after therapy. It is clear that some patients with cured Lyme disease may remain sero-positive for prolonged periods, just as some patients with ongoing disease can revert to seronegativity after antibiotic treatment.[35] Unfortunately, seropositivity is frequently misinterpreted as meaning active infection.

SLOWLY RESOLVING LYME DISEASE: NATURAL HISTORY

Many casual observers expect that the symptoms of Lyme disease should resolve during or shortly after therapy. This kind of prompt response has been described in early localized,[29] early disseminated,[5,9,23,27] and late[2,14,30] disease. However, it has been known since the initial studies of antibiotic therapy of Lyme disease that up to 50% of patients may develop nonspecific later complaints, including headache, fatigue, lethargy, and noninflammatory musculoskeletal pains after therapy of early or late manifestations of Lyme disease.[3,14,16,27,29] These compaints are, in general, refractory to further antibiotic therapy.

It is also known that, in some patients, ultimate resolution of symptoms may be quite delayed. Erythema chronicum migrans and associated symptoms usually resolve during the course of treatment.[29] In general, meningitis resolves promptly.[27] Cardiac disease may, however, linger for months, and occasional cases of residual first-degree atrioventricular block have been described.[23] In Lyme arthritis, the delay in ultimate resolution has been reported to be as long as 6 to 8 months after the termination of intravenous penicillin[26,27]; others have corroborated such delays in response.[7]

Gradual response to therapy in chronic neurologic damage has been the rule in Lyme disease.* Sensory and motor symptoms may persist for 6 months before resolution, and the delay until resolution may be 24 months in peripheral neuropathy and radiculitis.[27] The findings of late neuroborreliosis, the chronic neurologic damage of late Lyme disease, usually slowly resolve over the course of many months, often with some residual deficit as I and others have noted (Unpublished data).[2,14]

POST-LYME DISEASE: POSSIBLE REACTIVE PHENOMENA
Fibromyalgia

Nearly 200 patients have been referred to The Lyme Disease Center for evaluation of persistent Lyme disease who, in fact, have had fibromyalgia. Nearly

two thirds of these patients had Lyme disease before or coincident with the onset of their fibromyalgia. We believe that fibromyalgia may follow Lyme disease, perhaps related to the sleep disorder that can be seen during even mild early Lyme disease.[22] Oral antibiotic therapy for possible ongoing infection has not been effective in treating the fibromyalgia of any of these patients. Rather, these patients have responded to the standard therapy for fibromyalgia, which includes vigorous regular aerobic exercise and bedtime tricyclic antidepressant therapy, to modify sleep patterns.[22] Post–Lyme disease fibromyalgia represents a syndrome following Lyme disease but not due to ongoing infection. Thus, ongoing or repeated antibiotic therapy for this syndrome is not indicated, is not effective, and can result in significant side-effects. A chronic fatiguelike syndrome may also develop as a post-Lyme disease symptom. This is discussed further in Chapter 26.

Reactive arthritis

The immunopathogenesis of Lyme disease is likely the result of direct infection, with antigen-specific immune reactivity, both humoral and cellular, increased locally and systemically.[17,21,25] If this were the entire explanation for *B. burgdorferi*–induced disease, one would expect antibiotic therapy to be universally effective. It is known that immune function in patients with Lyme disease is also modified in a nonspecific fashion by the interaction with *B. burgdorferi*.[21] These immunologic phenomena may be part of the explanation of the recently proposed link between infection with *B. burgdorferi* and reactive arthritis. The lack of antibiotic response in eight of nine patients suggests that the joint inflammation is not due to ongoing infection.[33] This represents a second possible example of postinfectious complications of Lyme disease, neither of which can be expected to respond to further antibiotic therapy.

Rheumatoid arthritis

We have seen three patients who developed classic, rheumatoid factor positive rheumatoid arthritis *after* an episode of Lyme disease. This may represent mere coincidence of two relatively common diseases and an example of arthritis following Lyme disease, but not related to the infection. One of our non-Lyme disease patients with classic rheumatoid arthritis has had two episodes of erythema chronicum migrans; with each of these episodes, here previously well = controlled rheumatoid arthrits has flared, with quiescence once her early Lyme disease was treated with oral doxycycline. This may represent another coincidence. However, an altenative explanation is also plausible: infection

---

*References 2,4,14-16,31,34.

with *B. burgdorferi* may provide the nonspecific immunologic stimulus that serves as one of the causes of rheumatoid arthritis. Although Lyme arthritis can rarely affect joints in a distribution mimicking rheumatoid factor negative rheumatoid arthritis (termed *seronegative rheumatoid arthritis*), rheumatoid factor positivity is not a feature of Lyme arthritis.[28] Positive serologic tests both enzyme-linked immunosorbent assay (ELISA) and Western blot for Lyme disease have been reported in patients with rheumatoid arthritis, further confusing the issue.[32] Infection with *B. burgdorferi* causes Lyme arthritis; the antibiotic responses of this entity have been reviewed previously.[30] If the cause of arthritis is local, poorly uncontrolled nonspecific immunologic activity or persistence of local antigen-specific reactivity directed at residual, but dead, organism from antecedent infection,[21] one would predict that further antibiotic therapy would be ineffective. The antigen-induced arthritis animal model of rheumatoid arthritis may be of relevance to persistent Lyme arthritis. In the animal model, a systemic immune response to foreign protein (in the rat model, bovine serum albumin is used as the foreign protein) causes self-limited arthritis of the joint that has been previously injected with that protein. Intravenous injection with the same protein causes a flare of arthritis in that joint. This reinfusion of the protein causes an increase in the specific immune reactivity, which reactivates the inflammation where the protein persists. The intermittent arthritis of Lyme disease might be caused by episodic systemic release of borrelial proteins and likely represents a process that is not antibiotic-sensitive.[21]

Autoimmunity

Autoimmunity has been proposed as a mechanism of Lyme neurologic disease, predicated on molecular mimicry.[21,24] In this scheme, a component of the organism resembles a component of human tissue; the immune response to the organism elicits an immune reactivity, which can attack the human component, as well. Examples of this phenomenon in human disease include rheumatic fever and Chagas' disease. If such a mechanism were active in Lyme disease, antibiotic therapy would do nothing to dampen the immune reactivity that is causing ongoing neural tissue damage. Sera of patients with lyme neurologic disease bind to human nerve in indirect immunofluorescence assays (IFA); sera from normal controls and from Lyme disease patients with other than neurologic manifestations do not bind to nerve. We have found that the subunit of *B. burgdorferi's* flagella, a 41-kD protein known as flagellin, contains a structure that cross-reacts with a component of human nerve. Cross-reactivity

with human neuroblastoma cells has allowed the identification of a specific neural protein that accounts for this cross-reactivity. Certain of these findings have been corroborated by others.[1] Thus, molecular mimicry could be part of the immunopathogenesis of lyme disease. Were this to be establised as the case, further antibiotic therapy would not be expected to alter the natural history of the inflammation. Rather, immunomodulatory therapy (e.g., corticosteroids) might be useful. Although this is currently a matter for speculation rather than action, the fact remains that such a model would not include a role for further antibiotic therapy.

SYMPTOMS UNRELATED TO LYME DISEASE: INITIAL MISDIAGNOSIS

Many of the patients referred to The Lyme Disease Center at Robert Wood Johnson Medical School have complaints thought to result from the persistence of their preceding Lyme disease, which continue after antibiotic therapy. In many of these patients, we cannot verify the preceding diagnosis of Lyme disease. Often, the patient had a poorly defined illness and a positive serologic test for Lyme disease. It is quite clear that many normal people test positive for Lyme disease by ELISA or IFA and do not have the disease. In northwestern Wisconsin, 5.6% of the general population is seropositive,[3] whereas up to 20% of the population near Vienna, Austria, is reactive[12]; we estimate the rate to be 4% to 5% in our area of New Jersey. Unfortunately, many patients go from doctor to doctor (and often, laboratory to laboratory) being tested repeatedly until one test returns positive. Given the variation in testing and the statistical methods often used to determine the "normal" range, such repeated testing is virtually guaranteed to ultimately yield a positive test.[20] Many of these "false positives" may be defined as such by the use of Western blot analysis. In the absence of such confirmatory testing, many of these people may be incorrectly labeled with the diagnosis of Lyme disease as the explanation for their clinical complaints. A recent report of four cases of subacute bacterial endocarditis initially misdiagnosed as Lyme disease further documents the danger of misdiagnosis based solely on serologic reactivity.[11] Frequently, the diagnosis of Lyme disease was made despite a negative serologic test because the patient lived in an endemic area and had symptoms "compatible with Lyme disease." Increasingly, the diagnosis of Lyme disease is made by this intrinsically flawed process of exclusion. Our initial experience suggested that only about one third of patients referred to our Center actually had Lyme disease, either active or by history.[22] The directors of other Lyme disease referral centers have corroborated this estimate. At our Center, the remaining group of non-Lyme disease patients were found to have other maladies, including rheumatoid arthritis, seronegative spondylarthropathies, mechanical disease of the knee, osteoarthritis, and fibromyalgia, among other overlooked causes of the patients' complaints. The patients described in our study are likely not representative of the general population. Nonetheless, it is apparent that imprecise criteria have lead to the overdiagnosis of Lyme disease in many endemic areas. In these patients, the lack of response to therapy suggests initial misdiagnosis rather than persistent or resistant Lyme disease.

Since this initial published experience, we have seen patients with a number of other illnesses initially misdiagnosed as Lyme disease. These have included: the anticardiolipin antibody syndrome, toxic synovitis of the hip, multiple sclerosis, congenital leukoencephalopathy, amyotrophic lateral sclerosis, brain tumors, Wegener's granulomatosis, and many more cases of fibromyalgia. These misdiagnoses have often occurred because of patient adamancy that Lyme disease is the correct diagnosis with subsequent physican acquiescence. Occasionally, physicians have made Lyme disease the "diagnosis of exclusion," or physicians mistakenly think that in endemic areas Lyme disease is truly the cause of most ailments. Recent reports have documented the mischief that can be made by basing the diagnosis of Lyme disease merely on serologic testing.[11]

Perhaps the only unifying principle in all of these cases is that physician and patient have rushed to a diagnosis of Lyme disease with inattention to details or eschewing diagnostic tests that might have assisted in identifying the correct etiology (e.g., not doing a magnetic resonance imaging [MRI] scan in a patient with peculiar neurologic complaints and thereby missing the infiltrating medulloblastoma). This pressure to diagnose Lyme disease before permanent damage develops is a frequent phenomenon in endemic areas and should be discouraged.

CONCLUSION

Persisting complaints in a patient with prior diagnosis of Lyme disease should raise a number of questions in the mind of the clinician, but first among them should be: Was the initial diagnosis of Lyme disease correct? Inadequate prior therapy, slow resolution, permanence of tissue damage from the prior episode of *B. burgdorferi*–induced inflammation, and evolution of a "reactive" process or autoimmunity are also plausible explanations for the ongoing complaints. It is known that *B. burg-*

dorferi is capable of producing a wide range of immunologic changes, and perhaps molecular mimicry is part of this phenomenon. "Post-Lyme disease" syndromes of musculoskeletal complaints and fatigue have been described frequently after therapy of early disease. The clinician also must consider post-Lyme disease fibromyalgia as the explanation of the patient's complaints; this entity is potentially treatable, so making this diagnosis is of major clinical importance.

It might be valuable for clinicians to expand the definitiion of Lyme disease to include three "Lyme disease-related" clinical entities in her or his thinking. These are:

1. *Lyme borreliosis.* Symptoms are due to active infection with *B. burgdorferi*. Symptoms are usually antibiotic sensitive.

2. *Post-Lyme disease syndromes.* The antecedent infection is acknowledged; it is now likely bacteriologically cured. An understanding of the pathogenesis of these conditions allows the clinician to predict that the complaints will not respond to further antibiotic therapy. This category includes many of the conditions outlined above.

3. *Lyme anxiety.* There is concern that the current complaints are due to infection, evidence of which is absent. No infection, preceding or current, can be documented. Serologic evidence of exposure to *B. burgdorferi* may or may not be available. Antibiotic therapy is not indicated. Lyme disease is especially a problem in endemic areas.

With these entities in mind, and the previous discussion of the mechanisms underlying these phenomena, the clinician in areas endemic for Lyme disease can make a rational clinical decision. Furthermore, it is possible to predict the time course of response to therapy and warn the patient in advance of the likely clinical course. Thus forewarned, the patient is less likely to experience needless anxiety and concern about the natural history of resolving of Lyme disease.

REFERENCES

1. Aberer E et al: Molecular mimicry and Lyme borreliosis, *Ann Neurol* 26:732, 1989.
2. Ackermann R et al: Chronic neurologic manifestations of erythema migrans borreliosis, *Ann NY Acad Sci* 539:16, 1988.
3. Agger W et al: Lyme disease: clinical features, classification, and epidemiology in the upper Midwest, *Medicine* 70:83, 1991.
4. Broderrick JP, Sandok BA, Mertz LE: Focal encephalitis in a young woman 6 years after the onset of Lyme disease: tertiary Lyme disease? *Mayo Clin Proc* 62:313, 1987.
5. Clark JR et al: Facial paralysis in Lyme disease, *Laryngoscope* 95:1341, 1985.

6. Dattwyler RJ, Halperin JJ: Failure of tetracycline therapy in early Lyme disease, *Arthritis Rheum* 30:448, 1987.

7. Dattwyler RJ et al: Treatent of late Lyme borreliosis—randomized comparison of ceftriaxone and penicillin, *Lancet* i:1191, 1988.

8. Dattwyler RJ et al: Amoxicilin plus probenecid compared to doxycycline for the treatment of erythema migrans (EM), *Arthritis Rheum* 33:S85, 1990.

9. Halperin JJ et al: Lyme disease: cause of a treatable peripheral neuropathy, *Neurology* 37:1700, 1987.

10. Hyppertz H-I: Childhood Lyme borreliosis in Europe, *Eur J Pediatr* 149:814, 1990.

11. Kaell AT et al: Positive Lyme serology in subacute bacterial endocarditis: a study of four patients, *JAMA* 264:2916, 1990.

12. Kinigadner U et al: *Borrelia* infection as a possible cause of HLA-B27 negative sacroiliitis, *J Rheumatol* 18:484, 1991.

13. Kohler J et al: Chronic central nervous system involvement in Lyme borreliosis, *Neurology* 38:863, 1988.

14. Logigian EL, Kaplan RF, Steere AC: Chronic neurologic manifestations of Lyme disease, *N Engl J Med* 323:1438, 1990.

15. Pachner AR: Lyme borreliosis: presentation and therapy, *Neurology* 41:463, 1991.

16. Pachner AR, Duray P, Steere AC: Central nervous system manifestations of Lyme disease, *Arch Neurol* 46:790, 1989.

17. Pachner AR et al: Antigen specific proliferation of CSF lymphocytes in Lyme disease, *Neurology* 35:1642, 1985.

18. Rahn DW, Malawista SE: Lyme disease: recommendations for diagnosis and treatment, *Ann Intern Med* 114:472, 1991.

19. Reik Jr L et al: Demyelinating encephalopathy in Lyme disease *Neurology* 35:267, 1985.

20. Schwartz BS et al: Antibody testing in Lyme disease: a comparison of results in four laboratories, *JAMA* 262:3431, 1989.

21. Sigal LH: Lyme disease, 1988: immunologic manifestations and possible immunopathogenetic mechanismsm *Sem Arthritis Rheum* 18:151, 1989.

22. Sigal LH: Experience with the first one hundred patients referred to a Lyme Disease referral center, *Am J Med* 88:577, 1990.

23. Sigal LH: *Severe complications of Lyme disease: recognition and management.* In Mandell BF, editor: *Management of the critically ill patient with rheumatic or immunologic illness,* New York, 1992, Marcel Dekker.

24. Sigal LH, Tatum AH: Molecular mimicry in Lyme neurologic disease: cross-reactivity between *Borrelia burgdorferi* and neuronal antigens, *Neurology* 38:1439, 1988.

25. Sigal LH et al: Proliferative responses of mononuclear cells in Lyme disease: concentration of *Borrelia burgdorferi*-reactive cells in joint fluid, *Arthritis Rheum* 29:761, 1986.

26. Steere AC: Pathogenesis of Lyme arthritis: implications for rheumatic disease, *Ann NY Acad Sci* 539:87, 1989.

27. Steere AC, Pachner AR, Malawista SE: Neurologic abnormalities of Lyme disease: successful treatment with high dose intravenous penicillin, *Ann Intern Med* 99:767, 1983.

28. Steere AC, Schoen RT, Taylor E: The clinical evolution of Lyme arthritis, *Ann Intern Med* 107:725, 1987.

29. Steere AC et al: Treatment of the early manifestations of Lyme disease, *Ann Intern Med* 99:22, 1983.

30. Steere AC et al: Successful parenteral penicillin therapy of established Lyme arthritis, *N Engl J Med* 312:869, 1984.

31. Weder B et al: Chronic progressive neurological involvement in *Borrelia burgdorferi* infection, *J Neurol* 234:40, 1987.

32. Weiss NL et al: False positive seroreactivity to *B. burgdorferi* in rheumatic disease: the value of immunoblotting, *Arthritis Rheum* 33:R35, 1990.

33. Weyand CM, Goronzy JJ: Immune responses to *Borrelia burgdorferi* in patients with reactive arthritis, *Arthritis Rheum* 32:1057, 1989.

34. Wokke JHJ et al: Chronic forms of *Borrelia burgdorferi* infection of the nervous system, *Neurology* 37:1031, 1987.

35. Zoller L et al: Spontaneous and post-treatment antibody kinetics in late Lyme borreliosis, *Serodiag Immunother Infect Dis* 3:345, 1989.

25 Seronegative Lyme Disease

Steven E. Schutzer

DEFINITION OF THE PROBLEM

The number and percentage of seronegative Lyme disease cases remain controversial. At some academic centers the estimate is 5%, and in certain private settings the number may be higher. There is little question that seronegative Lyme disease can exist.[6,11] For the clinician to decide what course to follow with a patient suspected of Lyme disease, but who is seronegative, an understanding of the terminology and mechanisms of seronegativity is imperative. This chapter offers approaches that the clinician might follow.

Seronegative antibody tests may refer to different circumstances and must be defined. For this review, seronegative is defined as an antibody test that is reported as negative yet the patient is infected with *Borrelia burgdorferi,* the causative agent of Lyme disease.[2,12]

It may be an apparent seronegative result because the level of antibody is far below a conventional assay's ability to detect reactive antibody, or it may be reported negative because even the level detected is below a defined criteria for a test to be called positive, or it may be truly negative because no specific antibody has been produced. Table 25–1 and Fig. 25–1 illustrate these points.

SEQUENCE OF EVENTS FROM INITIAL INFECTION

To understand why each of these variations can occur, it is useful to review the immune response to *B. burgdorferi* and its antigens from the moment of infection.

After a tick bite, *B. burgdorferi* enters the skin and comes in contact with the immune system. After antigen processing and T-cell presentation to B cells, antibody is produced and binds to epitopes of the antigens of the infectious agent. When the antigenic binding sites are saturated, one can find antibody in excess of antigen. Depending on the sensitivity of the assay, this antibody may be detectable (Fig. 25–1). It usually takes a B cell more than 4 days to begin differentiation into a plasma cell and subsequently begin production of antibody.

The total quantity may be very low and then build up. In a new infection, the first antibody to be produced is IgM. Some of the B cells responsible for IgM production eventually undergo a genetic switch and become committed to produce IgG. The IgG may be produced well after the organism has been eliminated. The levels of specific IgM usually taper down toward undetectable. Early after infection, and later in certain instances, the circulating antibody is not in excess and may not be detected by conventional probes, but may be detected by techniques that liberate the antibody from its bound immune complex (IC) form. Specifically in Lyme disease, even a person who eventually seroconverts to positive requires a relatively long lag period before this occurs. The IgM response may peak at 2 to 4 weeks after infection, then wane off.[8] In certain cases, a reappearance of IgM occurs.[5] The IgG response often peaks 6 weeks after infection. The levels of specific IgG may either begin to wane or persist.[8] As is described in Chapters 2, 14, and 22, *B. burgdorferi* is composed of several different antigenic components, some more immunogenic than others.[1,3,7,10] It should not be surprising to see variability in the isotypic immunoglobulin levels reactive to each component. For example, early in the infection, antibody may be detected against the flagellar component of 41 kD. The first antibody is likely to be IgM, followed by IgG. Later, IgM and IgG may be detected to the OspA (31 kD) and OspB (34 kD) antigens.

A variety of other *B. burgdorferi* antigens are encountered, as described in the other chapters. Some of these are specific to *B. burgdorferi,* whereas others are common to other bacteria. Therefore, a positive or negative result must also be considered in the context of the target antigen used in a test. The quantity of the antigen may be important as well. In the enzyme-linked immunosorbent assay (ELISA) described by Golightly,[6] sonicates of whole *B. burgdorferi* are used. This gives a potpourri of antigens that are coated on the ELISA plate. A positive result is above the mean plus three standard deviations determined from a

Table 25–1 Types of seronegativity in a patient with Lyme disease

True seronegativity	The B cells/plasma cells are not producing specific antibody.
Apparent sero-negativity	Specific absolute antibody is lower than the minimum amount detectable by the assay.
Laboratory sero-negativity	Specific antibody is present, but the level is below the cutoff criteria for a result to be called positive.
Borderline or inde-terminate	The level of antibody is between the particular laboratory's cutoff values of negative and positive results.
False positive	The level of reactive antibody exceeds the defined cutoff value for a positive test but may not be specific antibody. The antibody may be cross-reactive, or its production may have been stimulated by a polyclonal B cell trigger.
False negative	The antibody may be present as in clinically apparent seronegativity but is not detected for a variety of reasons.

Figure 25–1 Examples of antibody responses to antigen over time. Illustration of the window period before free antibody reaches a threshold detectable by the laboratory assay.

group of healthy uninfected controls. It is conceivable that cutoff thresholds would vary according to reactivity of the control group. For example, dental conditions related to treponemal species may cause cross-reactive antibody to the 41-kD flagellar protein. Although the levels may be relatively low, they could mathematically push up the cutoff needed for a positive result. Usually a careful history will avoid this. Likewise, the use of a single recombinant antigen may result in a negative value, whereas another one might have detected a positive reaction.

CASE ILLUSTRATION

Several different situations are described here to illustrate these concepts more clearly.

A patient is bitten by a tick in an endemic area, and a few days later he develops erythema migrans (EM); a few days after that he develops a bilateral facial nerve palsy. A skin biopsy is positive for B. burgdorferi *by histopathology and polymerase chain reaction (PCR). On clinical grounds alone, this case is very likely to be Lyme disease. The additional laboratory data confirm it. Therefore, we can consider that this patient has Lyme disease and examine different scenarios that might occur. Imagine that a serum sample were taken every week for 2 years.*

A sample from the first week most likely will be negative in almost any clinical laboratory or kit. This is because the patient's humoral immune system has not had enough time to produce sufficient antibody that could be detected. A sample at 4 weeks assayed for IgM may be called positive by one laboratory and negative or

Table 25–2 Predictive values of detection of complexed anti–*B. burgdorferi* antibody with sensitivity of 98.2% and specificity of 98% and varying prevalence

	Prevalence					
	1%	10%	20%	30%	40%	50%
Positive predictive value (%)	33.2	84.5	92.5	95.5	97.0	98.0
Negative predictive value (%)	100	99.8	99.5	99.2	98.8	98.2

borderline by others. This is because the limitations of sensitivity and numerical cutoff ranges become magnified between tests and test sites. A sample at 8 weeks is analyzed for IgG at three different laboratories. All come back positive. This can happen because the immune system has responded with a level of specific anti-B. burgdorferi antibody that should be detected by most ELISA or immunofluorescent assay (IFA) tests. Any number of results may occur from here on. The patient may recover, and the antibody level may wane or persist.

Consider that the same patient begins treatment the day of the rash. It has been reported that early antibiotic therapy may abrogate the humoral immune response. Other data support this appearance of a diminished response but note that the antibody may be detected in immune complexes. The level of detectable antibody may appear so low as to suggest the immune response has been dampened. This prolonged apparent seronegative state has been estimated to occur in at least 5% of Lyme disease cases.

If the same patient never developed EM, as may happen in 30% to 40% of cases, and did not have even a subtle unilateral facial nerve palsy, the clinician and the patient might remain in the dark until the laboratory test had become positive at 6 to 8 weeks. This would represent an unwanted delay in deciding whether to treat. Or if treatment is given right after the tick bite, follow-up tests might be negative. Ordinarily, this would not be a problem except if a later or systemic symptom of Lyme disease, such as arthritis or cognitive dysfunction, occurred. Antibiotics may have interfered with a diagnostic response. It might be very difficult to differentiate Lyme disease from another arthritic disorder or neurologic condition.

ANTIBODY ASSAY SYSTEMS

The most commonly used test is the ELISA,[6] which measures antibody to the Lyme disease spirochete. However, the mere presence of antibody does not mean that the patient is actually infected. It only indicates past infection has occurred.[4,11] Its use can be improved by obtaining two or more blood samples several weeks apart and running them side by side in the same test plate. This eliminates much of the variables that can affect tests on a daily basis and eliminates differences that may occur when the tests are run separately in different laboratories. It is still indirect evidence of infection. The Western

blot is a picture model of what is happening in the ELISA and, therefore, by itself cannot distinguish between active and past infection.

A new research test is the immune complex Lyme disease test.[11] In a series of experiments in which the samples were coded, this test picked out every bona fide case of Lyme disease and was not falsely positive in any sample that came from another disease or healthy person. More experiments showed that almost all active cases were positive and that recovered cases were negative. This indicates that it may be able to determine when someone is infected and when the infection is gone. It could also establish the diagnosis much earlier than the regular tests for the reasons explained above. Identification of the target (antigen) provides even more proof of the infection. This has also been accomplished with this test.

It is common to assess a diagnostic test by looking at how useful it is in a given population. The usefulness may be described statistically in terms of positive predictive values, which indicate how often the test is able to pick up the disease in those who truly have the disease among the particular population. The negative predictive value indicates how often it can exclude the disease in uninfected people in the particular population. Using a representative population in an endemic area, we calculated the following. The assay was positive in 98.2% of seropositive symptomatic Lyme disease patients. It was negative in all of 50 healthy controls and 96% of other disease controls from the endemic area. Combining the latter two groups, we can use a specificity of 98%, and from the first group a sensitivity of 98.2%. If one assumes that the population to be studied includes not just anyone from the endemic area but those with at least one major compatible sign or several less specific signs, one can conservatively assume a prevalence of 10% to 20% of the disease. As can be seen in Table 25–2, given this prevalence one has a good positive predictive value and an excellent negative predictive value. Therefore, as an adjunct to the history and physical examination, the assay can help decide whether someone has the disease or not.

Table 25–3 Types of suspected seronegative cases and approaches to diagnosis

True seronegative	Search for antigen[R] or DNA by PCR[R]
Apparent seronegative	Send specimen to another laboratory with a high proficiency. Send serial samples of serum to be run simultaneously in the same assay. Look for a rising titer over time. Immune complex antibody[R], antigen[R], PCR[R].
Laboratory seronegative	As above for apparent seronegative. Discuss criteria with laboratory director.
Borderline or indeterminate	As above.
False positive	History and evidence for Epstein-Barr virus infection, treponemal or other borreliae infections, VDRL.

[R], research assay.

APPROACHES TO THE SERONEGATIVE SUSPECTED CASE

Even in the best assays, seronegativity must be taken in the context of the patient's history and disease chronology.[6]

A physician can follow a number of approaches when a "seronegative" case of Lyme disease is suspected. If the time period is early, a repeat sample several weeks later might become positive. The simultaneous analysis of two or more samples taken over a period of time in the same assay would give an indication of a rising titer, suggesting recent infection. The best way to store a serum sample is at $-70°$ C or colder, but for the length of time usually involved in nonresearch situations, even 4° C (refrigerator temperature) may be acceptable. Of course the early period patient falls into a group with an acceptable explanation. Other situations may be more perplexing.

If the patient was treated and develops a new set of symptoms, a single conventional antibody test is not helpful. A paired sample pair over weeks might show a rise in titer and lead the clinician to suspect reinfection. A positive test with no rise in titer might mean that the patient is or has remained at the plateau. A complexed antibody test, although a research tool at present, would indicate an active process. Nonantibody research assays, such as PCR[9] or antigen detection would indicate a reinfection or continued infection. These are summarized in Table 25–3.

REFERENCES

1. Benach JL, Coleman JL, Golightly MG: A murine IgM monoclonal antibody binds an antigenic determinant in Osp A, immunodominant basic protein of the Lyme disease spirochete, *J Immunol* 140:265, 1988.
2. Benach JL et al: Spirochetes isolated from the blood of two patients with Lyme disease, *N Engl J Med* 308:740, 1983.
3. Coleman JL, Benach JL: Identification and characterization of an endoflagellar antigen of *Borrelia burgdorferi*, *J Clin Invest* 84:322, 1989.
4. Coyle PK et al: Cerebrospinal fluid immune complexes in patients exposed to *Borrelia burgdorferi:* detection of *Borrelia* specific and non-specific complexes, *Ann Neurol* 28:739, 1990.
5. Craft JE et al. Antigens of *Borrelia burgdorferi* recognized during Lyme disease: appearance of a new immunoglobulin M response and expansion of the immunoglobulin G response late in the illness, *J Clin Invest* 78:934, 1986.
6. Dattwyler RJ et al: Seronegative Lyme disease. Dissociation of specific T- and B-lymphocyte responses to *Borrelia burgdorferi*, *N Engl J Med* 319:1441, 1988.
7. Luft BJ et al: Immunologic and structural characterization of the dominant 66- to 73 kDa antigens of *Borrelia burgdorferi*, *J Immunol* 146:2776, 1991.
8. Rahn DW, Malewista SE: Lyme disease: recommendations for diagnosis and treatment, *Ann Intern Med* 114:472, 1991.
9. Rosa PA, Schwan TG: A specific and sensitive assay for the Lyme disease spirochete *Borrelia burgdorferi* using the polymerase chain reaction, *J Infect Dis* 160:1018, 1989.
10. Schubach WH et al: Mapping antibody binding domains of the major outer surface protein (Osp A) of *Borrelia burgdorferi*, *Infect Immun* (in press).
11. Schutzer SE et al: Sequestration of antibody to *Borrelia burgdorferi* in immune complexes in seronegative Lyme disease, *Lancet* 335:312, 1990.
12. Steere AC et al: The spirochetal etiology of Lyme disease, *N Engl J Med* 308:733, 1983.

26 Fatigue

Lauren B. Krupp, Joseph E. Schwartz, and Lina Jandorf

Overwhelming fatigue is a well-recognized clinical feature of Lyme disease. However, because fatigue is so nonspecific a symptom, it has not been extensively investigated and little is known regarding the impact of fatigue on Lyme disease patients. The purpose of this review is to summarize the clinical characteristics of fatigue in Lyme disease, analyze the relationship of fatigue to other disease manifestations including cognitive dysfunction and depression, and provide a rational approach to its differential diagnosis and treatment.

DEFINITION OF FATIGUE

Fatigue is defined as an overwhelming sense of tiredness, lack of energy, or feeling of exhaustion. It is distinguished from symptoms of depression, which include lack of self-esteem, despair, or a sense of hopelessness. Fatigue is also distinct from limb weakness. It is most easily conceptualized as an exhausted feeling that in healthy people may transiently develop during mild viral illnesses. Unfortunately, some patients with Lyme disease may experience disabling fatigue, which persists for many months.

FATIGUE DURING DIFFERENT STAGES OF *BORRELIA BURGDORFERI* INFECTION

Fatigue can develop during all stages of *B. burgdorferi* infection. It may occasionally continue after antibiotic therapy and resolution of other Lyme disease manifestations (Table 26–1). Fatigue has been well-documented in patients with early disease. In one study, 80% of 314 Lyme disease patients with erythema migrans (EM) experienced fatigue, lethargy, or malaise.[36] Fatigue was noted both before and after the onset of the rash. Unlike other disease manifestations, which often fluctuated in severity, fatigue and lethargy tended to be constant.[36] Symptoms often associated with fatigue during early infection include malaise, chills, fever, headache, and stiff neck.[35]

Fatigue occurs among Lyme disease patients with early stages of *B. burgdorferi* infection throughout Europe and North America.[16,39,42] For example, 74% of 90 Lyme disease patients with

EM from Russia reported fatigue and malaise.[9] In fact, fatigue appears to be a nearly universal characteristic of the early illness.

Several longitudinal studies have examined the natural history of untreated Lyme disease and the development of fatigue.[19,34] In one North American series of EM patients who never received antibiotics, 40% (18 of 44) of the patients who developed late rheumatologic manifestations experienced persistent fatigue.[34] Fatigue was particularly associated with chronic arthritis.[34] In contrast to these North American findings, a European study demonstrated infrequent sequelae in 72 untreated patients with neuroborreliosis.[19] The patients were examined 5 to 27 years after their initial presentation and only radicular nerve root pain (35%) or mild weakness (10%)[19] were noted. There was no mention of persistent fatigue or related symptoms such as cognitive difficulty.[19] The reasons for the differences between these two studies are unclear but may relate to strain differences in *B. burgdorferi* between Europe and North America, variations in the immune response, patient selection, or other methodologic differences between the clinical investigations.

Fatigue is not limited to patients with early Lyme disease. It is also a frequent finding during late infection. In patients with late rheumatologic and neurologic manifestations, 39% to 85% list fatigue among their symptoms.[4,16] Other related minor symptoms include headache, sweating, and tachycardia.[16]

Fatigue is particularly common in patients with late central nervous system (CNS) complications of *B. burgdorferi* infection.[39] For example, between 60% and 74% of patients with mild encephalopathy experience fatigue.[24,30,39] In addition, late infection encephalopathy patients with more dramatic CNS syndromes such as focal or diffuse encephalitis also suffer from fatigue, but this symptom is usually overshadowed by their other neurologic findings.*

After active Lyme disease has subsided, some

---

*References 1, 10, 25, 26, 30, 42.

196

Table 26–1 Frequency of fatique during stages of Lyme disease

	Prevalence (%)	References
Fatigue during active infection		
Early disease	70-80	9,36
Late disease	39-86	7,16,34
Fatigue after treatment		
Treated localized EM*	8	8
Treated EM with constitutional symptoms	16	8
Treated late disease†	23-60	7,16

*Fatigue resolved entirely within 6 months.
†Refers only to patients who reported fatigue before antibiotic therapy. Follow-up was 6 to 9 months, and incidence of fatigue was less in cephalosporin- versus penicillin-treated groups.

Table 26–2 Fatigue and depression in chronic medical illness

	Lyme disease (LYME)	Multiple sclerosis (MS)	Chronic fatigue syndrome (CFS)	Healthy controls (CTRL)
*n**	42	57	67	40
Age	37 ± 12	44 ± 10	38 ± 15	35 ± 9
Depressive symptoms†	17 ± 11	16 ± 11	21 ± 10	9 ± 7.0
Fatigue severity‡	4.8 ± .9	5.1 ± 1.4	6.1 ± 0.8	2.8 ± 0.7

*n refers to number of subjects.
†Depressive symptoms are measured by the Center for Epidemiologic Studies Depression Scale (CES-D; scored 0 to 60 with >15 indicating elevated depressive symptoms).[28] CES-D for Lyme disease patients and all patient groups is significantly higher than in healthy controls, $p < 0.0001$, CES-D for Lyme disease significantly lower than for CFS, $p < 0.04$, but not different from MS.
‡Fatigue is measured by the fatigue severity scale (FSS) scored 1 to 7 (1 signifies no fatigue and 7 signifies severe fatigue).[21] FSS for Lyme disease patients and all patient groups significantly greater than healthy controls, $p < 0.001$ and FSS in Lyme disease significantly lower than in CFS, $p < 0.0001$, but not significantly different than MS.

people continue to experience fatigue. Persistent fatigue may accompany a post-Lyme syndrome. Although the post-Lyme syndromes are covered more fully in Chapter 24, later in this chapter we review the relationship between prior antibiotic therapy and post-Lyme fatigue and the overlap between post-Lyme fatigue and chronic fatigue syndrome (CFS).

FATIGUE CHARACTERISTICS

To examine the nature of fatigue during active Lyme disease, we analyzed fatigue characteristics in 42 Lyme disease patients with late infection, who included fatigue among their symptoms. Their fatigue characteristics were compared to those reported by 40 healthy controls. A 29-item fatigue questionnaire and severity scale (in which each item is scored from 1 through 7) were administered to all subjects.

As expected, Lyme disease patients had much more severe and persistent fatigue. Lyme disease patients, compared to controls, indicated that their fatigue came on more easily ($p<.0001$); interfered with physical functioning ($p<.0001$), interfered with their family, work, and social activities ($p<.0001$), and prevented them from meeting certain responsibilities ($p<.0001$).[31] Half of the Lyme disease patients reported that fatigue was their most disabling symptom. As shown in Table 26–2, Lyme disease patients had significantly higher mean fatigue severity ratings than the control group (4.8 ± 1.4 versus 2.8 ± 1.2, $p<.0001$) as measured by a previously validated fatigue severity scale.[21]

Although these findings demonstrate that fatigue is distinct in Lyme disease patients compared to healthy controls, it is unclear whether fatigue in Lyme disease differs from fatigue in other diseases. To address this question, 42 Lyme disease patients with complaints of fatigue were compared to 57 patients with multiple sclerosis (MS), a CNS disorder frequently associated with profound fatigue, and 62 patients referred for CFS.[17,20] As shown in Table 26–2, Lyme disease patients and MS patients had nearly identical fatigue severity scores. However, fatigue in MS was made worse by stress and temperature to a significantly greater degree as compared to Lyme patients.[31] Despite these qualitative differences, the impact of fatigue on activities of daily living was similar in the two disease groups.[31]

In contrast to the findings with the MS group, when Lyme disease patients were compared to patients referred for CFS, dramatic differences emerged. Compared to the Lyme disease group, patients referred for CFS rated their fatigue as more severe on almost every self-report measure. CFS patients reported to a significantly greater degree that fatigue made other symptoms worse and that fatigue was their most disabling disease symptom. As shown in Table 26–2, Lyme disease patients had significantly lower fatigue severity ratings compared to the CFS group (4.8 ± 1.4 versus 6.1 ± 0.8, $p<.0001$). It is clear that, although fatigue in Lyme disease patients is a severe problem that does interfere with activities of daily living, it does not reach the level of fatigue seen in CFS. We have also observed that fatigue has a better prognosis among Lyme disease patients compared to those with CFS.

FATIGUE AND COGNITIVE DYSFUNCTION

The concurrence of Lyme encephalopathy and fatigue presents certain questions. For example, what is the relationship between cognitive function and fatigue? How do depressive symptoms in Lyme disease patients affect cognitive performance? These questions are important because a mild to moderate encephalopathy is particularly frequent during late stages of the disease in North America.[11–14,24,30] Such patients often perform poorly on

neuropsychological testing.[12,22,24] Cognitive abnormalities are more fully covered in Chapter 27, but we have recently looked at the relative role of fatigue and depressive symptoms on cognitive functioning in Lyme encephalopathy. We evaluated the cognitive ability of 25 Lyme disease patients compared to 17 healthy controls matched in aggregate for age and education. All Lyme disease patients had received treatment for Lyme disease but continued to complain of persistent intellectual difficulty and fatigue 3 to 18 months after antibiotic therapy. Many also had depressive symptoms.

As shown in Table 26–3, the neuropsychological testing revealed objective cognitive deficits among the Lyme disease patients. Compared to controls, Lyme disease patients had significantly lower scores on tests of memory, verbal learning, verbal fluency, and attention. However, other tests of cognitive function, which included measures of visual-spatial ability, general intelligence, and abstract reasoning were not impaired (data not shown in Table 26–3). Lyme disease patients also showed a significant elevation in depressive symptoms. However, even after the depressive symptoms were controlled for (by analysis of covariance [AN-COVA] for group differences), the Lyme disease patients had demonstrable cognitive impairment compared to healthy controls. These findings suggest that fatigue may be associated with objective deficits in cognitive functioning and that these abnormalities are not simply the result of depressive symptomatology.

In a prior study, we found that not all treated Lyme disease patients who complain of cognitive difficulty had abnormalities on neuropsychological testing.[22] In fact, despite their subjective com-

Table 26–3 Neuropsychological measures in treated Lyme disease patients with fatigue and healthy controls (mean ± standard error)*

Cognitive measure (neuropsychological test)	Lyme disease $n = 25$	Control $n = 17$	p
Attention and concentration (WAIS-R digit span[40])	9.5 ± 0.7	12.0 ± 0.7	<0.04
Verbal fluency (Controlled Oral Word Association Test[23])	39.4 ± 2.6	52.9 ± 2.6	<0.001
Verbal memory learning (Selective Reminding Test Consistent Retrieval[2])	27.5 ± 2.7	43.4 ± 3.6	<0.003
Verbal memory (Wechsler Memory Scale Paired Associate Learning[41])	18.7 ± 0.8	22.7 ± 1.0	<0.001

*Lyme disease refers to seropositive Lyme borreliosis patients with objective evidence of late Lyme disease who underwent neuropsychological evaluation a mean of 8 months after antibiotic therapy; healthy control subjects were drawn from the same geographic area as the patients and were matched in aggregate on age and education; all means are adjusted for group differences on CES-D depression scores[28] by analysis of covariance.

plaints of memory difficulty and poor concentration, 6 of 15 (40%) patients had entirely normal performance on their neuropsychological evaluation.[22] One possibility raised was that depressive symptoms were contributing to the patients' false perception of cognitive difficulty. To determine this, patients were divided into cognitively intact and impaired groups based solely on their neuropsychological profile. When the depression symptom scores between the two subgroups were compared, the cognitively normal group had significantly higher mean depression symptom scores than the cognitively impaired group.[22] This finding would suggest that fatigued patients who perceive difficulties in cognitive function that are *not* confirmed on neuropsychological testing may have elevated depressive symptoms. In contrast, if neuropsychological testing confirms objective cognitive loss, it is likely that a Lyme disease–associated encephalopathy accounts for their symptoms.

FATIGUE AND DEPRESSION

Any evaluation of fatigue in Lyme disease must consider the possible contribution of psychological factors, such as depression. However, in evaluating the possible role of depression, it is important to distinguish between depressive symptoms and a clinical diagnosis of major depression. Whereas depressive symptoms are common in Lyme disease and overlap with fatigue, clinical major depression is infrequent.

As shown in Table 26–2, Lyme disease patients do have significantly greater depressive symptoms (as measured by a standard assessment tool, the Center for Epidemiologic Studies Depression Scale [CES-D][28]) than healthy controls. However, Lyme disease patients do not have significantly elevated depression symptoms compared to patients with other chronic illnesses such as MS or patients with systemic lupus erythematosus.[21] Thus, although depressive symptoms are common in Lyme disease, their severity is similar to that of other chronic medical disorders. However, as shown in Table 26–2, Lyme disease patients have significantly lower levels of depressive symptomatology than patients evaluated for CFS.

Few Lyme disease patients meet diagnostic criteria for major depression. Of 42 Lyme disease patients evaluated for fatigue and depression symptoms, most were not considered by their primary physician to have clinical depression. Furthermore, when 12 Lyme disease patients with elevated depressive symptomatology underwent a structured psychiatric interview, only 2 (17%) met diagnostic criteria for current major depression or dysthymia. Thus, although depressive symptomatology is present in Lyme disease patients, it is usually not severe enough for psychiatric diagnosis.

PERSISTENT FATIGUE AFTER ANTIBIOTIC TREATMENT FOR LYME DISEASE

It is not uncommon for some patients to experience persistent fatigue for many months after adequate antibiotic treatment for Lyme disease. The reasons for this are not known. In initial studies involving tetracycline or penicillin treatment, persistent minor complications including fatigue were frequent.[37] Subsequently, newer antibiotic regimens were shown to be more efficacious in preventing long-term complications.[7,8,27] However, some patients treated with modern cephalosporins or newer penicillins continue to experience fatigue months after completing antibiotic therapy.[7,22,28]

Persistent fatigue is less prevalent in patients promptly treated for localized early infection than in those treated for late disease. Dattwyler et al[8] found that only 8% of patients treated with either amoxicillin and probenecid or doxycycline for early disease, as manifested by EM, experienced persistent severe fatigue. However, if the subset of their patients with complicated EM (single skin lesion associated with constitutional symptoms) or multiple EM are analyzed, persistent fatigue is noted in 16% of the patients.[8]

Patients treated for late Lyme disease experience persistent fatigue at even higher rates. In a study comparing penicillin to ceftriaxone treatment for late Lyme borreliosis, 21% of the ceftriaxone group and 62% of the penicillin group who experienced fatigue before antibiotics still had fatigue on follow-up 6 to 9 months after therapy.[7] Although newer cephalosporins may be more effective than penicillin for late Lyme disease and associated fatigue, additional research is required to determine why some patients, despite such treatment, continue to experience fatigue months to years later.

POST-LYME DISEASE CHRONIC FATIGUE SYNDROME

To evaluate whether post-Lyme disease patients with fatigue meet the Centers for Disease Control (CDC) case definition for CFS,[17] we identified 15 patients with clinical evidence (by history, physical examination, and serologic testing) of past Lyme disease who had received appropriate antibiotic therapy but were still experiencing severe fatigue at least 6 months after treatment. The mean age of these "post-Lyme" patients was 39 ± 11 years, and 73% were women. Patients were queried regarding the symptoms listed in the CDC case definition of CFS.[17]

To meet the CDC case definition for CFS, a

patient must satisfy 2 major criteria and 8 of 11 minor criteria. The two major criteria are that (1) they must have severe debilitating fatigue for at least 6 months and (2) there must be no other concurrent medical disorder that accounts for this symptom. Minor symptom criteria include headache, myalgia, arthralgia, sore throat, painful lymph nodes, muscle weakness, prolonged fatigue after exercise, neuropsychological symptoms, sleep disturbance, and an acute to subacute onset of the symptom complex.[17]

All 15 post–Lyme disease patients met both major criteria for CFS (i.e., they had severe fatigue that could not be explained by any other medical illness [with the exception of having had Lyme disease]) and 9 (67%) reported 8 or more of the 11 minor symptoms. All patients had at least five minor symptoms. Thus, these post-Lyme patients resemble CFS patients with respect to many of their symptoms. Despite their severe fatigue, the post-Lyme disease group had a mean depression symptom score below the cut-off suggestive of depression, a finding that implies that concurrent depressive symptoms were unlikely to explain fully their fatigue.

The pathogenesis for persistent fatigue and related symptoms in post-Lyme disease patients is unknown. However, some of these patients have *B. burgdorferi*–specific immune complexes and elevated levels of IgM and IgM immune complexes, implying a persistent state of immune activation.[5] Thus, a factor possibly contributing to persistent fatigue in post–Lyme disease patients is a state of ongoing immune stimulation. Further investigations, including prospective studies incorporating psychological and immunologic evaluations of Lyme disease patients, are needed to determine the basis for persistent fatigue and other post–Lyme disease syndromes.

Because of the high prevalence of fatigue in Lyme disease patients, the question has been raised whether *B. burgdorferi* may trigger CFS in the absence of other evidence of Lyme disease. Persistent fatigue without other associated symptoms of Lyme disease has been anecdotally described in patients seropositive for *B. burgdorferi*.[25] However, clinical details regarding such cases are limited.[25] Others have failed to show intrathecal antibody synthesis to *B. burgdorferi* in seropositive patients whose only symptom was persistent fatigue.[33]

Two studies examining *B. burgdorferi* exposure in association with CFS have revealed intriguing results. In a preliminary report, Coyle et al noted increased levels of circulating *B. burgdorferi*–specific immune complexes in CFS patients compared to other neurologic disease controls from the same endemic geographic area.[4] Wright and colleagues

screened 60 persistent fatigue patients for antibodies to *B. burgdorferi* and found that 10% had both antibodies to *B. burgdorferi* and unique antibodies not found in either Lyme disease or neurologic disease controls.[44] These findings need to be expanded before concluding an association other than coincidence between CFS and *B. burgdorferi* exposure. However, many CFS patients demonstrate elevated antibodies to a wide range of viruses, suggesting an activated immune response. Because pneumonia, influenza, other viral infections, and stress may in a susceptible person trigger CFS, it is conceivable that *B. burgdorferi* exposure might have a similar effect.

MANAGEMENT

Managing fatigue in Lyme disease depends on assessing the patient's stage of infection, the temporal relationship of fatigue to antibiotic therapy, the association of other related symptoms of Lyme disease, and the contribution of possible psychosocial factors. Several specific questions are relevant to treatment.

1. *Should a seropositive patient in whom fatigue is the only symptom of* B. burgdorferi *infection be considered to have Lyme disease and receive antibiotic therapy?*

Choosing the appropriate treatment for a seropositive patient with fatigue depends on accurate diagnosis and determining whether the symptom is due to *B. burgdorferi* infection or some other cause. In patients with other manifestations of Lyme disease (facial palsy, EM, or other neurologic, cardiac, or rheumatologic findings), the diagnosis of Lyme disease is straightforward and antibiotic therapy is appropriate. In most cases, fatigue eventually resolves after antibiotic therapy, although occasionally this may take many months.

The management of seropositive patients with fatigue is complicated by the fact that many Lyme disease patients lack classic manifestations of infection.[29] Approximately 20% to 40% of Lyme disease patients do not develop the pathognomonic rash.[36] In these patients, additional evaluation is necessary to determine if their fatigue is caused by *B. burgdorferi* infection. For example, if fatigue is associated with cognitive complaints, a neurologic work-up is appropriate. If a diagnosis of CNS neuroborreliosis is established, parenteral antibiotic treatment should be administered.[11,43]

If fatigue is of recent onset and if it occurred in association with a flulike illness with symptoms of fever, meningeal irritation, or arthralgia, it is appropriate to consider Lyme disease as a possible cause. This is particularly true if there is a history of probable exposure to *B. burgdorferi* (by tick bite or travel to a highly endemic area) or documented seroconversion. In such patients, a single course of antibiotic treatment is appropriate. However, there is no evidence that repeated courses of antibiotic therapy are of any value for patients whose only symptom is persistent fatigue.[25]

On the other hand, not all patients with documented seropositivity to *B. burgdorferi* have clinical evidence of Lyme disease. In two prospective studies involving people who seroconverted to *B. burgdorferi* antibody, there were as many asymptomatic subjects as there were patients with clinical manifestations of Lyme disease.[15,38] In a prospective European study, only 4% of army personnel who had documented seroconversion to *B. burgdorferi* 6 weeks after a tick bite developed EM. Furthermore, none developed additional manifestations.[32] Thus, documentation of seropositivity to *B. burgdorferi* is not sufficient for a diagnosis of Lyme disease. In seropositive patients with fatigue and no other clinical findings, the clinical history becomes extremely important. For example, patients who give a history of having had fatigue all their life, particularly if in association with other vague psychosomatic symptoms, are unlikely to have Lyme disease, even if they are seropositive. Other possible explanations for the fatigue should be sought including other medical disorders such as hypothyroidism, collagen vascular disease, endocrine disorders, and psychosocial factors such as family discord or mild depression. Additional psychological or psychiatric evaluation may be helpful.

2. What route and type of antibiotic therapy is appropriate for an untreated Lyme disease patient with clinical evidence of infection whose CNS symptoms include fatigue and cognitive loss?

The most direct way to determine the appropriate treatment in a seropositive Lyme disease patient with suspected cognitive dysfunction and fatigue is to assess CNS involvement with a careful neurologic examination including tests of higher cor-

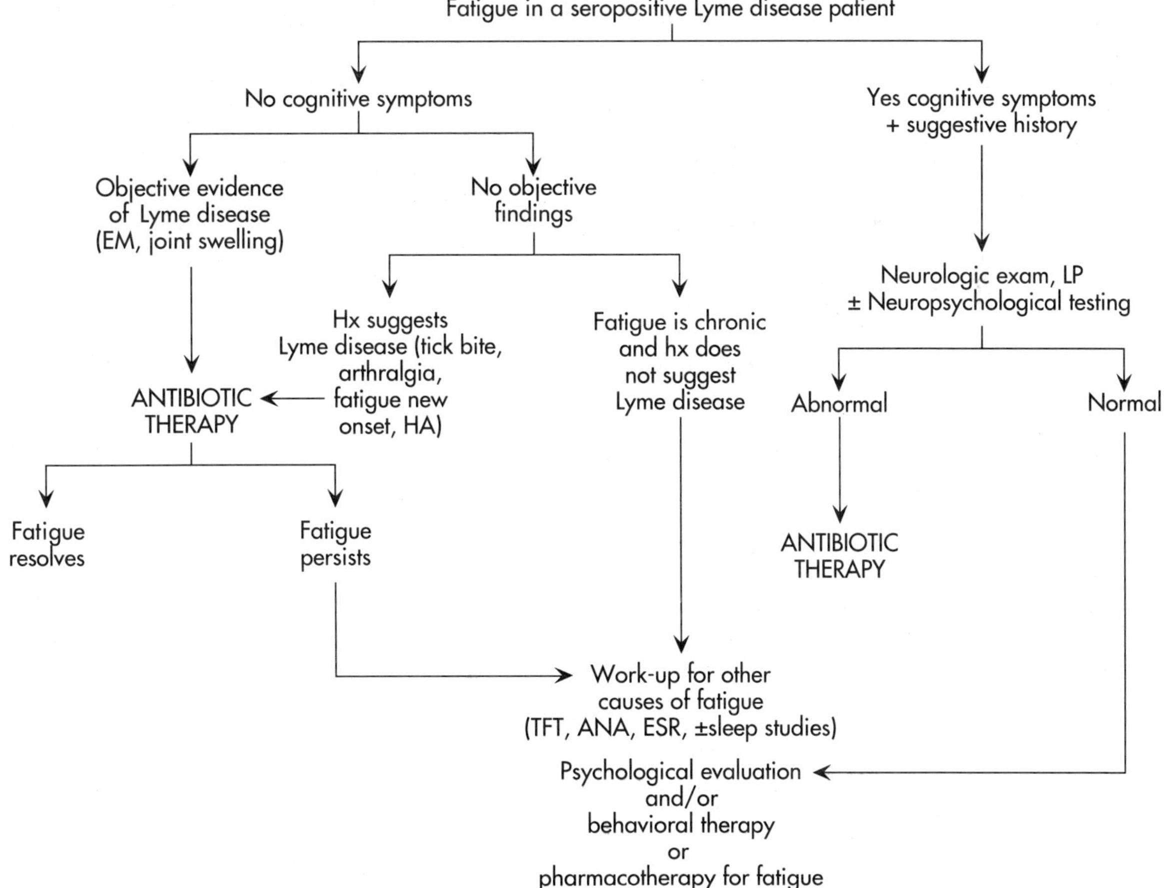

Figure 26–1 Management of fatigue in a seropositive Lyme disease patient. ANA, antinuclear antibodies; EM, erythema migrans; ESR, erythrocyte sedimentation rate; HA, headache; hx, history; LP, lumbar puncture; TFT, thyroid function tests.

tical function, lumbar puncture, and, in selected cases, neuropsychological evaluation. Neuropsychological testing provides an objective measure of cognitive functioning and establishes a basis for future comparisons.[22] Lumbar puncture is essential to determine whether there is direct CNS infection as evidenced by antibodies to *B. burgdorferi,* *B. burgdorferi*–specific immune complexes,[6] CSF pleocytosis, or intrathecal antibody synthesis.[13] If encephalopathy is demonstrated in association with CSF abnormalities, parenteral antibiotic therapy (usually a cephalosporin) is appropriate.

3. Does persistent fatigue after oral or intravenous antibiotic therapy imply continued infection? If not, are there more appropriate therapeutic options than repeated administration of antibiotic drugs?

Fatigue that persists despite antibiotic treatment for Lyme disease in the absence of any other clinical findings suggestive of continued infection should not be treated with multiple course antibiotics. There is no evidence that this treatment approach is effective.[25] More rewarding treatments are those directed toward ameliorating the fatigue and related symptoms. For example, if pain or mood disturbance accompany fatigue, antidepressant medications with mild energizing and analgesic properties may be helpful. Some post-Lyme disease patients with fatigue are plagued by sleep disturbance. Instruction regarding good sleep hygiene or, in some cases, medical treatment of insomnia may be beneficial. Occasionally, patients with fatigue associated with major disruption of sleep require evaluation with polysomnography.[20]

Another treatment approach to chronic fatigue after Lyme disease involves behavioral modification therapy. Such programs have been used extensively for chronic pain and have recently been successfully applied to patients with postviral CFS.[3] Select post–Lyme disease patients with severe fatigue, who are psychologically stable, may also respond well to a self-limited course of a mild CNS stimulant. An algorithm for the management of fatigue in the seropositive Lyme disease patient is presented in Fig. 26–1.

SUMMARY

Fatigue occurs during early and late disease and may cause disability. In some Lyme disease patients treated with antibiotic therapy, fatigue persists for many months. Fatigue appears to be more common in patients treated for late or disseminated disease than early localized infection. Although persistent fatigue after antibiotic treatment is unlikely to represent continued infection, it may result in part from an altered host immune response to the infection.

Treatment for persistent fatigue should involve a comprehensive evaluation with attention to possible associated neurologic and psychological symptoms. In patients who have received appropriate antibiotic therapy for Lyme disease, additional therapeutic modalities for fatigue include simple reassurance and support, behavioral therapy, and in some cases, antidepressant medication or mild CNS stimulants. Fortunately, in the majority of Lyme disease patients, fatigue eventually resolves.

REFERENCES

1. Broderick J, Sandok BA, Mertz LE: Focal encephalitis in a young woman 6 years after the onset of Lyme disease: tertiary Lyme disease? *Mayo Clin Pro* 62:313, 1978.
2. Buschke H, Fuld PA: Evaluating storage, retention, and retrieval in disordered memory and learning, *Neurology* 24:1019, 1974.
3. Butler S et al: Cognitive behavior therapy in chronic fatigue syndrome, *J Neurol Neurosurg Psychiatry* 54:153, 1991.
4. Coyle PK, Krupp LB: *Borrelia burgdorferi* infection in chronic fatigue syndrome, *Ann Neurol* 28:243, 1990.
5. Coyle PK, Krupp LB, Belman AL: Immune correlates of cognitive impairment in Lyme disease, *Neurology* 40 (suppl):333, 1990.
6. Coyle PK et al: CSF immune complexes in patients exposed to *Borrelia burgdorferi* detection of *Borrelia* specific and non specific complexes, *Ann Neurol* 28:739, 1990.
7. Dattwyler RJ et al: Treatment of late Lyme borreliosis—randomized comparison of ceftriaxone and penicillin, *Lancet* 1:1191, 1988.
8. Dattwyler RJ et al: Amoxicillin plus probenecid versus doxycycline for treatment of erythema migrans borreliosis, *Lancet* 336:1404, 1990.
9. Dekoenenko EP et al: Lyme borreliosis in the Soviet Union: a cooperative US-USSR report, *J Infect Dis* 158:748, 1988.
10. Diringer MN, Halperin JJ, Dattwyler RJ: Lyme meningoencephalitis: report of a severe penicillin-resistant case, *Arthritis Rheum* 30:705, 1987.
11. Halperin JJ: Nervous system manifestations of Lyme disease, *Rheum Dis Clin North Am* 15:635, 1989.
12. Halperin JJ et al: Nervous system abnormalities in Lyme disease, *Ann NY Acad Sci* 593:24, 1988.
13. Halperin JJ et al: Lyme neuroborreliosis—central nervous system manifestations, *Neurology* 39:753, 1989.
14. Halperin JJ et al: Lyme borreliosis-associated encephalopathy, *Neurology* 40:1340, 1990.
15. Hanrahan JP et al: Incidence and cumulative frequency of endemic Lyme disease in a community, *J Infect Dis* 150:489, 1984.
16. Hassler D et al: Cefotaxime versus penicillin in the late stage of Lyme disease—prospective, randomized therapeutic study, *Medizin Verlag GmbH Munchen* 18:16, 1990.
17. Holmes GP et al: Chronic fatigue syndromes: a working definition, *Ann Intern Med* 108:385, 1988.
18. Kohler J et al: Chronic central nervous system involvement in Lyme borreliosis, *Neurology* 38:863, 1988.
19. Kruger H et al: Meningoradiculitis and encephalomyelitis due to *Borrelia burgdorferi:* a follow-up study of 72 patients over 27 years, *J Neurol* 236:322, 1989.
20. Krupp LB, Mendelson WB, Friedman R: An overview of chronic fatigue syndrome, *J Clin Psychiatry* 52:403, 1991.

21. Krupp LB et al: The fatigue severity scale applied to patients with multiple sclerosis and systemic lupus erythematosus, *Arch Neurol* 46:1121, 1989.
22. Krupp LB et al: Cognitive functioning in Lyme borreliosis, *Arch Neurol* 48:1125, 1991.
23. Lezak MD: *Neuropsychological assessment,* New York, 1983, Oxford University Press.
24. Logigian EL, Kaplan RF, Steere AC: Chronic neurologic manifestations of Lyme disease, *N Engl J Med* 323:1438, 1990.
25. Pachner AR: Spirochetal diseases of the CNS, *Neurol Dis Clin North Am* 4:207, 1986.
26. Pachner AR, Steere AC: The triad of neurologic manifestations of Lyme disease, *Neurology* 35:47, 1985.
27. Pfister H-W et al: Cefotaxime vs. penicillin G for acute neurologic manifestations in Lyme borreliosis, *Arch Neurol* 46:1190, 1989.
28. Radloff LS: CES-D scale: a self-report depression scale for research in the general population, *Appl Psychol Meas* 1:385, 1977.
29. Reik L, Burgdorfer W, Donaldson JO: Neurologic abnormalities in Lyme disease without erythema chronicum migrans, *Am J Med* 81:73, 1986.
30. Reik L et al: Neurologic abnormalities of Lyme disease, *Medicine* 58:281, 1979.
31. Schwartz J, Krupp LB: Unpublished data, 1991.
32. Stanek G et al: European Lyme borreliosis, *Ann NY Acad Sci* 539:274, 1988.
33. Steere AC et al: Evaluation of the intrathecal antibody response to *Borrelia burgdorferi* as a diagnostic test for Lyme neuroborreliosis, *J Infect Dis* 161:1203, 1990.
34. Steere AC, Schoen R, Taylor E: The clinical evolution of Lyme arthritis, *Ann Intern Med* 107:725, 1987.
35. Steere AC et al: Erythema chronicum migrans and Lyme arthritis: the enlarging clinical spectrum, *Ann Intern Med* 86:685, 1977.
36. Steere AC et al: The early clinical manifestations of Lyme disease, *Ann Intern Med* 99:76, 1983.
37. Steere AC et al: Treatment of the early manifestations of Lyme disease, *Ann Intern Med* 99:22, 1983.
38. Steere AC et al: A longitudinal assessment of the clinical and epidemiological features of Lyme disease in a defined population, *J Infect Dis* 154:295, 1986.
39. Stiernstedt G et al: Clinical manifestations and diagnosis of neuroborreliosis, *Ann NY Acad Sci* 539:46, 1988.
40. Wechsler D: *WAIS-R Manual,* New York, 1981, Psychological Corporation.
41. Wechsler D: *Memory Scale-Revised,* San Antonio, 1987, Psychological Corporation.
42. Wokke JHJ et al: Chronic forms of *Borrelia burgdorferi* infection of the nervous system, *Neurology* 37:1031, 1987.
43. Wormser GP: Treatment of *Borrelia burgdorferi* infection, *Lab Med* 21:316, 1990.
44. Wright DJM et al: Postviral fatigue and borrelial antibodies, *Ann NY Acad Sci* 593:507, 1988.

27 Cognitive and Psychiatric Aspects

Harold L. Pass and Avraham Calev

Lyme disease, a tickborne disease caused by the spirochete *Borrelia burgdorferi*, was first recognized in the United States in 1975 as the result of an unusual clustering of children with arthritic symptoms in the vicinity of Lyme, Connecticut.[24] Initially, Lyme disease (Lyme arthritis) was thought to be a new disease entity. However, a very similar disease with many of the same clinical manifestations, including the large, round, expanding erythematous skin rash, was recognized in Europe as Bannwarth's disease in the early 1940s. Early research emphasized the arthritic and other physical symptoms.[24] However, as more clinical data became available, it became evident that Lyme disease affected multiple organic systems, including the central nervous system (CNS), resulting in both cognitive and neuropsychiatric manifestations[20] thought to be related to the presence of meningeal and encephalopathic involvement.

This chapter discusses these aspects of Lyme disease in both the early acute and late chronic stages of this illness.

COGNITIVE IMPAIRMENT IN LYME DISEASE

Few studies describe the cognitive manifestations of Lyme disease. We were able to locate 19 published reports that mentioned cognitive impairment associated with this disease (Table 27–1). Only five studies used formal psychometric testing[5,10-12,18] to document cognitive deficits and to assess the response to antibiotic treatment.

Early phase

During the initial period of infection with *B. burgdorferi*, when 50% to 75% of patients may develop the characteristic skin lesion, erythema migrans (EM), up to 80% of all patients have reported experiencing malaise, fatigue, and lethargy consistent with nervous system involvement early in the course of the infection.[22,25,26] Approximately 15% of patients in one sample developed the triad of acute neurologic symptoms including meningitis, cranial neuritis, and painful radiculitis.[22,25,26]

Acute phase

During the period of acute infection, which can last from several weeks to several months, patients have described various cognitive impairments, including decreased attention and concentration and impaired memory.* For the majority of patients, cognitive disturbance during the early acute stage of Lyme disease tends to be relatively mild. However, Diringer et al[4] reported a case study of a 33-year-old man who was infected for only a few months when he developed severe meningeal and encephalopathic symptoms, including slurred speech and a mild dementia, which ultimately resolved after antibiotic therapy. This study suggests that even in the early acute stage of Lyme disease, there may be considerable variability in the severity of cognitive disturbances observed.

Late chronic phase

During the later period of infection with Lyme disease, more severe cognitive disturbances have been reported. In addition to impaired recent and long-term memory, attention and concentration, other disturbances of cognitive functioning have been described.[16] These deficits include impaired conceptual ability,[5] language difficulties, including dysphasia and aphasia,[2] general cognitive impairment and confusional states,[7] memory loss,[11] and general intellectual deterioration.[9] A drop in school grades in children with Lyme disease was reported by Pachner and Steere.[16] Ackermann et al[1] reported that in a sample of patients who were ill for a mean of 2.8 years, two patients demonstrated disorientation and severe dementia. Only one of these patients improved with antibiotic treatment. Szer et al,[28] in a prospective study, followed 46 children who were diagnosed with Lyme disease and who received no antibiotic therapy for at least the first 4 years of their illness. Two children (4%) were found to have a subtle encephalopathy with memory impairment, headache, and fatigue. Serologic

---

*References 5, 18, 20, 22, 25, 26.

Table 27–1 Cognitive deficits in Lyme disease

Study year	Duration of illness	Cognitive symptoms
Ackermann et al 1988[1]	7 months-12 years, mean = 2.8 years	Poor memory and concentration
Broderick et al 1987[2]	6 years	Language difficulties, aphasia
Dattwyler et al 1988[3]	17-39 months	Subjective memory impairment
Halperin et al 1988	More than 4 weeks	Deficiencies in memory, attention, concentration, mental speed, conceptual ability
Halperin et al 1989[6] and Pass et al 1987[18]	At least 1 month, mean = 32.6 months	Deficits in remote and recent memory, orientation, fund of knowledge, calculations, construction, concentration, confusion
Halperin and Pass 1989[5]	At least 4 weeks	Deficits in memory, conceptual ability, attention, concentration, speed
Halperin et al 1990	Not specified	Deficits in concentration, orientation, language, remote and recent memory, fund of knowledge, calculation, construction; confusion also seen
Kollikowski et al 1988[9]	2½ years	Poor logical thinking, flight of ideas, impaired short- and long-term memory, impaired general mental functioning
Krupp et al 1989[10] and 1991[11]	3-12 months after treatment	Modest cognitive deficits with neuropsychological testing in memory, and verbal fluency
Logigian et al 1990[12]	3 months-14 years	Subacute encephalopathy, impaired memory, concentration, and language
Pachner and Steere 1984[15]	1 month after treatment for ECM began	Poor concentration and memory
Pachner and Steere 1985[16]	1-8 years	Poor concentration and memory
Pachner and Steere 1985[17]	Several months to years	Drop in school grades
Pachner et al 1989[14]	1 month-5 years	Confusion, disorientation, drop in school grades
Reik et al 1979[20]	1 week-7 months	Impaired memory and concentration
Reik et al 1985[21]	4 years	Memory deterioration, periods of poor insight and judgment
Reik et al 1986[19]	Several weeks to 2 years	Deficits in memory and concentration, disorientation, confusion, poor calculation and attention
Steere et al 1983[22]	Several weeks	Memory deficits
Szer et al 1991[28]	Greater than 4 years	Subtle encephalopathy, memory impairment, fatigue, headache

testing indicated evidence of intrathecal production of antibodies to the Lyme spirochete, consistent with previous findings.[7,12] However, a major methodologic omission in the study by Szer et al[28] is the absence of a comparable control group. It is not unusual to find cognitive impairment exceeding 5% in a sample of children randomly drawn from the general population. The presence of intrathecal antibody production in the affected children warrants further investigation to identify better the relationship between CNS involvement and the cognitive impairment in more chronic Lyme disease.

Another significant methodologic deficiency in most of these studies has been a lack of standardized measurement of cognitive and intellectual impairment. Most studies used a standard mental status examination to describe the presence of a cognitive deficit. We were able to find only five studies[5,10-12,18] reporting the use of neuropsycho-

logical psychometric assessment of their patients. The first of these studies[5,18] used a comprehensive battery of neuropsychological tests to examine 17 patients with Lyme disease before and after treatment with antibiotics. The mean duration of symptomatic Lyme disease was 32.6 months. Compared to a control group that was matched for age, education, and sex, the patients with Lyme disease clearly showed a generalized, mild deterioration in most aspects of cognitive and intellectual functioning, including attention, concentration, verbal learning, recent and long-term memory, motor speed, and conceptual ability. Each patient was interviewed and also completed a Beck Depression Inventory, which demonstrated that the deficits observed could not be explained by the presence of a depressive disorder (mean pretreatment score was 7.63; the usual cut-off indicating mild depression is greater than 10). After treatment with antibiotic therapy, this sample of patients demonstrated significant improvement in their cognitive functioning.

Absence of CNS involvement. Although measurable CNS involvement appears to explain the cognitive pathology for some of the patients with late chronic Lyme disease, this explanation fails to account for those patients who do not demonstrate direct evidence of CNS involvement, yet present with impaired cognitive functioning. An alternative explanation for the presence of decreased cognitive functioning may be inferred from the results obtained by Krupp et al[10,11] and Logigian et al.[12] Krupp et al[10] reported cognitive deficits similar to those reported by Pass et al[18] and Halperin and Pass.[5] However, Krupp et al,[10] in a small group of subjects, noted that the neuropsychological deficits in their Lyme disease patients were not significantly greater than in their control group of patients with chronic fatigue syndrome (CFS). They suggested that the subjective complaints as well as the psychometric deficits might be associated with depressed mood, fatigue, and the psychological distress related to Lyme disease and CFS. In a later study in which significant cognitive impairment was observed in late Lyme disease patients, they suggested that immune or metabolic factors might be responsible, because patients lacked evidence of intrathecal antibody synthesis. Logigian et al[12] replicated the neuropsychological findings of Pass et al[18] and Halperin et al[7] in a group of 27 patients with chronic neurologic symptoms associated with Lyme disease. Using standard neuropsychological tests, they found that 24 of 27 patients had cognitive deficits consistent with a subacute encephalopathy. The most significant impairments involved memory and language. However, their findings also lend some support to the presence of depressed mood contributing to the cognitive difficulties observed. Approximately one third of their patients with mild encephalopathy had elevated depression scores (scale 2) on the Minnesota Multiphasic Personality Inventory.

It is well established that depressed mood can produce cognitive impairment. However, it is not known whether the depression observed by Logigian et al[12] and Krupp et al[10] is a direct result of CNS involvement or a psychological reaction to the presence of a chronic debilitating illness in this sample. It should be noted that Pass et al[18] and Halperin and Pass[5] did not observe the presence of depression, as measured by a Beck Depression Scale, in their sample of patients with Lyme disease, despite the presence of cognitive impairment that improved after antibiotic therapy. Further research is necessary to determine how the psychological and organic factors interact in producing the cognitive disturbances observed in Lyme disease.

Other studies have suggested that possible direct CNS involvement may be the cause of observed cognitive deficits. It has been reported that the cognitive deficits observed in late Lyme disease may be related to the structural, multifocal white matter lesions in the brain observed on magnetic resonance imaging (MRI).[7,12] However, these lesions were present in only a small percentage of the patients in both studies. Halperin et al[7] concluded that chronic Lyme disease may be associated with a mild, low-grade inflammatory process in the CNS, which is reversible with antibiotic therapy. Antibiotic treatment resulted in improved cognitive functioning as well as resolution of the white matter lesions observed on MRI.

Presence of CNS involvement. Another finding that supports the relationship between CNS involvement and cognitive impairment is the relationship between deficits in memory and concentration as measured by mental status examination, and the presence of intrathecal antibody production to *B. burgdorferi*. However, it is clear that not all patients have such antibody production, despite objective deficits. It has been reported that the majority of patients with intrathecal antibody production to the spirochete seem to improve after antibiotic therapy.[5,7,12] These findings would suggest that the cognitive impairments reported in Lyme disease patients may be directly related to CNS pathology. However, others[10,11] have suggested that other factors, such as immune or metabolic abnormalities, or depression, may be responsible for these deficits. Further research in this area needs to be conducted to explain the underlying factors involved in the sometimes profound cognitive impairment that can be present in Lyme disease patients. The precise role of spirochetal brain infection, versus spirochete-triggered immune and inflammatory processes, needs to be examined. It is conceivable that related cytokine production, immune complex deposition, autoantibody production, or other indirect mechanisms could be playing a role in cognitive disturbance. Such mechanisms might ideally require treatment modalities other than, or in addition to, antibiotics to produce optimal recovery.

NEUROPSYCHIATRIC ASPECTS OF LYME DISEASE

Early studies of patients with Lyme disease observed, in addition to the arthritic, cardiac, and neurologic-neuropsychological findings, that patients also presented with psychiatric symptoms (Table 27–2). During the acute-early phase of their

Table 27–2 Psychiatric aspects of Lyme disease

Study year	Duration of illness	Behavioral psychiatric symptoms
Ackermann et al 1988[1]	7 months-12 years, mean = 2.8 years	Slight alteration in affect, dementia, altered consciousness, loss of orientation
Broderick et al 1987[2]	6 years	Apraxia, restlessness, agitation, personality change
Dattwyler et al 1988[3]	17-39 months	Headache, fatigue
Diringer et al 1987[4]	1-4 months	Fatigue, increased thirst, agitation, paranoia, seizures, lethargy
Halperin et al 1988	More than 4 weeks	Fatigue, psychomotor and perceptual-motor impairment
Halperin et al 1989[7]	At least 1 month	Recurrent depression, schizoaffective symptoms
Halperin and Pass 1989[5] and Pass et al 1987[18]	Mean = 32.6 months	No evidence of depressed mood
Kahan et al 1985[8]	~1 month	Emotional lability
Kollikowski et al 1988[9]	2½ years	Incoherent speech, euphoria, emotional lability, vertigo, nocturnal seizures
Krupp et al 1989[10] and 1991[11]	3-12 months after treatment	Mild depression, fatigue
Logigian et al 1990[12]	3 months-14 years	Elevated depression scale on Minnesota Multiphasic Personality Inventory
Meissner et al 1982[13]	2 weeks	Headaches, dizziness, loss of consciousness
Pachner and Steere 1984[15]	1 month after treatment for ECM began	Fatigue, irritability, emotional lability, transient bladder and bowel dysfunction
Pachner and Steere 1985[17]	1-8 years	Emotional lability, sleep disturbance, irritability
Pachner and Steere 1985[16]	Several months to years	Irritability, mood swings, seizures, auditory hallucinations, sleep disturbance, anorexia, fatigue, loss of friends
Pachner et al 1989[14]	1 month-5 years	Agitation, inappropriate laughter, violent outbursts, fatigue, withdrawal, depression, anorexia, compulsive exercising
Reik et al 1979[20]	1 week-7 months	Headache, somnolence, lethargy, emotional lability, irritability, depression, dizziness
Reik et al 1985[21]	4 years	Olfactory hallucinations, seizures, dirty/disheveled, apathy, incontinence

illness, the following signs and symptoms have been reported: headaches, fatigue, lethargy, emotional lability, irritability, and depressed mood.* Diringer et al,[4] in a case study, reported that, in addition to significant cognitive changes, a 33-year-old male patient also developed paranoid thinking, agitation, lethargy, and confusion approximately 4 months after being infected with Lyme disease.

Early acute phase

Based on these studies, it appears that the early acute phase of Lyme disease is typically characterized by relatively mild neuropsychiatric symptoms including headaches, fatigue, and slight alterations of mood. Only in rare cases do more severe symptoms, which are more frequently seen in psychosis, manifest themselves. In fact, we were able to find only one case report of psychotic-like

---

*References 1, 4, 6-8, 13-17, 20, 22, 25-27.

symptoms.[4] Interestingly, this patient's condition worsened after treatment with two separate courses of high-dose intravenous penicillin. The patient's condition improved after the administration of chloramphenicol, suggesting the usefulness of this drug in treating the more severe CNS manifestations that might not respond to penicillin. It is still unclear what the optimal treatment regimen should be during the acute stage of Lyme disease, because a small percentage of patients go on to develop a more resistant chronic disorder.

Late chronic phase

During the late chronic phase of Lyme disease, more severe neuropsychiatric symptoms have been observed. Reik et al,[21] in a single case report, described olfactory hallucinations and personal neglect of appearance and hygiene as well as the development of seizures. Pachner and Steere[16,17] found that, in 5 of 15 patients with late infection, psychiatric symptoms were observed 1 to 5 years after the diagnosis of Lyme disease was established. Two of the patients in the sample developed irritability, mood swings, social withdrawal, and a deterioration in school performance. Another patient developed auditory hallucinations, and yet another patient developed personality changes and a sleep disturbance. Additionally, one patient developed an anorexia-like syndrome. This patient recovered completely after 2 weeks of high-dose intravenous penicillin. Broderick et al[2] described a single case report of a 19-year-old woman who developed a personality change accompanied by agitation and restlessness. A computed tomography (CT) scan of her brain did not reveal any lesions. After 2 weeks of treatment with high-dose intravenous penicillin-G, the patient fully recovered. Kollikowski et al[9] also reported a single case report of a 57-year-old man with late chronic Lyme disease who developed incoherent speech in the presence of euphoric mood and emotional lability. High-dose intravenous penicillin therapy improved his symptoms. Ackermann et al[1] reported observing slight affective instability, loss of orientation, and alterations of consciousness in 12 of 18 patients. Pachner et al[14] reported that two of six patients with late-chronic Lyme disease developed significant behavioral and emotional changes, including inappropriate laughter, emotional lability, violent outbursts, agitation, compulsive exercising, and anorexic behavior. Others[3] have reported that, during the late chronic stage, some patients may only manifest mild neuropsychiatric symptoms, including fatigue, irritability, and headaches.

The above studies suggest that the late chronic phase of Lyme disease seems to be characterized by more severe neuropsychiatric symptoms as compared to the early acute stage. However, this conclusion is confounded by several methodologic problems. Histories provided by patients are often vague and unreliable, especially in the absence of EM, in determining when the patient was first exposed to the spirochete. Therefore, the distinction between early and late Lyme disease is often arbitrarily established so that there may be considerable variability in establishing the time course when neuropsychiatric symptoms appear in patients. Additionally, unless a careful psychiatric history is obtained, patients with previous histories of psychiatric problems may be erroneously diagnosed as having psychiatric manifestations of Lyme disease, when, in fact, they may be displaying a primary psychiatric disorder, an exacerbation of a previously existing psychiatric disorder, or another unrelated disorder. For example, in a sample of 72 schizophreniform patients experiencing their first psychotic episode, 2 patients were identified as

having definite Lyme disease. However, a detailed history revealed an extensive psychiatric illness before infection with *B. burgdorferi* (DeLisi and Calev, personal communication). Krupp et al[10] suggest that CFS may share certain features with Lyme disease and, therefore, this disease entity also needs to be considered among the list of differential diagnoses.

CONCLUSIONS

In our review of the available literature presented in this chapter, it seems clear that the cognitive and neuropsychiatric manifestations of Lyme disease vary greatly. The majority of patients who receive early treatment with antibiotics do not appear to develop any significant cognitive impairment or psychiatric symptoms. However, there does appear to be a small number of patients who go on to develop cognitive deficits and behavioral-emotional changes that can range from minimal impairment to very profound encephalopathy-like syndromes. These more disturbing aspects of Lyme disease typically occur in the late-chronic stage of patients who were not treated or who received inadequate early treatment. In very rare cases, more severe cognitive and psychiatric symptoms can appear in the early acute stages of Lyme disease, even when patients receive high-dose antibiotic therapy.[4]

More prospective longitudinal research needs to be conducted to understand the course of both untreated and treated Lyme disease.[28] To define and understand the cognitive pathology of this disease, well-designed, prospective studies, using objective neuropsychological tests before and after treatment, are needed to quantify changes in mental status as a function of treatment. Such studies also need to assess which treatment regimens produce the most favorable outcomes. For those patients who relapse and go on to develop late chronic Lyme disease, serial testing would enable the physician to monitor carefully either deterioration or improvement over the course of the illness. MRI results and intrathecal antibody production have been shown to perhaps correlate with cognitive impairment, at least in some cases, and therefore further studies of this kind might help to understand the relationship between focal CNS pathology and specific cognitive deficits. More intensive immunologic assessments of the spirochete-related host immune responses would also be of interest in these patients.

The above statements also apply to the neuropsychiatric manifestations of this disease. The physician should obtain a careful history of previous psychiatric illness from patients who describe mental status abnormalities such as fatigue and depression. It is important to try to determine whether preexisting psychiatric disorders are being exacerbated by Lyme disease, or whether the patient's symptoms might be directly attributable to putative CNS involvement. For some patients, a psychiatric referral may be indicated to treat specific disabling changes in mood, thought, and behavior. For those patients who develop more persistent and disabling symptoms associated with chronic Lyme disease, treatment with individual psychotherapy or participation in a support group may be helpful to assist them to better cope with having a chronic illness. We hope that future research will help to define these often profoundly disturbing manifestations of Lyme disease, as well as identify more specific and efficacious treatments.

REFERENCES

1. Ackermann R et al: Chronic neurologic manifestations of erythema migrans borreliosis, *Ann NY Acad Sci* 539:16, 1988.
2. Broderick JP, Sandok BA, Mertz LB: Focal encephalitis in a young woman 6 years after the onset of Lyme disease: tertiary Lyme disease, *Mayo Clin Proc* 62:313, 1987.
3. Dattwyler RJ et al: Treatment of late Lyme borreliosis— randomized comparison of ceftriaxon and penicillin, *Lancet* 1191, 1988.
4. Diringer MN, Halperin JJ, Dattwyler RJ: Lyme-meningoencephalitis: report of a severe penicillin resistant case, *Arthritis Rheum* 30:705, 1987.
5. Halperin JJ, Pass HL: Abnormalities of the nervous system in Lyme disease: response to antimicrobial therapy, *Rev Infect Dis* II (Suppl 6):S1499, 1989.
6. Halperin JJ, Pass HL et al: Nervous system abnormalities in Lyme disease, *Ann NY Acad Sci* 539:24, 1987.
7. Halperin JJ et al: Lyme neuroborreliosis: central nervous system manifestations, *Neurology* 39:753, 1989.
8. Kahan A et al: Meningoradiculitis associated with infections by *Borrelia burgdorferi*, *Lancet* p 148, July 20, 1985.
9. Kollikowski HH et al: Chronic *Borrelia* encephalomyeloradiculitis with severe mental disturbance: immunosuppressive vs. antibiotic therapy, *J Neurol* 235(3):140, 1988.
10. Krupp LB et al: Comparison of neurologic and psychologic findings in patients with Lyme disease and chronic fatigue syndrome, *Neurology* 39(3, Suppl 1): 44, March 1989.
11. Krupp LB et al: Cognitive functioning in late Lyme borreliosis, *Arch Neurol* 84:1125, 1991.
12. Logigian EL, Kaplan RF, Steere AC: Chronic neurologic manifestations of Lyme disease, *N Engl J Med* 323:1438, 1990.
13. Meissner HC, Gelliss E, Milliken JF: Lyme disease first observed to be aseptic meningitis, *Am J Dis Child* 136:465, 1982.
14. Pachner AR, Duray P, Steere AC: Central nervous system manifestations of Lyme disease, *Arch Neurol* 46(7):790, 1989.
15. Pachner AR, Steere AC: Neurological findings of Lyme disease, *Yale J Bio Med* 57:481, 1984.
16. Pachner AR, Steere AC: Tertiary Lyme disease—central nervous system manifestations of long-standing infection with *B. burgdorferi*. Second International Symposium on Lyme Disease and Related Disorders, Vienna, Austria, September 1985, p 38.
17. Pachner AR, Steere AC: The triad of neurologic manifestations of Lyme disease: meningitis, cranial neuritis and radiculoneuritis, *Neurology* 35:47, 1985.
18. Pass HL et al: Neuropsychological measures of a reversible dementia in Lyme disease, *J Clin Exper Neuropsychol* 9:75, 1987 (abstract).
19. Reik L, Burgdorfer W, Donaldson JO: Neurologic abnormalities in Lyme disease without erythema chronicum migrans, *Am J Med* 81:73, 1986.
20. Reik L et al: Neurologic abnormalities of Lyme disease, *Medicine* 58(4):281, 1979.
21. Reik L et al: Demyelinating encephalopathy in Lyme disease, *Neurology* 35:267, 1985.
22. Steere AC, Pachner AR, Malawista SE: Neurological abnormalities of Lyme disease: successful treatment with high dose IV penicillin, *Ann Intern Med* 99:767, 1983.
23. Steere AC et al: Erythema chronicum migrans and Lyme arthritis: the enlarging clinical spectrum, *Ann Intern Med* 86:685, 1977.
24. Steere AC et al: Lyme arthritis: an epidemic of oligoarticular arthritis in children and adults in three Connecticut communities, *Arthritis Rheum* 20:7, 1977.
25. Steere AC et al: The early clinical manifestations of Lyme disease, *Ann Intern Med* 99:76, 1983.
26. Steere AC et al: Treatment of the early manifestations of Lyme disease, *Ann Intern Med* 99:22, 1983.
27. Sterman AB, Nelson S, Barclay P: Demyelinating neuropathy accompanying Lyme disease, *Neurology* 32:1302, 1982.
28. Szer IS, Taylor E, Steere DC: The long-term course of Lyme arthritis in children, *N Engl J Med* 325:3:159, 1991.

Anita L. Belman

Lyme disease was recognized as a separate entity in the United States in 1975 because of an unusual geographic clustering of children with inflammatory arthropathy in eastern Connecticut.[67] In fact, it was two mothers from Old Lyme, Connecticut, who alerted the epidemiologists of the Connecticut State Health Department and the rheumatologists at Yale University School of Medicine to an inordinate number of children in their community who had what was then thought to be newly diagnosed juvenile rheumatoid arthritis. Of the 51 patients subsequently identified with this condition, 39 were children. All lived in three contiguous towns on the Connecticut River—Old Lyme, Lyme, and East Hadden.

This new illness, initially called Lyme arthritis, was characterized by the acute onset of pain and swelling in a few large joints. Remissions and recurrences were common. Approximately 25% of the patients recalled a skin rash that was often accompanied by systemic symptoms of fever, headache, malaise, and myalgias.[66,67] It soon became apparent that multisystem involvement was common; the name Lyme disease was adopted.[62,66,68,69] Evidence accumulated over the next several years that Lyme disease was similar to a well-described tickborne illness in Europe, Garin-Bujadoux Bannworth's syndrome.[6,16,33,38] Shortly thereafter, *Borrelia burgdorferi*, an arthropodborne spirochete, was identified as the etiologic agent of the North American disease, and a closely related *Borrelia* species was identified as the cause of the European illness.[17] The term *borreliosis* was adopted.

It is now well-recognized that Lyme borreliosis is a complex multisystem illness. The disease has emerged from a local concern to become the leading arthropod-transmitted disease in the United States.[19,48] As such, it represents an increasing health risk for children, especially those living in endemic areas. This chapter focuses on the spectrum of manifestations associated with pediatric Lyme disease.

EPIDEMIOLOGY

Lyme borreliosis has become the leading reported tickborne disease in the United States and Europe.[19,48] In 1982, the Centers for Disease Control (CDC) established a national surveillance for Lyme borreliosis. Approximately 13,700 cases were reported in the next 7 years (1982 to 1988) documenting a progressive increase in reported cases. In 1988, there were 4572 cases, representing a ninefold increase since 1982, and a doubling of cases from 1987.[23,24,48] Preliminary data from 1989 show a further increase with 8516 cases reported. Of these cases, 23% were in children and adolescents. There were 444 children between the ages of 0 and 4 years; 674 children between the ages of 5 and 9 years of age; 474 children between the ages of 10 and 14 years; and 380 adolescents between the ages of 15 and 19 years. The overall incidence in children and adolescents is 2.2/100,000, with an incidence by age group of 1.6/100,000 (0 to 4 years); 2.5/100,000 (5 to 9 years); 1.7/100,000 (10 to 14 years); and 1.4/100,000 (15 to 19 years; personal communication, Roy Campbell, M.D., Ph.D., Division of Vector-Borne Infectious Diseases, CDC, Atlanta).

The rising incidence of Lyme disease is undoubtedly due in part to increased recognition and better reporting. However, entomologic surveys are consistent with epidemiologic observations. The increased populations and spread of *Ixodes dammini* have been documented in national field studies and parallel regional infection rates in *Ixodes* ticks.[48]

Transmission of Lyme disease has been reported in 43 states, with an average annual incidence for 1987/1988 of 1.4/100,000.[48] As would be expected, rates vary according to geographic location, and focal areas of endemic transmission account for the majority of cases. Approximately 80% of cases reported nationally occurred in the mid-Atlantic and northeastern states. The second focus of hyperendemic transmission is in the upper midwest, notably Minnesota and Wisconsin, and the third principal area includes California, coastal Oregon, and Washington. Not unexpectedly, the incidence in children in some endemic areas is quite high. Forty percent of cases reported in Westchester County, New York, were children. In Connecticut, another endemic region, the incidence of Lyme disease in children aged 5 to 9 years was greater than in adults ages 20 to 24 years.[18,19]

CLASSIFICATION AND DISEASE STAGING

As in other spirochetal infections, Lyme disease may manifest in distinct stages. However, clinical experience in Europe and the United States has shown that stages may overlap or even be skipped, and manifestations may undergo remissions and exacerbations. For these reasons the terms *early* and *late* infection have been adopted.[26,64] For surveillance purposes, the CDC in Atlanta has recently revised the case definition for Lyme disease. "A case of Lyme disease is defined as (1) a person with erythema migrans; or (2) a person with at least one late manifestation and laboratory confirmation of infection."

As further information is gained and more precise diagnostic tests become available, it can be expected that classification and disease staging will be further defined.

CLINICAL CHARACTERISTICS

Lyme disease is a multisystem disease of varying severity. The skin, joints, heart, eye, and nervous system may be affected. Manifestations may be protean, and the clinical spectrum may be wide. The illness may range in severity from a mild "flu-like illness" to a more severe and chronic condition with rheumatologic, cardiac, ocular, and neurologic complications.

Dermatologic

Erythema migrans. Erythema migrans (EM), the pathognomic skin lesion of Lyme disease, was first described in Europe by Afzelius in 1909.[3] Classically, EM begins as a red macule or papule at the site of the tick bite, then expands to form an erythematous, annular lesion with partial clearing. The lesion is usually flat; however, the centrifugally migrating edges may be indurated or elevated.[4,14,46] EM is found most commonly on body areas where ticks feed. Children have EM on the face and neck more frequently than adults.[4,5,41,46] Other sites include the ankles, the intertriginous areas (axilla, groin, thigh, and buttocks), and the thorax. Size is variable. Because of the circular appearance of the lesion, many parents have mistaken EM for ringworm.

Less classical EM lesions described include homogeneous erythematous lesions; lesions with alternating rings of clearing and erythema (large target lesions); lesions with central areas of induration, vesiculation, discoloration, necrosis, or ulceration; and lesions with oval, triangular, or linear configurations.[14,46]

EM generally occurs 3 to 30 days after a tick bite and is usually nonpruritic and asymptomatic. However, dysesthesia, burning, and pruritus have been reported. The lesion may be warm to touch and may appear more erythematous after a warm bath. Fever (which may be high in children), malaise, headache, neck pain, and lymphadenopathy may be associated with the cutaneous lesion. If untreated, EM fades over a period of days to months, with an average duration of 1 month.

EM may be less frequent in children with North American Lyme disease than in adults, occurring in only approximately one third of patients.[76]

Secondary erythema migrans. Secondary or multiple EM lesions may appear several days to weeks after the initial EM lesion, during dissemination of disease, resulting from spirochetemia or lymphatic spread.[45,46] These lesions may appear at the original (primary) site or in areas distinct from the original EM lesion. The appearance may be similar to the primary EM or may be smaller, may lack indurated centers, or may become confluent. In general, they are asymptomatic. In untreated patients, the lesions usually resolve within 1 month, but relapses with recurrent EM have been described, as have persistent lesions. When treated, secondary lesions are reported to resolve within days.[46]

Acrodermatitis chronica atrophicans. Acrodermatitis chronica atrophicans (ACA), a chronic cutaneous lesion leading to sclerosis and atrophy of the skin (see Chapter 9), has not as yet been reported in children in the United States or Europe.[5,41]

Borrelia *lymphocytoma.* *Borrelia* lymphocytoma, a form of B-cell pseudolymphoma, is characterized histopathologically as a dense dermal nodular lymphocytic infiltrate with well-delineated lymphoid follicles or pseudogerminal centers. The infiltrate is composed of an admixture of B and T lymphocytes, plasma cells, and occasional eosinophils and macrophages. Using silver stain, spirochetes have been identified in the lesion, and *B. burgdorferi* has been cultured from biopsy specimens. The term *Borrelia* lymphocytoma is reserved for lesions in which *B. burgdorferi* is identified by culture or staining.

In children, there is a predilection for the lesion to develop on the pinna of the ear, or ear lobe, and less frequently, on mamilla or scrotum. Although *Borrelia* lymphocytoma has been well-described in European children with borreliosis, it seems to be a rare complication in children in the United States.[41]

Musculoskeletal

Arthralgias and myalgias. The musculoskeletal system may be involved early in the illness.

Myalgias and arthralgias often accompany nonspecific systemic symptoms of fever, malaise, lymphadenopathy, headache, neck stiffness, and pharyngitis.[67] Symptoms of musculoskeletal involvement may also develop in some patients during or after this first stage. Typically, there is a pattern of migratory musculoskeletal pain that can involve joints, tendons, muscles, bursa, or bone, without objective signs of swelling, tenderness, or erythema.[27,66,67] Pain and discomfort tend to affect one or two sites at a time, may last for a few hours to several days, resolve at a given site, and recur in another site.[57]

Arthritis. Arthritis may begin within months (median of 3.4 months, range 2 weeks to 2 years)[73] after the onset of Lyme disease or may be the presenting symptom. Of 46 children with Lyme arthritis followed by Szer and colleagues, 72% had EM at the beginning of the illness.[73] However, other investigators have reported EM in fewer than 50% of children with North American Lyme disease and arthritis.[27,28,31,63]

Typically, Lyme arthritis involves the large joints, with oligoarticular or pauciarticular involvement.[31,57,66,67,70] The knee is the most common joint affected in children, followed by the elbow, ankle, wrist, shoulder, and hip. The temporomandibular joint, sternoclavicular joint, and small joints of the hands and feet may also be involved, but less frequently, and symmetric and migratory patterns may occur, but in a minority of patients, and usually adults.[57,67] Fever associated with acute arthritis is common in children.

In general, arthritic attacks last for a few weeks to a few months but may be as short as 3 days or as long as 2 years.[28,73] Untreated patients may have recurrences, and, when they do, attacks occur at longer and longer intervals (i.e., frequency of attacks diminishes after the first year of illness). However, the duration of each flare-up of arthritis may increase.[73] Duration of arthritic attacks in younger children appears to be shorter than in adolescents and adults. Unlike adults, most children are asymptomatic and well during the intervals between attacks. In contrast to children with pyogenic arthritis, children with Lyme arthritis involving the hip or knee were able to walk on the affected extremity without excessive pain.[28]

The most common sign is articular swelling. Other signs include articular tenderness, usually at the extremes of motion; decreased range of motion, often proportional to the extent of effusion; and local elevation of the temperature of the skin. Erythema is uncommon.

Szer et al reported that the course of Lyme disease in children initially untreated may include acute infection followed by attacks of arthritis.[73] However, a low rate of relapse after antibiotic therapy was noted. Of 39 patients followed longitudinally, 12 (31%) had occasional brief episodes of joint pain. By the fourth year of follow-up, 10 children had a mean of two episodes of arthritis per year. By year six, five children had recurrent arthritis, but only one of these children continued to have brief attacks (lasting several days) during the seventh and eighth years of follow-up. Chronic arthritis seems a more common problem in adults than in children. However, children with more severe arthritis, as adults with Lyme arthritis, are also more likely to have the DR4 allele.[65]

Analysis of synovial fluid reveals a polymorphonuclear leukocytosis with a protein content ranging from 3 to 8 g/dl. Cryoglobulins may be present.[57]

Synovitis and popliteal cysts. In addition to frank arthritis, children may also have recurrent attacks of synovitis.[29] Popliteal cysts have also been described.

Cardiac

Cardiac abnormalities associated with borreliosis are estimated to occur in 8% to 10% of patients,[44,68,73] manifesting within several weeks to few months after the onset of illness. The most common cardiac complication reported is atrioventricular block, which may fluctuate in degree and may be transient. Complete heart block has been reported in children as well as adults, although less frequently. Presenting symptoms included syncope, dizziness, chest pain, and fatigue.[44] In a series of 20 (young adult) patients, more than half also had evidence of more diffuse cardiac abnormalities including myopericarditis, left ventricular dysfunction, and cardiomegaly. In a recent literature review of 105 cases of Lyme carditis, the overall prognosis was found to be favorable.[74]

Ophthalmologic

Ophthalmologic complications of Lyme disease are increasingly being recognized. Reported associations in children include conjunctivitis, uveitis, choreoretinitis, interstitial keratitis, optic neuritis, and papilledema.[1,42,77] Ophthalmologic complications of Lyme disease are discussed in detail in Chapter 12.

Conjunctivitis, the most common ocular complication in children, usually occurs during the early phase of the disease. Keratitis is a late complication. In one series, keratitis, characterized by multiple focal opacities of the corneal stroma, complicated the course of the illness in 2 of 46 (4%) children.[73]

Neurologic

Neurologic involvement may complicate the course of Lyme disease in children as well as in adults. In adult patients with North American Lyme neuroborreliosis, lymphocytic meningitis, cranial neuritis, radiculoneuritis, and peripheral neuropathy are the most frequent complications (see Chapter 13).* Review of the American and European literature, as well as our own experience at University Hospital Stony Brook, suggests that the most frequent complications in children include lymphocytic meningitis, meningoencephalitis, cranial neuropathy, and a "pseudotumor cerebri-like" syndrome.† In contrast to adult patients, Bannwarth's syndrome and syndromes of radiculoneuropathy and peripheral neuropathy are rare in pediatric patients.

Incidence. The true incidence of neurologic involvement in pediatric Lyme disease is not known. Reik estimates that approximately 15% of patients have early ("stage 2") neurologic involvement (i.e., lymphocytic meningitis, facial palsy, or facial palsy with lymphocytic meningitis).[60] The incidence of neurologic complications may be higher in children with more severe Lyme disease (e.g., those that go on to develop disseminated disease and Lyme arthritis). In one longitudinal series of 46 children with Lyme arthritis, 10 children (22%) also had aseptic meningitis or facial palsy.[73]

Manifestations. In our series of 71 children with neurologic problems and Lyme disease who were referred for evaluation to our center, the most frequent manifestations of neurologic involvement included headache (67%), behavioral changes (54%), facial palsy (11%), disturbance in sleep patterns (7%), and papilledema (6%). Paresthesias (3%), focal motor deficits (1%), and peripheral neuropathy (1%) occurred, but less frequently.[11,12] Ataxia, chorea, transverse myelitis, vertigo, seizures, and a Guillian-Barré-like syndrome have also been reported in case reports and in small series.[13,20,32,40]

Symptoms and signs

Headaches. Headaches are most often frontal or occipital in location, intermittent, and not associated with nausea or vomiting. Throbbing, bitemporal, and vertex headaches occur, but less frequently. Headaches may occur early in the illness associated with fever, malaise, myalgias, and neck pain. Headaches may resolve only to recur weeks to months later.[10,11,15,60,62]

Behavioral changes. Behavioral changes including irritability, emotional lability, worsening of attention deficit disorders (in children with pre-existing, previously diagnosed attention deficit hyperactivity disorders), or decline in school performance were the next most common signs in our patients.[10,11]

Disturbance of sleep patterns. Disturbance in sleep patterns, especially excessive daytime sleepiness, was another fairly frequent complaint.[10] Parents of the younger children reported a resumption of daytime naps or an increase in the number of daytime naps required. School-age children and teenagers related coming home from school, taking a nap before dinner, and then retiring for the night at an hour earlier than usual. (It is possible that these signs and symptoms described by the children and their parents are the same as the "fatigue" described by adults.) The new onset of nightmares or night terrors, or frequent nighttime awakenings, were reported for some children. In general, these disturbances in sleep patterns resolved spontaneously or after parenteral antibiotic treatment. Excessive daytime sleepiness was the reason for neurologic referral in one preadolescent girl, who was subsequently found to have narcolepsy in addition to Lyme disease.

Cranial nerve involvement. Facial nerve palsy (cranial nerve VII) followed by involvement of the optic nerve and the nerves that innervate the extraocular eye muscles, especially the abducens (cranial nerve VI), are the most common cranial nerve abnormalities in children.*

CRANIAL NERVE II—OPTIC NERVE. Papilledema (optic disc edema), associated with increased intracranial pressure, has been well-described in children with Lyme disease and is the most common optic nerve abnormality reported.[15,42,58,77] In some cases, cerebrospinal fluid (CSF) analysis has revealed a pleocytosis, with or without a mild elevation in protein content, compatible with the diagnosis of chronic meningitis. However, CSF analyses in other children have been normal, suggesting a "pseudotumor cerebri-like" syndrome.[10,42,58] Optic disk edema with normal CSF pressure has also been described and most likely represents optic perineuritis presumably caused by inflammation along the meninges of the optic nerve. Optic neuritis presenting as the acute onset of visual loss may also occur, but will do so with less frequency. Papilledema with increased intracranial pressure, optic perineuritis, or optic neuritis may be the presenting sign of Lyme disease in children.[10,42,58,77]

---

*References 34, 35, 51, 52, 60-62, 71.
†References 10, 11, 20-22, 39, 40, 47, 49, 55, 56, 58, 62, 70, 73.

---

*References 9-10, 15, 20, 22, 40, 55, 60.

CRANIAL NERVES III, IV, VI. Abnormalities of cranial nerves III, IV, and VI (the nerves that innervate the extraocular muscles of the eye) may occur, and, when they do, they typically result in diplopia. Diplopia resulting from a sixth cranial nerve palsy associated with increased intracranial pressure is the most common abnormality, and involvement may be bilateral.[10,43,60]

NERVE V. Trigeminal neuralgia has been described in adults but does not appear to be a common complication in children.[60]

NERVE VII. Facial palsy (Bell's palsy) is the most frequent cranial nerve abnormality in children with Lyme disease, as it is in adults. In our series of 71 children, 8 (11%) developed facial palsy, with bilateral involvement in 3. Clark et al[25] also reported a prevalence of 11% in their large series that included both children and adults. Bilateral involvement occurred in 23% of their patients. Facial palsy associated with Lyme disease occurs in a distinct seasonal pattern, from May to November, with the peak incidence in the summer months.[22,25] Facial palsy may be the presenting sign of Lyme disease.

When a preceding tick bite is recalled, or there is EM on the face or neck, the facial palsy is usually on the same side. Interestingly, one of our patients had striking facial erythema in the distribution of the facial paresis.

Lyme disease is also the single largest cause of "idiopathic" facial palsy in children. Of 84 consecutive children with facial palsy studied by Christen et al, 31% had Lyme borreliosis diagnosed by detection of specific IgM antibodies in the CSF by enzyme-linked immunosorbent assay (ELISA).[22]

CSF analysis in children with facial palsies often shows a mild to moderate pleocytosis, even in the absence of meningismus or meningeal signs.[22] Prognosis for recovery is excellent with a 99.2% rate reported by Clark et al in their large series.[25]

NERVE VIII. Sensorineural hearing loss and vertigo with or without hearing loss have been reported as complications of neuroborreliosis, but infrequently.[13,37,60] Involvement may be on a peripheral (neuropathic) or central (brain stem) basis, or both. Symptoms usually remit. However, severe sequelae have been described when, for example, involvement is associated with a destructive progressive meningoencephalitis due to *B. burgdorferi*.[13]

CRANIAL NERVES IX, X, XII. Involvement of the glossopharyngeal, vagus, and hypoglossal nerves is uncommon, but it has been reported in patients with other cranial neuropathies or brain stem dysfunction.[60]

Focal motor deficits. Focal motor deficits including monoparesis, hemiparesis, and quadriparesis may complicate the course of Lyme disease.[13,32,60,62] These more severe complications of Lyme disease reflect central nervous system (CNS) parenchymal involvement, meninogencephalitis, focal encephalitis, or myelitis (see below). In some cases, vasculopathy or demyelinating conditions have been implicated.[60]

Ataxia. Cerebellar dysfunction resulting in ataxia has also been a well-described complication of Lyme disease in children, although it is not a frequent complication.[60,62] In most instances, it is preceded by, or occurs concomitantly with, other signs of meningoencephalitis or encephalitis. Manifestations may include an ataxic gait, truncal ataxia, or limb ataxia.

Movement disorders. Abnormalities of movement including chorea, dystonia, and tremor have been described in children with neuroborreliosis encephalitis or meningoencephalitis.[60,62]

Myelitis. Myelitis may complicate the course of Lyme disease in children, as it does in adults. It may present acutely or in a subacute fashion, and, most often, manifests as a spastic paraparesis with a sensory level, or in a milder form, manifesting with signs of paraparesis.[20,60]

Peripheral neuropathy. In contrast to adult Lyme disease, peripheral neuropathy is not a frequent complication of pediatric Lyme disease. One of our teenage patients (1%) had a carpal tunnel syndrome associated with arthritis of the wrist. Two younger children (2.8%) described intermittent paresthesias. One of these children recounted "pins and needles" in his legs, and the other, "bugs crawling" on her back and arms. In both cases, symptoms were intermittent and resolved spontaneously, and electrophysiologic studies were not performed. Another patient had a Guillain-Barré-like syndrome, an infrequent complication of Lyme disease that has been reported by others.[20,60] Polyradiculoneuritis with lymphocytic meningitis has recently been reported by Pieterski-Rigler and Zbacnik in 1 of 76 children (1%) followed at their institution.[55]

Painful radiculitis. Painful radiculoneuropathies do not seem to occur in children with Lyme disease, or, if they do, it would seem to be a rare complication. To our knowledge, this complication has not been reported in children. In our cohort, no children had signs or symptoms of painful radiculitis. This has also been true in Christen and colleagues' experience. They did not observe a single case of Bannwarth's syndrome in their large series of patients.[22]

Cerebrospinal fluid findings. CSF findings are similar in children and adults and are reviewed in Chapters 13 and 17.

Neuroimaging studies. Computed tomography (CT) of the head in children with neuroborreliosis is usually normal. However, as in adults, there have been case reports describing abnormalities such as focal white matter low-density lesions, or low-density lesions in cerebral cortical areas that enhanced with contrast material.[13,32,60] Not surprisingly, patients with these findings had clinical signs and symptoms of severe CNS parenchymal disease.

Magnetic resonance imaging (MRI), a more sensitive neuroimaging technique than CT, may at times demonstrate abnormalities not imaged on CT. Twelve of 40 (30%) of our children with neurologic problems associated with *B. burgdorferi* infection had abnormalities on brain MRI.[10] Findings were located predominantly in the deep white matter, were best visualized on T 2-weighted images, and could be classified into three subtypes based on size, location, and presence or absence of abnormal signal intensity on proton density images.[12] Further studies, in progress, will be required to correlate neurologic syndromes with MRI findings.

Neuroborreliosis summary. A wide range of neurologic abnormalities may occur in children with *B. burgdorferi* infection. The most common complications are lymphocytic meningitis, a mild meningoencephalitis, facial palsy, and a "pseudotumor cerebrilike" syndrome. Bannwarth's syndrome and peripheral neuropathy are rare. It appears that the clinical course in most children with these syndromes may be both milder and shorter than in adults.

However, a subtle encephalopathy and chronic meningoencephalitis may occur as late complications.[11,36,56,60] The most frequent manifestations of these syndromes also include headache, behavioral changes, cranial neuropathy, and a "pseudotumor cerebrilike" syndrome.[15,53] In addition, focal CNS symptoms and signs, and progressive encephalomyelitis, have been reported as late manifestations, but these occur infrequently.[2,13,36,53,60]

The pathogenetic mechanisms of pediatric neuroborreliosis syndromes are unclear. Some neurologic complications are a direct consequence of CNS infection, whereas others may include a direct or indirect spirochete-triggered immune process.

DIAGNOSIS

The diagnosis of Lyme disease in children is similar to that in adults. Diagnosis is based on clinical, epidemiologic, and laboratory criteria. If the child presents with EM, the diagnosis presents little problem. If the child presents with musculoskeletal, neurologic, or cardiac involvement and has a well-documented history of EM, with or without a preceding "flu-like" illness, the diagnosis is also straightforward and strengthened by presence of serum anti-*B. burgdorferi* antibodies. However, in the child with isolated joint, neurologic, or cardiac involvement, or multisystem involvement, without an antecedent history of EM, the diagnosis may be more difficult. The physician must rely on the recognition of clinical features of the illness, clinical judgment, epidemiologic data, and laboratory evidence supportive of exposure to *B. burgdorferi.*

In differentiating Lyme arthritis from juvenile rheumatoid arthritis, it may be helpful to keep the following points in mind. To fulfill the diagnostic criteria for juvenile rheumatoid arthritis, arthritis must be present for 6 or more consecutive weeks at onset. Joint involvement in most children with Lyme disease usually begins with migratory arthralgias, followed by brief attacks of frank arthritis. Iritis, a typical feature of pauciarticular rheumatoid arthritis, is uncommon in pediatric Lyme disease. Antinuclear antibodies, however, may be present in both illnesses.

Although Lyme disease may, at times, be difficult to distinguish from rheumatic fever, especially initially, it should be kept in mind that arthritis in rheumatic fever is usually polyarticular and migratory; heart involvement is valvular; and there is an antecedent history of streptococcal infection.[57]

In the absence of EM, Lyme meningitis may be indistinguishable from aseptic (viral) meningitis. In both conditions, patients may have severe headache, neck stiffness, and fever; in both conditions, the CSF findings (cell count and chemistries) are identical. If the child lives in an endemic area or has recently traveled to an endemic area, or Lyme disease is suspected, CSF and serum anti-*B. burgdorferi* antibody titers may be helpful.

Lyme disease should be considered in the differential diagnosis of a child who presents with facial nerve palsy, especially if the child lives in an endemic area. Again, anti–*B. burgdorferi* antibody titers in CSF and serum should be obtained. If negative, it is our custom to repeat serologic studies in 6 to 8 weeks. This is also our policy in the child who presents with optic nerve edema (papilledema), with or without increased intracranial pressure, in whom a mass lesion has been ruled out by appropriate neuroimaging studies.

TREATMENT

The goal of therapy is to eradicate the causative organism. Current recommendations are based on clinical experience and the fact that, in general, spirochetal illnesses are most responsive to antibiotic therapy early in the course of the disease. Treatment for late manifestations, disseminated disease, and more severe complications, is generally longer. Treatment strategies have varied and are still evolving. The treatment regimens presented here represent guidelines from clinical experience. Most have not been subjected to controlled clinical trials. It can be assumed that recommendations will continue to be refined as further information is gained when clinical trials, now in progress in the United States and Europe, are completed.

EM and early Lyme disease

The treatment of choice for EM (and early disease) is oral antibiotic therapy, amoxicillin 40 to 50 mg/kg/day for 2 to 3 weeks. Erythromycin is the drug of choice for the penicillin-allergic child, 30 to 40 mg/kg/day for 2 to 3 weeks.

If the child is older than 9 years of age, tetracycline may be used, 250 mg qid for 2 to 3 weeks. However, clinical experience has shown that doxycycline achieves better tissue levels, causes fewer gastrointestinal side-effects, and may be given twice or three times a day, 100 mg bid for 2 to 3 weeks.[26,57]

Arthritis

Oral antibiotics are recommended as the preferred treatment: amoxicillin 50 mg/kg/day (not less than 1 g/day and not to exceed 2 g/day). Some clinicians also recommend the addition of probenecid 40 mg/kg/day for 30 days. In the child older than 9 years, oral doxycycline 100 mg bid or tid for 30 days may be used.[8,26,57]

While the joint is acutely inflamed, weight bearing should be restricted.

Neurologic

Facial palsy associated with Lyme disease without evidence of CSF inflammation may be treated with a 3-week course of oral antiotics (as in EM).

The recommendation for Lyme meningitis, encephalitis, or facial palsy associated with evidence of inflammation in the CSF is intravenous antibiotic therapy: penicillin G 250,000 to 500,000 U/kg/day for 2 to 3 weeks, or ceftriaxone 50 to 100 mg/kg/day for 2 to 3 weeks. The dose for older children is the same as for adults: penicillin G 20 million U/day for 2 to 3 weeks or ceftriaxone 2 g/day for 2 to 3 weeks. Many clinicians prefer ceftriaxone because of its greater penetration into the CNS and the easier dosage schedule, q24h, or divided q12h.[8,26,57] This permits outpatient therapy. A recent prospective clinical trial from Europe compared the two drugs for treatment of neuroborreliosis in children and found no difference.[50]

A minority of patients (estimates range from 10% to 14%)[57,66] with Lyme disease may experience a Jarisch-Herxheimer type reaction, usually within the first 24 hours of treatment. In general, these reactions are more likely to occur in patients with severe early symptoms. The characteristic feature of this reaction is an intensification of symptoms and signs that were present before initiation of therapy. Headache and neck stiffness may get worse, the fever may rise, myalgias may worsen, and the rash may become more erythematous. In addition to the Jarisch-Herxheimer reaction, Belani and Regelman reported another possible complication of therapy. They described a child with encephalomyelitis who developed transient cerebral edema one day after initiation of ceftriaxone. Symptoms responded to steroid therapy.[8]

ACKNOWLEDGMENTS

This article was supported in part by grant AR 40470 from the National Institutes of Health.

REFERENCES

1. Aaberg TM: The expanding ophthalmologic spectrum of Lyme disease, *Am J Ophthalmol* 107:77, 1989.
2. Ackermann R et al: Chronic neurologic manifestations of erythremia migrans borreliosis, *Ann NY Acad Sci* 539:16, 1988.
3. Afzelius A: Verhandlungen der Dermatologischen Gesellshaft zu Stockholm, *Arch Dermatol Syphilol* 101:404; 1910.
4. Asbrink E, Hovmark A: Early and late cutaneous manifestations in *Ixodes*-borne borreliosis (erythema migrans borreliosis, Lyme borreliosis), *Ann NY Acad Sci* 539:4, 1988.
5. Asbrink E, Hovmark A, Hederstedt B: The spirochetal etiology of acrodermatitis chronica atrophicans Herxheimer, *Acta Derm Venereol* 64:506, 1984.
6. Bannwarth A: Zur Klinik und Pathogenese der 'chronischen lymphozytaren Meningitis,' *Arch Psychiatr Nervenkr* 117:161, 1944.
7. Baumhackl U et al: Intrathecally synthesized antibodies to *Borrelia burgdorferi* in facial plasy. A multicenter study, Fourth International Conference on Lyme Borreliosis, 1990, Stockholm. Abstract W/TH-P-59.
8. Belani K, Regelmann WE: Lyme disease in children, *Rheum Dis Clin North Am* 15(4):679, 1989.
9. Belman AL, Coyle PK: *B. burgdorferi* specific immune complexes in children with neurologic involvement associated with Lyme disease, *Ann Neurol* 30:506A, 1991.
10. Belman AL, Iyer M, Coyle PK: Neurologic involvement in children with North American Lyme disease, *Neurology* 42:371A, 1992.
11. Belman AL et al: Neurologic involvement in pediatric Lyme disease, *Ann Neurol* 26:476, 1989.
12. Belman AL et al: MRI findings in children infected by *B. burgdorferi*, *Pediatric Neurology* (in press).
13. Bensch J, Olcen P, Hagberg L: Destructive chronic *Borrelia* meningoencephalitis in a child untreated for 15 years, *Scand J Infect Dis* 19:697, 1987.
14. Berger BW: Erythema chronicum migrans of Lyme disease, *Arch Dermatol* 120:1017, 1984.
15. Berger BW, Clemmensen OJ, Ackerman AB: Lyme disease is a spirochetosis: a review of the disease and evidence for its cause, *Am J Dermatopathol* 5:111, 1983.
16. Bjornstad RT, Mossige K: Erythema chronicum migrans med meningopolyradiculitis T norske laegefor, 75:264, 1955.

17. Burgdorfer W et al: Lyme disease—a tick-borne spiro-chetosis? *Science* 261:1317, 1982.
18. CDC Lyme Disease. Connecticut, *MMWR* 37A:1, 1988.
19. CDC: Lyme disease—United States, 1987 and 1988, *MMWR* 38:668, 1989.
20. Christen HJ, Hanefeld F: Neurologic complications of ery-thema-migrans-disease in childhood—clinical aspects, *Zentrolbl Bakteriol Mikrobiol Hyg [A]* 263:337, 1986.
21. Christen HJ et al: Lyme borreliosis in children, *Ann NY Acad Sci* 539:449, 1988.
22. Christen HJ et al: Facial palsy and aseptic meningitis caused by *Borrelia burgdorferi:* report on an ongoing prospective study in childhood, Abstract TU-L-12, p 30, Fourth Inter-national Conference on Lyme Borreliosis, 1990, Stock-holm.
23. Ciesielski CA et al: The geographic distribution of Lyme disease in the United States, *Ann NY Acad Sci* S39:283, 1988.
24. Ciesielski CA et al: Lyme disease surveillance in the United States 1983-1986, *Rev Infect Dis* 12:S1435, 1989.
25. Clark JR et al: Facial paralysis in Lyme disease, *Layrn-goscope* 95:1341, 1985.
26. Conference: Diagnosis and treatment of Lyme disease, NIH state of the art, NIAMS, NIAID, *Clinical Courier* 9:1, 1991.
27. Cristofaro RL et al: Musculoskeletal manifestations of Lyme disease in children, *J Pediatr Orthop* 7:527, 1987.
28. Culp RW et al: Lyme arthritis in children, *J Bone Joint Surg* 69A:96, 1987.
29. Davidson RS: Orthopaedic complications of Lyme disease in children, *Biomed Pharmacother* 43:405, 1989.
30. Edwards K et al: Lyme disease presenting as hepatitis and jaundice in a child, *Pediatr Infefct Dis J* 9(8):592, 1990.
31. Eichenfield AH et al: Childhood Lyme arthritis: experience in an endemic area, *J Pediatr* 109(5):753, 1986.
32. Feder HM, Zalneraitis EL, Reik L: Lyme disease: acute focal meningoencephalitis in a child, *Pediatrics* 82(6):931, 1988.
33. Garin-Bujadoux C. Paralysie par les tiques, *J Med Lyon* 71:765, 1922.
34. Halperin JJ: Lyme neuroborreliosis, *Lab Med* 21(5):310, 1990.
35. Halperin JJ et al: Lyme neuroborreliosis: central nervous system manifestations, *Neurology* 39:753, 1989.
36. Halperin JJ et al: Lyme neuroborreliosis, peripheral ner-vous system manifestations, *Brain* 113:1207, 1990.
37. Heininger U et al: Simultaneous palsy of facial and ves-tibular nerve in a child with Lyme borreliosis, *Eur J Pediatr* 149:781, 1990.
38. Hellerstrom S: Erythema chronicum migrans afzelius with meningitis, *Acta Derm Venereol* 31:227, 1951.
39. Huppertz HI: Childhood Lyme borreliosis in Europe, *Eur J Pediatr* 149:814, 1990.
40. Huppertz HI, Sticht-Groh V: Meningitis due to *Borrelia burgdorferi* in the initial stage of Lyme disease, *Eur J Pediatr* 148:428, 1989.
41. Hurwitz S: Erythema chronicum migrans and Lyme dis-ease, *Pediatr Dermatol* 2:266, 1985.
42. Jacobson DM, Frens DB: Pseudotumor cerebri syndrome associated with Lyme disease, *Am J Ophthalmol* 107:81, 1989.
43. Johnston YE et al: Lyme arthritis: spirochetes found in synovial microangiopathic lesions, *Am J Pathol* 118:26, 1985.
44. Kishaba RG et al: Lyme disease presenting as heart block, *Clin Pediatr* 27:291, 1988.
45. Leff RD, Akre SP: Late stage Lyme borreliosis in children, *South Med J* 82(8):954, 1989.
46. Malane MS et al: Diagnosis of Lyme disease based on dermatologic manifestations, *Ann Intern Med* 114:490, 1991.
47. Meissner HC, Gellis SE, Milliken JF: Lyme disease first observed to be aseptic meningitis, *Am J Dis Child* 136:465, 1982.
48. Miller GL et al: The epidemiology of Lyme disease in the United States 1987-1988, *Lab Med* 21:285, 1990.
49. Millner M et al: Lyme borreliosis in children, *Eur J Pediatr* 148:527, 1989.
50. Mulleger RK et al: Penicillin G and ceftriaxone in the treatment of neuroborreliosis in children—a prospective study, *Infection* 19:279, 1991.
51. Pachner AR, Duray P, Steere AC: Central nervous system manifestations of Lyme disease, *Arch Neurol* 46:790, 1989.
52. Pachner AR, Steere AC: The trial of neurologic manifes-tations of Lyme disease: meningitis, cranial neuritis and radiculoneuritis, *Neurology* 35:47, 1985.
53. Pachner AR, Steere AC: CNS manifestations of third stage Lyme disease, *Zentrolbl Bakteriol Mikrobiol Hyg [A]* 263:301, 1986.
54. Peter G: Q & A: diagnosis of Lyme arthritis, *Pediatr Infect Dis J* 9(10):753, 1990.
55. Pleterski-Rigler D, Zbacnik M: Neurological manifesta-tions of *Borrelia burgdorferi* infection in children (Borrelia 90), abstract W/TH-P-679, p105, Fourth International Conference on Lyme Disease Borreliosis, 1990, Stock-holm.
56. Psister H et al: Bannwarth's syndrome and the enlarged neurological spectrum of anthropod-borne borreliosis, *Zen-trolbl Bakteriol Mikrobiol Hyg [A]* 263:343, 1986.
57. Rahn DW, Malawista SE: Lyme disease, *West J Med* 154:706, 1991.
58. Raucher HS et al: Pseudotumor cerebri and Lyme disease: a new association, *J Pediatr* 107:931, 1985.
59. Deleted in proof.
60. Reik L: Lyme disease and the nervous system, New York, 1991, Thieme Medical.
61. Reik L, Burgdorfer W, Donaldson JO: Neurologic abnor-malities in Lyme disease without erythema chronicum mig-rans, *Am J Med* 81:73, 1986.
62. Reik L et al: Neurologic abnormalities of Lyme disease, *Medicine* 58:281, 1979.
63. Sagransky SM: Lyme disease masquerading as juvenile rheumatoid arthritis, *NJ Med* 83:951, 1986.
64. Steere AC: Lyme disease, *N Engl J Med* 321:586, 1989.
65. Steere AC, Feld J, Winchester R: Association of chronic Lyme arthritis with increase frequencies of DR4 and 3, *Arthritis Rheum* 31:S98, 1988.
66. Steere AC et al: Erythema chronicum migrans and Lyme arthritis: the enlarging clinical spectrum, *Ann Intern Med* 86:685, 1977.
67. Steere AC et al: Lyme arthritis, an epidemic of oliogarti-cular arthritis in children and adults in three Connecticut communities, *Arthritis Rheum* 720:7, 1977.
68. Steere AC et al: Lyme carditis: cardiac abnormalities of Lyme disease, *Ann Intern Med* 93:8, 1980.
69. Steere AC et al: The spirochetal etiology of Lyme disease, *N Engl J Med* 308:733, 1983.
70. Steere AC et al: The clinical spectrum and treatment of Lyme disease, *Yale J Biol Med* 57:453, 1984.
71. Steere AC et al: Unilateral blindness caused by infection with Lyme disease spirochete, *Borrelia burgdorferi*, *Ann Intern Med* 103:382, 1985.
72. Sterman AB, Nelson S, Barclay P: Demyelinating neurop-athy accompanying Lyme disease, *Neurology* 32:1302, 1982.

73. Szer IS, Taylor E, Steere AC: The long term course of Lyme arthritis in children, *N Engl J Med* 325:159, 1991.
74. Van der Linde MR: Lyme carditis: clinical characteristics of 105 cases, TU-L-4, p 23 W/TH-P87, Fourth International Conference on Lyme Borreliosis, 1990, Stockholm.
75. von Horsten B, Repp R, Wolf H: Borreliosis in childhood over a 3 year period in the area of Giessen [FRG] p 87, 123 W/TH-P87, Fourth International Conference on Lyme Borreliosis, 1990, Stockholm.
76. Williams C et al: Lyme disease, pregnancy and congenital malformations: a cordblood serosurvey, p 129 W/TH-P87, Fourth International Conference on Lyme Borreliosis, 1990, Stockholm.
77. Wu G et al: Optic disc edema and Lyme disease, *Ann Ophthalmol* 18:252, 1986.

29 European Lyme Disease

Juan Carlos Garcia-Monco

Lyme disease was named for the place where it was first described in the United States by Steere and colleagues.[72] With the discovery of the etiologic agent, it soon became evident that this disorder had been present in Europe for a long time. Although primarily considered a rheumatic disorder in the United States and a neurologic one in Europe, those differences now seem less prominent. However, certain clinical manifestations do vary in frequency on both sides of the Atlantic, and the organism shows certain genetic and antigenic variability that could be of relevance.

This chapter focuses on those aspects that are rather distinctive of the infection by *Borrelia burgdorferi* in Europe. The review of the different aspects leads unavoidably to some overlap with earlier chapters in this book.

HISTORICAL OVERVIEW

The pathognomonic skin lesion, erythema migrans (EM), was recognized for the first time in 1909 in Sweden by Azfelius.[10] He demonstrated to the Swedish dermatologic society a migrating annular lesion that had developed at the site of a bite by *Ixodes ricinus,* the sheep tick. Lipschutz in 1913 gave clinical criteria for the recognition of EM and suggested a role for ticks as vectors.[54] At that time, it was proposed that either a toxin or an infectious agent was the etiologic agent.

In 1922 Garin and Bujadoux,[32] in France, gave the first descriptions of neurologic complications after a tick bite and of a skin lesion that, although not recognized as such, was compatible with EM. They reported on a patient with a painful unilateral brachial plexopathy with amyotrophy of the deltoid muscle. In the 1930s, Hellerstrom[40] and other authors[27,33,36,87] established a link between the occurrence of meningitis and prior EM. Hellerstrom injected tick salivary gland extracts into the skin of patients and healthy people and noted an intense reaction in the former, whereas only a weak response was produced in the later. Between 1941 and 1944, Bannwarth in Germany reported several patients who suffered meningitis with evidence of cranial or peripheral neuropathy.[11-13]

In the 1950s, the beneficial effect of penicillin in treating EM was noted by Hollstrom, supporting the idea of an infectious organism as the causative agent of this disorder.[44] In fact, Lenhoff had reported, a few years before, the presence of spirochetelike elements in sections of skin from EM patients.[53] Binder and colleagues in 1955 transplanted pieces of skin from EM lesions into volunteers who developed erythema chronicum migrans (ECM) lesions, thus providing strong evidence for an infectious etiologic agent. Moreover, the "new" lesions disappeared after penicillin therapy.[22]

However, most of the investigators thought that a viral etiology was more likely, perhaps similar to that of another well-known tickborne disease in Europe, Central European encephalitis. Had the bacterial (spirochetal) theory been pursued, the etiology of this disorder would probably have been elucidated much sooner. Meanwhile, in Europe the neurologic complications after tick bite and EM were increasingly recognized under the denomination of meningopolyneuritis of Garin-Bujadoux-Bannwarth or Bannwarth's syndrome.

Since the 1970s, Horstrup and Ackermann[46] have reviewed the manifestations of this entity. They, and others,[80] insisted on an infectious etiology even before Lyme disease was discovered.

The final answer to the question of etiology would come many years later when, after the description of a new epidemic of arthritis by Steere and colleagues, a spirochete *(Borrelia burgdorferi)* was isolated from *Ixodes dammini*[24] and afterwards from patients with Lyme disease.[18,73]

After the spirochetal etiology of the disorder was established, two other entities well known in Europe for years were clearly linked to infection by *Borrelia burgdorferi:* acrodermatitis chronica atrophicans (ACA) and lymphadenosis benigna cutis.* The availability of serologic methods and the ability to demonstrate the spirochete in tissues and to cultivate this organism allowed this link to be established.

---

*References 2, 8, 48, 59, 65, 69, 82, 83.

ACA was first described by Buchwald[23] in 1883. Herxheimer and Hartmann[41] named the condition in 1902. Therefore, long before the description of EM, this late manifestation of Lyme borreliosis had been described. Of interest is the fact that the beneficial effects of penicillin were also noted for ACA[77,78] and that it could be transmitted from human to human.[34] A spirochetal etiology had also been proposed for this disease.[35]

EPIDEMIOLOGY

Lyme disease has been described in most of the countries of Europe.[68] It has traditionally been well recognized in places where it is particularly frequent, such as Germany, Scandinavia, Austria, and France. The recent increasing awareness of the disease has considerably enlarged the number of cases reported, as well as the number of countries reporting. It has been described in England, Hungary, Czechoslovakia, Yugoslavia, Switzerland, Italy, the Netherlands, Belgium, Rumania, Russia, and Spain.

The main vector of *Borrelia burgdorferi* in Europe is *Ixodes ricinus,* the sheep tick. The tick is widely distributed throughout most of Europe.[68] *Ixodes ricinus* ticks feed on a wide range of vertebrates. The immature stages attack primarily small- and medium-sized animals such as lizards, ground-frequenting birds, rodents, insectivores, carnivores, domestic and wild pigs, as well as humans. The adult ticks prefer large animals such as deer, cattle, dogs, and humans. They need an environment with a high constant relative humidity in the air, near saturation in the soil, and temperature fluctuations between $-10°$ C and $35°$ C, with extreme values for short periods only. Therefore, all stages develop in deciduous forests, brush and transitional vegetation bordering woodland, and grassland.[25]

Another member of the *Ixodes ricinus* complex, *Ixodes persulcatus,* the main vector in Asia, can be found in some parts of eastern Europe.

The life cycle is considered to be 2 to 3 years, although in northern climates it may be 5 or 6 years.[6] In Austria, nymphs and adults become active in the spring, particularly in May and June; large numbers also seek hosts in September and October. Larvae also become active after nymphs and adults have emerged from hibernation.[66]

Several studies have addressed the infection rate of ticks with *Borrelia burgdorferi* in Europe. In Czechoslovakia, for instance, between 3% and 30% of *Ixodes ricinus* ticks were found to be infected.[50] In Austria, about 20% of surveyed ticks were infected, including both the adult and nymph stages.[71] In Germany, between 3% and 35% were infected, particularly the adult forms.[85] In Switz-erland, ticks are infected at rates between 5% and 34%. Uninfected populations of ticks have not been found in Switzerland.[5] In England, 8% of ticks are infected,[58] and in northern Spain, a recent study showed an infection rate of 11% for *Ixodes ricinus.* Of possible relevance is the finding by the authors of the presence of spirochetes in *Ixodes hexagonus* and *Ixodes canisuga,* because these ticks prefer a dry climate.[61] It should be noted, however, that this study was performed using indirect immunofluorescence. It would be interesting to confirm these findings with direct immunofluorescence.

A study was carried out in Germany on 41 persons bitten by ticks infected with *Borrelia burgdorferi* to assess the risk of infection after a tick bite.[64] Only one person developed ECM, but 19 developed a high titer of antibodies to *Borrelia burgdorferi.* However, none of them developed clinical manifestations of borreliosis over a 2-year follow-up period. In the United States, the risk of infection has also been found to be low, with an approximate incidence even in endemic areas of 1 in 1000 per person per year.

The frequency of antibodies in people without clinical evidence of Lyme disease—the asymptomatic infection rate—has also been studied in different countries. Some factors influence the different results and need to be taken into account before different studies are compared. The first involves whether a population at high risk is being analyzed. In general, outdoor activity is the main factor associated with a carrier state. Workers in rural environments (forestry workers, farmers) may have an increased risk as a result of increased exposure, although sometimes this is not the case because of their higher awareness of the tick bite danger. A second factor involves the type of region studied, in terms of climate, density of wild animals, and so forth. Certain endemic areas have been found in several countries such as Germany, Austria, Northern Italy, and Switzerland, among others. Finally, the diagnostic test and titer used to define seropositivity also influence the results. It is well known that serologic tests are still far from ideal for Lyme disease.

Thus, seroprevalence also varied from 2% to 3% to more than 30% in the different studies performed in Europe.

No other vector has been confirmed in Europe other than *Ixodes* ticks, although Stanek et al reported in a large series of EM patients that 18% of them recalled an insect bite at the site where later EM developed.[71]

ORGANISM VARIABILITY

Antigenic differences have been noted by some authors when comparing European and North

American strains of *Borrelia burgdorferi*.[15-17,84,86] Outer surface protein B (OspB) and, less frequently, outer surface protein A (OspA) are absent in diverse European strains. These two proteins are prominent components of the outer envelope of this organism. Some differences have also been found when human isolates were compared with tick isolates. We have compared an isolate from Spain with several American strains, and have found some differences in the electrophoresis SDS-polyacrylamide gel (SDS-PAGE) profile and in the reactivity to several monoclonal antibodies.[31] A major protein in the 20-kD range, designated pC by Wilske et al, has also been found in some European strains.[86]

Genetic heterogeneity within the *Borrelia* species has also been recently shown using direct analysis of plasmid and DNA.[14,26,29,52]

This heterogeneity could be relevant when performing diagnostic serologies. Wilske et al described a European patient in whom the serology performed with American antigens had been negative.[84] Whether these differences translate into clinical differences is unknown.

CLINICAL SPECTRUM

As mentioned before, ever since the etiologic agent of Lyme disease was discovered there has been the question of whether clinical manifestations of the disorder were similar on both sides of the Atlantic.[70] After the description of the new epidemics of arthritis in the United States, Lyme disease (initially Lyme arthritis) was viewed mainly as a rheumatologic disorder. However, the connection was soon made with what had been a predominantly neurologic disorder in Europe. The initial cutaneous manifestations (EM) of both diseases were similar. It is conceivable that an important selection bias has existed both in Europe and North America.[28] Moreover, until a biologic marker exists or the etiology of a disorder is elucidated, it is difficult to delineate the complete clinical spectrum of any disorder.

However, it does seem clear that at least two cutaneous disorders, ACA and lymphadenosis benigna cutis (lymphocytoma), are extremely rare in the United States.

In the next section, the main clinical manifestations of Lyme disease are reviewed by systems to see whether major differences appear substantiated.

Cutaneous manifestations

A clinical marker of this disease, EM is an erythematous skin lesion that appears at the site of the tick bite (primary lesion) and usually heals in several weeks. Although it was named *chronicum* by

Lipschutz,[54] the designation by Azfelius,[10] older and shorter, seems more adequate. It has been suggested that the term *chronicum* be reserved for those cases lasting more than 4 weeks.[81]

This lesion has been observed also in the United States with similar characteristics. It is present in about 50% to 60% of patients on both continents.

Perhaps the most important difference with regard to EM is in the appearance of multiple skin lesions, which are present more frequently in the United States: 25% and 50% of patients develop multiple lesions, according to Berger and Steere, respectively.[19,72] In Europe, they occur in less than 10% of patients.[7]

Clear differences have also been found regarding two other lesions: ACA and lymphocytoma.

A late manifestation, ACA is initially inflammatory and followed by an atrophic phase. It is frequently accompanied by peripheral neuropathy, often most pronounced in the limb with the cutaneous involvement.[7,9,45,51] ACA has only exceptionally been described in North America. However, the peripheral nerve involvement could have some correlate with the chronic peripheral neuropathy described in late Lyme infections from the United States.

Lymphadenosis benigna cutis or *Borrelia* lymphocytoma is a bluish nodule that develops at the site of a tick bite or at a distance from it. It shows a predilection for the ear lobe and the nipple. The lesion usually appears during the early (second) stage of the infection, weeks or months after onset.[7,48] Again, this lesion is frequent in Europe and clearly linked to *Borrelia burgdorferi* infection, whereas no case to date has been described in North America.

Several reports have appeared in Europe suggesting a possible relationship between *Borrelia* infection and localized scleroderma (morphea).[1,39,60] However, sclerotic skin lesions may develop in patients with ACA and lymphocytoma, making it difficult to distinguish these lesions from morphea and lichen sclerosus et atrophicus.[7]

Neurologic manifestations

Neurologic involvement is considered to be more frequent in Europe. In the United States, 15% to 20% of patients are said to develop neurologic abnormalities during early infection (stage 2).[62,67] Aseptic meningitis, painful radiculitis, and cranial neuritis have been recognized as the classic triad.[62] These features are compatible with those described in Europe under the denomination of *Garin-Bujadoux, Bannwarth syndrome,* or *Bannwarth's syndrome.* Neurologists in Europe were familiar with this syndrome, which consisted of a painful meningoradiculitis after a tick bite, and accompanied by lymphocytic pleocytosis and increased protein levels in the cerebrospinal fluid (CSF). Despite this pleocytosis, patients in Europe generally do not show meningeal symptoms. In the United States, most patients do have meningeal symptoms of headache and slight neck stiffness,[62,67] and additionally they may have subtle encephalitic signs such as somnolence, poor memory, and mood change.

The availability of serologic methods to diagnose *Borrelia* infection led on both continents to a significant enlargement of the clinical neurologic spectrum associated with this infection. Thus, late central nervous system involvement was described by Ackermann et al in Germany under the term of *Borrelia* encephalomyelitis.[3,4] Soon thereafter it was described in the United States.[55,63] CSF abnormalities are known to be less frequent in American patients than they are in European patients, in whom inflammatory changes are almost universal. In a recent study, it was shown that European patients with neuroborreliosis had significantly higher CSF:serum ratios of specific antibody both early and late in the illness as compared to American patients. Intrathecal antibody production was found to be specific for the diagnosis of neuroborreliosis in Europe, but it was an inconsistent finding in American patients with late neurologic manifestations.[75] Recently, many reports have illustrated the protean neurologic manifestations of this disease, including myopathies, plexopathies, neuropathies, pseudotumor cerebri, encephalitis, psychiatric disorders, neuroophthalmologic abnormalities, and nervous system vasculitis, among others.

Before serology was available, many of the cases may have been confused or intermingled with cases of tick paralysis, neuralgic amyotrophy, and others.

Thus, it seems likely that the extent of neurologic involvement may have been underestimated in both the United States and Europe. In fact, the spectrum is still enlarging. It is now known, for instance, that early invasion of the nervous system occurs,[30] much in the same way as it does in syphilis.[56] It occurs at a time when no clear neurologic symptoms are evident, although patients may complain of malaise or headache. From looking at the literature, symptomatic meningitis, late encephalopathy, and peripheral neuropathy appear to be more common neurologic manifestations in North America. Painful nerve root involvement is more common in Europe. The most striking neurologic difference, however, is the rarity of ACA in the United States and, therefore, its accompanying neuropathy.

Joint manifestations

Arthritis has been reported in 50% to 60% of American patients,[72] and it was a widely held opinion

that it was less frequent in Europe. It has been claimed that chronic involvement of the joint does not occur in Europe as frequently as it does in the United States. Analyzing 68 cases of Lyme disease in the United Kingdom and Ireland, Muhlemann and Wright found only one case of self-limited polyarthritis, which subsided without therapy. Seemingly, this finding supported the rarity of joint manifestations in Europe or at least in England.[58]

Several other studies have been performed in Europe to address this area, which have modified these opinions somewhat. Huaux et al found a prevalence of 47% for definite arthritis in Belgium.[49] Previously, the same group had reported a prevalence of only 27%, but this was in a series of predominantly isolated EM cases.[21] The authors proposed that their higher figures were the result of a careful search for arthritis, systematic serology in cases of arthritis of unknown origin, and a population with rather late diagnosis who had not received early treatment. Oligoarthritis was the most common pattern, and in most of the cases it appeared in the first 3 months of disease. Arthritis affected limbs where other features of Lyme disease were present, or had developed before the rheumatic manifestation. This contrasted with the initial reports from the United States where arthritis was migratory in the initial stages and chronic in only 10% of the cases, even though proper antibiotic therapy had not been given at that time. There are also some differences among various clinical manifestations, although not in the major organ systems that are involved in this spirochetal infection. However, it has become clear that the basic disease process underlying European and North American Lyme disease is the same.

Herzer in Germany has found arthritis to be the most frequent manifestation in a series of 79 patients, where it was noted in 50.[42] He emphasizes that antibiotic therapy has been given for EM in Europe for a long time, perhaps preventing the appearance of arthritis. In his opinion, lack of awareness of Lyme arthritis in Europe may have contributed to the low frequency of its diagnosis. He did not find, in contrast to Huaux et al, any fundamental differences in the clinical characteristics of Lyme arthritis in Europe and North America. In addition he pointed out that before the description by his group of enthesitis and dactylitis, these features of Lyme arthritis also had not been recognized in the United States. Soon thereafter they were reported from America.[74]

Rheumatologic manifestations were present in 48% of patients in a recent study from Italy.[20] Half of them had arthritis (24% of the total), and the other half had arthralgia. The pattern of articular involvement did not differ from the literature, being most frequently monoarthritis or oligoarthritis with polyarticular arthralgia.

In a series of patients from Spain, articular involvement was found to be present in 45% of cases and arthritis in 27%.[37]

Reports from northern Europe showed a low general prevalence of arthritis.[47,76] In a Swedish study following untreated EM lesions, only 1 out of 16 patients developed arthritis.[47] During the first year of *Borrelia* infection, arthritis was found to be less common than in the United States. Joint abnormalities were common, however, in patients with ACA. Subsequently, this same group has reported an increasing number of arthritis cases from Sweden. The most common clinical picture was of a monoarthritis in the knee.[43]

Arthritis is, together with myalgia, the most common manifestation of late Lyme borreliosis in Finland.[79] Monoarthritis of the knee joint has been described in Swedish children similar to what has been described in the United States.[38]

Therefore, there does not seem to be a significant difference in terms of the key aspects of rheumatic involvement between Europe and the United States. Initially, joint involvement appeared to be less frequent in Scandinavia, where cutaneous and neurologic disorders were prominent. The fact that the initial description of the cutaneous manifestations came from Sweden along with the familiarity with later neurologic manifestations may have biased against seeking rheumatologic complaints. In more Mediterranean countries, where Lyme borreliosis was recognized more recently, the clinical spectrum has been closer to the present North American idea of this disease.

Other manifestations

The rest of the clinical spectrum of Lyme borreliosis is basically similar in Europe and the United States, and on both continents this spectrum continues to enlarge. Even cardiac involvement, initially thought to be rare in Europe, seems to share similar frequency and characteristics with American cases.[78a]

CONCLUSION

There are perhaps some differences in DNA, antigens, and plasmids between European and North American strains of *B. burgdorferi*. There are differences in the frequency of inflammatory CSF changes seen with neurologic involvement. Further studies are needed to clarify how strain differences might translate into clinical variability in this infection.

REFERENCES

1. Aberer E et al: Evidence for spirochetal origin or circumscribed scleroderma (morphea), *Acta Derm Venereol (Stockh)* 67:225, 1987.
2. Ackermann R et al: Serum antikorpen gegen *Ixodes ricinus* spirochete bei achrodermatitis chronica atrophicans (Herxheimer), *Dtsch Med Wochenschr* 109:6, 1984.
3. Ackermann R et al: Progressive borrelien-enzephalomyelitis. Chronische manifestations der erythema-migranskankreit am nervensystem, *Dtsch Med Wochenschr* 110:1039, 1985.
4. Ackermann R et al: Chronic neurologic manifestations of erythema migrans borreliosis, *Ann NY Acad Sci* 539:16, 1988.
5. Aeschlimann A et al: *Borrelia burgdorferi* in Switzerland, *Zentralbl Bakteriol Mikrobiol Hyg [A]* 263:450, 1986.
6. Anderson JF: Epizootiology of *Borrelia* in ixodes tick vectors and reservoir hosts, *Rev Infect Dis* 11:S1451, 1989.
7. Asbrink E, Hovmark A: Early and late cutaneous manifestations in Ixodes-borne borreliosis (Erythema migrans borreliosis, Lyme borreliosis), *Ann NY Acad Sci* 539:4, 1988.
8. Asbrink E et al: The spirochetal etiology of acrodermatitis chronica atrophicans Herxheimer, *Acta Derm Venereol (Stockh)* 64:506, 1984.
9. Asbrink E et al: Clinical manifestations of acrodermatitis chronica atrophicans in 50 Swedish patients, *Zentralbl Bakteriol Mikrobiol Hyg [A]* 263:253, 1986.
10. Azfelius A: Verhandlungen der dermatologischer Gesellschaft zu Stockholm, *Arch Dermatol Syph* 101:404, 1910.
11. Bannwarth A: Chronische lymphocytare meningitis, entundliche polyneuritis und "rheumatismus." Eing beitrag zum problem "allergie und nervensystem," *Arch Psychiatr* 113:284, 1941.
12. Bannwarth A: Zur klinik und pathogenese der "chronischen lymphocytaren meningitis." I. Mitteilung, *Arch Psychiatr* 117:161, 1944.
13. Bannwarth A: Zur klinik und pathogenese der "chronische lymphocytaren meningitis." II. Mitteilung. Ein beitrag zum thema: serose und lymphocytare phasen bei den entzundlichen erkrankungen des peripheren nervensystems mit infektionsallergischer pathogenese, *Arch Psychiatr* 117:682, 1944.
14. Barbour AG: Plasmid analysis of *Borrelia burgdorferi*, the Lyme disease agent, *J Clin Microbiol* 26:475, 1988.
15. Barbour AG, Schrumpf ME: Polymorphisms of major surface proteins of *Borrelia burgdorferi*, *Zentralbl Bakteriol Mikrobiol Hyg [A]* 263:83, 1986.
16. Barbour AG, Heiland RA, Howe TR: Heterogeneity of major proteins of Lyme disease *borreliae:* a molecular analysis of North American and European isolates, *J Infect Dis* 152:478, 1985.
17. Barbour AG, Tessier SL, Hayes SF: Variation in a major surface protein of Lyme disease spirochetes, *Infect Immun* 45:94, 1984.
18. Benach JL et al: Spirochetes isolated from two patients with Lyme disease, *N Engl J Med* 308:740, 1983.
19. Berger BW: Erythema chronicum migrans of Lyme disease, *Arch Dermatol* 120:1017, 1984.
20. Bianchi G et al: Articular involvement in European patients with Lyme disease. A report of 32 Italian patients, *Br J Rheumatol* 29:178, 1990.
21. Bigaignon G et al: Lyme borreliosis in Belgium, *Lancet* 1:557, 1987.
22. Binder E et al: Experimentelle ubertragung des erythema chronicum migrans von mensch zu mensch, *Hautarzt* 6:494, 1955.
23. Buchwald A. Ein fall von diffuser idiopatischer haut—atrophie, *Arch Dermatol Syph* 10:553, 1883.
24. Burgdorfer W: Vector/host relationship of the Lyme disease spirochete, *Borrelia burgdorferi*, *Rheum Dis Clin North Am* 15:775, 1989.
25. Burgdorfer W et al: Lyme disease—a tick-borne spirochetosis? *Science* 216:1317, 1982.

26. Cinco M et al: Restriction endonuclease analysis of four *Borrelia burgdorferi* strains, *FEMS Microbiol Immunol* 47:511, 1989.

27. Dalsgaard-Nielsen T, Kierkegaard A: Allergic meningitis and chronic erythema migrans azfelii after bite by *Ixodes reduvius, Acta Allerg (Kbh)* 1:388, 1948.

28. Dattwyler RJ et al: Lyme disease in Europe and North America, *Lancet* 1:681, 1987.

29. Fattorini P et al: DNA homology comparison between American and European *Borrelia burgdorferi* strains, *FEMS Microbiol Immunol* (in press).

30. Garcia-Monco JC et al: *Borrelia burgdorferi* in the central nervous system: experimental and clinical evidence for early invasion, *J Infect Dis* 161:1187, 1990.

31. Garcia-Monco JC et al: Caracterizacion de una cepa española de *Borrelia burgdorferi, Med Clin (Barc)* 98:89, 1992.

32. Garin CH, Bujadoux M: Paralysie par les tiques, *J Med Lyon* 71:765, 1922.

33. Gelbjerg-Hansen G: Erythema chronicum migrans Azfelii and meningitis after a tick bite, *Acta Derm Venereol (Stockh)* 25:458, 1945.

34. Gotz H: Die acrodermatitis chronica atrophicans Herxheimer als infektionkrankheit, *Hautarzt* 5:491, 1954.

35. Gruneberg T: Zur frage der atiologie der acrodermatitis chronica atrophicans, *Dermatol Wochenschr* 126:1041, 1952.

36. Gsell O: Beitrage zur meningitis serosa und radikulitis, *Schweiz Arch Neurol Psychiat* 59:135, 1947.

37. Guerrero A et al: Joint manifestations of Lyme disease in Spain, *Br J Rheumatol* 30:71, 1991.

38. Hammers-Berggren S et al: Borrelia arthritis in Swedish children. IV International Conference on Lyme Borreliosis. Stockholm. Book B. Abstract W/TH-P-99, 1990.

39. Hansen K et al: Antibodies to *Borrelia burgdorferi* and localized scleroderma, *Lancet* 1:682, 1987.

40. Hellerstrom S: Erythema chronicum migrans Azfelii, *Acta Derm Venereol (Stockh)* 11:315, 1930.

41. Herxheimer K, Hartmann K: Uber acrodermatitis chronica atrophicans, *Arch Dermatol Syph* 61:255, 1902.

42. Herzer P: Lyme arthritis in Europe: comparisons with reports from North America, *Ann Rheum Dis* 47:789, 1988.

43. Hirsch U et al: Rheumatic manifestations of borrelia infection in Sweden. IV International Conference on Lyme borreliosis. Stockholm. Book B. Abstract W/TH-P-79, 1990.

44. Hollstrom E: Successful treatment of erythema chronicum migrans Azfelius, *Acta Derm Venereol* 31:235, 1951.

45. Hopf HC: Peripheral neuropathy in acrodermatitis chronica atrophicans, *J Neurol Neurosurg Psychiatry* 38:452, 1975.

46. Horstrup P, Ackermann R: Durch Zecken ubertragene Meningopolyneuritis (Garin-Bujadoux, Bannwarth), *Fortschr Neurol Psychiatr* 41:583, 1973.

47. Hovmark A et al: Joint and bone involvement in Swedish patients with *Ixodes ricinus*-borne borrelia infection, *Zentralbl Bakteriol Mikrobiol Hyg [A]* 263:275, 1986.

48. Hovmark A et al: The spirochetal etiology of lymphadenosis benigna cutis solitaria, *Acta Derm Venereol (Stockh)* 66:479, 1986.

49. Huaux JP et al: Pattern of Lyme arthritis in Belgium: report of 14 cases, Ann Rheum Dis 47:164, 1988.

50. Kmety E et al: Investigations of ticks for the presence of borrelia in Czechoslovakia, *Zentralbl Bakteriol Mikrobiol Hyg [A]* 263:468, 1986.

51. Kristoferitsch W et al: Neuropathy associated with acrodermatitis chronica atrophicans. Clinical and morphological features, *Ann NY Acad Sci* 539:35, 1988.

52. LeFebre RB, Perng GC, Johnson RC: Characterization of *Borrelia burgdorferi* by restriction endonuclease analysis and DNA hybridization, *J Clin Microbiol* 27:636, 1989.

53. Lenhoff C: Spirochaetes in aetiologically obscure diseases, *Acta Derm Venereol* 28:295, 1948.

54. Lipschutz B: Uber eine seltene Erythemform (Erythema chronicum migrans), *Arch Dermatol* 113:349, 1913.

55. Logigian EL et al: Chronic neurologic manifestations of Lyme disease, *N Engl J Med* 323:1438, 1990.

56. Lukehart SA et al: Invasion of the central nervous system by *Treponema pallidum:* implications for diagnosis and treatment, *Ann Intern Med* 109:855, 1988.

57. Deleted in proof.

58. Muhlemann MF, Wright DJM: Emerging pattern of Lyme disease in the United Kingdom and Irish Republic, *Lancet* 1:260, 1987.

59. Neubert U et al: Microbiological findings in erythema chronicum migrans, acrodermatitis chronica atrophicans and lymphadenosis cutis benigna, *Zentralbl Bakteriol Mikrobiol Hyg [A]* 263:237, 1986.

60. Neubert U et al: Serum antibodies to *Borrelia burgdorferi* in localized scleroderma and lichen sclerosus et atrophicans. Abstracts of the IV International Conference on Lyme Borreliosis. Stockholm. Book B 88, 1990.

61. Oteo JA et al: Enfermedad de Lyme en España, *Med Clin (Barc)* 96:599, 1991.

62. Pachner AR, Steere AC: The triad of neurological manifestations of Lyme disease: meningitis, cranial neuritis and radiculoneuritis, *Neurology* 35:47, 1985.

63. Pachner AR et al: Central nervous system manifestations of Lyme disease, *Arch Neurol* 46:790, 1989.

64. Paul H et al: Infectiousness for humans of *Ixodes ricinus* containing *Borrelia burgdorferi, Zentralbl Bakteriol Mikrobiol Hyg [A]* 263:473, 1986.

65. Preac-Mursic V et al: Acrodermatitis chronica atrophicans—eine borreliose? *Hautarzt* 36:691, 1985.

66. Radda A et al: Austrian hard ticks as vectors of *Borrelia burgdorferi,* overview, *Zentralbl Bakteriol Mikrobiol Hyg [A]* 263:79, 1986.

67. Reik L et al: Neurologic abnormalities of Lyme disease, *Medicine (Baltimore)* 58:281, 1979.

68. Schmid GP: The global distribution of Lyme disease, *Rev Infect Dis* 7:41, 1985.

69. Stanek G: Lyme disease and related disorders, *Microbiol Sciences* 2:231, 1985.

70. Stanek G et al: Differences between Lyme disease and European arthropod-borne borrelia infection, *Lancet* 1:401, 1985.

71. Stanek G et al: European Lyme borreliosis, *Ann NY Acad Sci* 539:274, 1988.

72. Steere AC et al: Lyme arthritis: an epidemic of oligoarticular arthritis in children and adults in three Connecticut communities, *Arthritis Rheum* 20:7, 1977.

73. Steere AC et al: The spirochetal etiology of Lyme disease, *N Engl J Med* 308:733, 1983.

74. Steere AC et al: The clinical evolution of Lyme arthritis, *Ann Intern Med* 107:725, 1987.

75. Steere AC et al: Evaluation of the intrathecal antibody response to *Borrelia burgdorferi* as a diagnostic test for Lyme neuroborreliosis, *J Infect Dis* 161:1203, 1990.

76. Stiernstedt G, Granstrom M: Borrelia arthritis in Sweden, *Zentralbl Bakteriol Mikrobiol Hyg [A]* 263:285, 1986.

77. Svartz N: Penicillinbehalding vid dermatitis atrophicans Herxheimer, *Nord Med* 32:2783, 1946.

78. Thyresson N: The penicillin treatment of acrodermatitis chronica atrophicans (Herxheimer), *Acta Derm Venereol (Stockh)* 29:572, 1949.

78a. Van Der Linde MR et al: Lyme carditis in Europe: clinical features of 66 documented cases. IV International Conference on Lyme borreliosis. Stockholm. Book B. Abstract W/TH-P-75, 1990.

79. Wahlberg P, Granlund H: Late Lyme borreliosis in the Aland islands (Finland): symptoms, signs and treatment. IV International Conference on Lyme borreliosis. Stockholm. Book B. Abstract W/TH-P-82, 1990.

80. Weber K: Erythema chronicum migrans meningitis—eine bakterielle infektionskankreit? *Munch Med Wochenschr* 116:1993, 1974.

81. Weber K: Remarks on the infectious disease caused by *Borrelia burgdorferi, Zentralbl Bakteriol Mikrobiol Hyg [A]* 263:206, 1986.

82. Weber K et al: Zur klinik und atiologie der acrodermatitis chronica atrophicans, *Hautarzt* 35:571, 1984.

83. Weber K et al: Das lymphozytom—eine borreliose? *Z Hautkr* 60:1585, 1985.

84. Wilske B et al: Immunochemical and immunological analysis of European *Borrelia burgdorferi* strains, *Zentralbl Bakteriol Mikrobiol Hyg [A]* 263:92, 1986.

85. Wilske B et al: Epidemiologische Daten zum Aufretechen von Erkrakungsfallen sowie zur Durchseuchung von Zecken *(Ixodes ricinus)* mit *Borrelia burgdorferi, Dtsch Med Wochenschr* 112:1730, 1987.

86. Wilske B et al: Antigenic variability of *Borrelia burgdorferi, Ann NY Acad Sci* 539:126, 1988.

87. Zellweger H: Uber die chronische allergische meningitis, *Helv Paediatr Acta* 1:417, 1946.

Index

A

Abducens nerve palsy, 97-98, 104
  in children, 213
Accesory nerve palsy, 104
Acoustic nerve palsy, 104
  in children, 214
Acrodermatitis chronica atrophicans, 3, 4-5, 52, 71,
    211, 219-220
  in European Lyme disease, 221
  peripheral neuropathy in, 108
Acute disease, treatment of, 163-165
Age groups, Lyme disease in, 34-35
Amikacin, susceptibility of *Borrelia burgdorferi* to,
    151
Amoxicillin, susceptibility of *Borrelia burgdorferi* to,
    151
Amoxicillin/probenecid, in Lyme arthritis, 81
Ampicillin, susceptibility of *Borrelia burgdorferi* to,
    151
Anetoderma, 71
Animal hosts of vector ticks, 22-24, 29
Ankylosing spondylitis, differential diagnosis of, 79
Antibiotics
  in acute and chronic disease, 163-165
  in carditis, 91
  in childhood, 216
  in Lyme arthritis, 80-81
  new agents, 167-170
  persistent fatigue after, 199
  susceptibility of *Borrelia burgdorferi* to, 150-153,
    167-168
Antibody assays, 115-119, 194
  ELISA, 117, 194
  immunofluorescent, indirect, 116-117
  interpretations of, 118-119
  western blot or immunoblot, 117-118
Antibody response in Lyme disease, 46
Antigen detection tests, 136-138
  clinical applications of, 137-138
Antiinflammatory agents, nonsteroidal, in rheumatic
    symptoms, 80
Arrhythmias in Lyme disease, 89
  treatment of, 91
Arthralgias, 74
  in children, 211-212
  differential diagnosis of, 78
Arthritis in Lyme disease, 55-56
  in children, 212
    treatment of, 216
  chronic, 75
  clinicoepidemiologic definition of, 73
  in European disease, 222-223
  immunogenetic basis of, 38-45

inflammatory, 74-75
laboratory tests in, 76-77
radiography in, 77
seronegative, 77-78
treatment of, 80-82
Ataxia in children, 214
Atrophoderma, 71
Autoimmunity in Lyme disease, 179-180, 189
Avian hosts of vector ticks, 24, 29
Azithromycin, susceptibility of *Borrelia burgdorferi*
    to, 151

B

B cell response in Lyme disease, 46
Bannwarth's syndrome, 3, 73, 219, 221
Behavioral symptoms, 206-209
  in children, 213
Behavioral therapy, in fatigue after Lyme disease, 202
Biopsies of lesions, 49-56
Birds as hosts of vector ticks, 24, 29
Blood tests in Lyme arthritis, 76
Borrelia burgdorferi, 64-65
  adherence to cells, 180
  chromosomes of, 9
  cytomorphology of, 50
  discovery of, 3-6
  gene structure of, 13-14
  genome features of, 8-11
  molecular typing of, 14-15
  outer membrane structure of, 168
  pathobiology in vector ticks, 21-22
  penicillin-binding proteins in, 168-169
  phagocytosis of, 180-181
  plasmids in, 9-11
  proteins of, 11-13
  structure and biology of, 8
  susceptibility to antibiotics, 150-153, 167-168
  transmission of, 22, 27
    direct contact between animals and humans, 36
    salivary, 21
    transovarial, 22
  variability of, in Europe, 220-221
Borrelia hermsii, 63
Borrelia recurrentis, 62, 63-64

C

Cardiac manifestations, 86-91
  arrhythmias in, 89
  in children, 212
  in chronic disease, 91

Cardiac manifestations—cont'd
  conduction system abnormalities in, 88-89
  diagnosis of, 89-90
  in myocardium and pericardium, 53-54, 88
  treatment of, 91
Carditis, 53-54, 88
  in children, 212
Carpal tunnel syndrome, 107
Cefotaxime, susceptibility of *Borrelia burgdorferi* to,
    151
Ceftriaxone
  in Lyme arthritis, 81
  susceptibility of *Borrelia burgdorferi* to, 151
Cefuroxime, susceptibility of *Borrelia burgdorferi* to,
    151
Cell-mediated immune response (CMI), measurements
    of, 121-125
Central nervous system abnormalities
  and cognitive impairment, 206
  in early disease, 101-103
  in late disease, 105-107
  latent infection in, 107
Cerebral symptoms, 102-103
Cerebrospinal fluid studies, 138-143
  antibody titers in neurologic disorders, 108, 110
  in children, 214
  in cranial neuropathy, 142
  in encephalomyelitis, 142
  in encephalopathy, 142
  indications for, 139-140
  intrathecal antibody production in, 140, 141,
    206
  in meningitis, 102, 141-142
  normal findings in, 142-143
  in peripheral neuropathies, 142
Childhood, Lyme disease in, 210-216. *See also* Pedi-
    atric Lyme disease
Chloramphenicol, susceptibility of *Borrelia burgdor-
    feri* to, 151
Choroiditis, 94
Chromosomes of *Borrelia burgdorferi*, 9
Chronic disease. *See also* Persisting symptoms
  treatment of, 163-165
Ciprofloxacin, susceptibility of *Borrelia burgdorferi*
    to, 151
Clarithromycin, susceptibility of *Borrelia burgdorferi*
    to, 151
Clinical features of Lyme disease, 27, 64-65
Cognitive dysfunction
  in fatigue, 198-199
  in Lyme disease, 204-206
    in absence of CNS involvement, 206
Computed tomography of head, 103
  in children, 215

Conduction system abnormalities, 88-89
Conjunctivitis, 93
  in children, 212
Corticosteroid therapy, in heart block, 91
Cranial neuropathies, 97-98, 103-104
  cerebrospinal fluid in, 142
  in children, 213-214
Cutaneous lesions, 51-54, 69-71
  in children, 211
  in European Lyme disease, 221
Cysts, popliteal, in children, 212
Cytokine response in Lyme disease, 47, 49

D

Deer as hosts of vector ticks, 24, 29
Definition of Lyme disease, 31-32
Depression, and fatigue, 199
Dermatitis, spongiotic, 53
Dermatologic lesions, 51-54, 69-71
  in children, 213-214
  in European Lyme disease, 221
Diagnostic techniques
  antibody assays, 115-119, 194
  antigen detection, 136-138
  cellular immune assays, 121-125
  cerebrospinal fluid studies, 138-143
  in childhood, 215
  immune complex test, 194
  nucleic acid detection, 127-134
Differential diagnosis of rheumatic manifestations,
    78-80
DNA
  of *Borrelia burgdorferi* chromosomes, 9
  polymerase chain reaction for, 128-133
Doxycycline
  in Lyme arthritis, 81
  susceptibility of *Borrelia burgdorferi* to, 151

E

83-kD protein in *Borrelia burgdorferi*, 13
Electrophysiologic testing, 105, 108
ELISA, 117, 194
Encephalitis, 103
Encephalomyelitis
  cerebrospinal fluid in, 142
  progressive *Borrelia*, 105-106
Encephalopathy
  cerebrospinal fluid in, 142
  in late disease, 106-107
Endocarditis, subacute bacterial, arthritis in, 79

Enzyme-linked immunosorbent assays (ELISA), 117, 194
Epidemiology, 27-36
  age, sex, and racial distribution, 34-35
  ecologic factors in, 28-29
  of European Lyme disease, 220
  geographic distribution, 33-34, 86
    global, 28
    in U.S. and Canada, 28-30
  incidence trends, 30-33
  national surveillance statistics, 30-35
  occupational and recreational risk factors, 35-36
  outbreaks of disease, 29
  in pediatric Lyme disease, 210-211
  state and regional emergence, 29-30
  temporal distribution, 34
  transmission cycle in, 22, 27
Episcleritis, 93
Erythema migrans, 3-4, 51, 69-70
  clinical appearance of, 69
  in European Lyme disease, 221
  extracutaneous features of, 70
  histopathology of, 70
  microbiology of, 70
  in pediatric Lyme disease, 211
  serologic tests in, 70
  treatment of, 149-159
    historical aspects of, 149-150
Erythema nodosum, 71
Erythromycin, susceptibility of *Borrelia burgdorferi* to, 151
European Lyme disease, 219-223
  clinical features of, 221-223
  epidemiology of, 220
  historical review of, 219-220
  rheumatic manifestations in, 75-76
  variability of *Borrelia* strains in, 220-221
Eye disorders. *See* Ophthalmic manifestations

F

Facial hemiatrophy, progressive, 71
Facial nerve palsy, 103-104
  in children, 213, 214
Fasciitis
  eosinophilic, 71
  subcutaneous, 53
Fatigue, 196-202
  after antibiotics in Lyme disease, 199
  characteristics of, 197-198
  chronic syndrome after Lyme disease, 199-200
  and cognitive dysfunction, 198-199
  and depression, 199
  management of, 200-202
  during stages of Lyme disease, 196-197
Fibromyalgia, after Lyme disease, 188
Fibrositis, treatment of, 81
Flagellin, in *Borrelia burgdorferi*, 12

G

Gene structure of *Borrelia burgdorferi*, 13-14
Genetic factors in chronic Lyme disease, 38-45
Gentamicin, susceptibility of *Borrelia burgdorferi* to, 151
Geographic distribution
  of *Ixodes* ticks, 18-19, 28-30
  of Lyme disease, 86
    in U.S. and Canada, 33-34
Glossopharyngeal nerve palsy, 104
  in children, 214
Gonorrhea, arthritis in, 79
Gout, differential diagnosis of, 78
Granuloma annulare, 71

H

Headaches in children, 213
Heart, in Lyme disease, 53-54, 86-91. *See also* Cardiac manifestations
Heart block, 88-89
  in children, 212
  treatment of, 91
Heat shock proteins, in *Borrelia burgdorferi*, 13
Hemophiliac arthropathy, differential diagnosis of, 80
Henoch-Schönlein purpura, 71, 79
Hepatitis, 55
Histopathology, 49-57
  musculoskeletal system, 55-56
  nervous system, 54-55
  reticuloendothelial system, 55
  skin and soft tissue, 51-54
History of Lyme disease, 3-6
HLA-DR4 markers
  in Lyme disease, 27, 41, 76
  in rheumatoid arthritis, 38
Hypoglossal nerve palsy, 104
  in children, 214

I

Imipenem, susceptibility of *Borrelia burgdorferi* to, 151
Immune complex Lyme disease test, 194

Immune response in Lyme disease, 46-48, 180-182
  B cells in, 46
  in clinical cases, 47-48
  cytokines in, 47, 49
  T cells in, 46, 50, 121-125
Immunoblot test, 117-118
Immunofluorescent assays, indirect, 116-117
Immunogenetic basis of Lyme arthritis, 38-45
Immunosorbent assay, enzyme-linked, 117, 194
Incidence trends, 30-33
Infectious arthritis, differential diagnosis of, 79
Inflammatory arthritis, treatment of, 81-82
Interleukin levels in Lyme disease
  IL-1, 179
  IL-2, 49
Intrathecal antibody production, 140, 141, 206
Iridocyclitis, 94
Ixodes
  dammini, 18-22, 33, 86
  pacificus, 19, 22, 33, 86
  persulcatus, 19, 22, 86
  ricinus, 18, 22, 86
  scapularis, 19, 22, 33

J

Jarisch-Herxheimer reaction to treatment, in children,
  216

K

Keratitis, 94
  in children, 212

L

Leptospirosis, 65-66
  heart in, 86-87
Lichen sclerosus et atrophicus, 71
Life cycle of ticks, 19-21, 27
Lincomycin, susceptibility of *Borrelia burgdorferi* to,
  151
Liver disease, 55
Lupus erythematosus, differential diagnosis of, 80
Lyme disease, surveillance case definition of,
  31-32
Lymph node biopsies, 55
Lymphocyte response in Lyme disease, 46, 50, 121-
  125
Lymphocytoma, borrelial, 52, 70-71
  in children, 211
  in European Lyme disease, 221
Lymphoma, cutaneous B-cell, 71

M

Magnetic resonance imaging of head, 103
  in children, 215
Mast cells in Lyme disease, 50
Meningitis, 101-102
  cerebrospinal fluid in, 141-142
  differential diagnosis of, 215
  treatment of, in childhood, 216
Meningoencephalitis, 54
  optic neuropathy in, 96
Mezlocillin, susceptibility of *Borrelia burgdorferi* to,
  151
MHC class II, association with rheumatoid arthritis,
  38-39
Migratory arthritis, differential diagnosis of, 79
Minocycline, susceptibility of *Borrelia burgdorferi* to,
  151
Misdiagnosis of Lyme disease, 189-190
Morphea
  cutaneous, 51-52, 71
  in European Lyme disease, 221
Motor neuron disease, and Lyme disease, 107
Movement disorders in children, 214
Multiple sclerosis
  fatigue in, 197-198
  and Lyme disease, 107
  ophthalmic manifestations of, 98-99
Musculoskeletal symptoms, 55-56, 73-74
  in children, 211-212
Myalgia, 105
  in children, 211-212
  differential diagnosis of, 78
Myelitis, 102
  in children, 214
Myocarditis, 53-54, 88
Myositis, 53, 105, 108
  orbital, 98

N

Neisserial infections, arthritis in, 79
Neurologic disorders, 101-111
  in childhood, 213
    treatment of, 216
  and cognitive impairment, 206
  diagnosis of, 109-110
  in early disease, 101-105
  in European Lyme disease, 221-222

in late disease, 105-109
pathology and pathogenesis of, 108-109
treatment of, 110-111
Neuropathies
   cranial, 97-98, 103-104
     cerebrospinal fluid in, 142
     in children, 213-214
   optic, 95-97
   peripheral, 54-55
     cerebrospinal fluid in, 142
     in early disease, 103-105
     in late disease, 107-109
Neuropsychiatric aspects of Lyme disease, 206-209
Nucleic acid detection, 127-134
   amplification methods in, 128-134
   direct, 127-128
   ligase chain reaction in, 134
   polymerase chain reaction in, 128-133
   Q-beta replicase system in, 134
   transcript amplification system in, 133-134

O

Occupation, and Lyme disease incidence, 35-36
Oculomotor nerve palsy, 97, 104
   in children, 214
Ofloxacin, susceptibility of *Borrelia burgdorferi* to, 151
Ophthalmic manifestations, 93-99
   in children, 212, 213
   intraocular inflammation in, 94-95
   keratitis in, 94
   in ocular surface, 93-94
   oculomotor palsy in, 97-98
   optic neuropathy in, 95-97
   orbital myositis in, 98
   pupillary abnormalities in, 98
Optic neuritis, 104
   in children, 213
Orbital myositis, 98
OspA and OspB proteins of *Borrelia burgdorferi*, 11-12, 169, 181
Oxacillin, susceptibility of *Borrelia burgdorferi* to, 151

P

P22A protein in *Borrelia burgdorferi*, 13
P39 protein in *Borrelia burgdorferi*, 12-13
Panniculitis, 53
Papilledema, 95, 96
   in children, 213

Paresthesias, 107
Pathogenesis of Lyme disease, 179-182
pC protein in *Borrelia burgdorferi*, 13
Pediatric Lyme disease, 210-216
   classification and staging of, 211
   clinical features of, 211-215
   dermatologic lesions in, 211
   diagnosis of, 215
   epidemiology of, 210
   musculoskeletal system in, 211
   neurologic disorders in, 213-215
   ophthalmic manifestations of, 212
   treatment of, 215-216
Penicillin
   binding proteins in *Borrelia burgdorferi*, 168-169
   in Lyme arthritis, 81
   susceptibility of *Borrelia burgdorferi* to, 151
Pericarditis, 53, 88
Peripheral neuropathies, 54-55
   cerebrospinal fluid in, 142
   in children, 214
   in early disease, 103-105
   in late disease, 107-109
Persisting symptoms, 187-190
   from inadequate therapy, 187
   and initial misdiagnosis, 189-190
   permanent tissue damage in, 187-188
   post-Lyme disease, 188-189
   in slowly resolving disease, 188
Phagocytosis of *Borrelia burgdorferi*, 180-181
Plasmids in *Borrelia burgdorferi*, 9-11
Polymerase chain reaction, 128-133
   applications of, 130-132
   false negative results in, 130
   false positive results in, 129-130
   in human and animal infections, 132-133
   in studies of vectors, 133
Polymyalgia rheumatica, differential diagnosis of, 78
Polyneuropathy, in late disease, 107-108
Popliteal cysts, in children, 212
Pregnancy, Lyme disease in, 184-186
   treatment of, 185-186
     in early disease, 159
Prevention of Lyme disease, recommendations for, 156-157
Proteins of *Borrelia burgdorferi*, 11-13, 169, 181
Psoriatic arthritis, differential diagnosis of, 79
Psychiatric aspects of Lyme disease, 206-209
Psychogenic rheumatism, differential diagnosis of, 78
Pupillary abnormalities, 98
Purpura, Schönlein-Henoch, 71, 79

R

Race, and Lyme disease incidence, 35
Radiculitis, 54, 104-105, 107
  in children, 214
Radiography, in Lyme arthritis, 77
Reactive arthritis
  after Lyme disease, 188
  differential diagnosis of, 79
Reiter's syndrome, differential diagnosis of, 79
Relapsing fever, 62-64
  heart in, 87
Reticuloendothelial system, 55
Rheumatic fever, differential diagnosis of, 79, 215
Rheumatic manifestations, 73-82
  arthritis in. *See* Arthritis in Lyme disease
  blood tests in, 76
  differential diagnosis of, 78-80
  early, 73-74
  in Europe and other countries, 75-76
  late, 74-75
  pathogenesis of, 76
  radiography in, 77
  serologic assays in, 77
  synovial fluid in, 76-77
  synovial pathology in, 77
  treatment of, 80-82
  unusual, 75
Rheumatism, psychogenic, differential diagnosis
    of, 78
Rheumatoid arthritis
  after Lyme disease, 188-189
  juvenile
    diagnosis of, 79-80
    differential diagnosis of, 215
    predisposition to, and susceptibility to chronic Lyme
      arthritis, 38-45
  seronegative, differential diagnosis of, 79
Rifampin, susceptibility of *Borrelia burgdorferi* to,
    151
RNA, polymerase chain reaction for, 128-133
Roxithromycin, susceptibility of *Borrelia burgdorferi*
    to, 151

S

Sarcoidosis, differential diagnosis of, 80
Schönlein-Henoch purpura, 71, 79
Scleroderma, focal, 51-52, 71
  in European Lyme disease, 221
Sclerosis, multiple. *See* Multiple sclerosis
Serologic assays, in Lyme arthritis, 77
Seronegative Lyme disease, 77-78, 192-195

Sex, and Lyme disease incidence, 35
Skin lesions, 51-54, 69-71
  in children, 211
  in European Lyme disease, 221
Sleep disorders in children, 213
Soft tissue lesions, 51-54
Spirochetal infections, 61-66
  leptospirosis, 65-66
  Lyme disease, 64-65
  relapsing fever, 62-64
  syphilis, 66
Spleen studies, 55
Spondylitis, ankylosing, differential diagnosis
    of, 79
Spongiotic dermatitis, 53
Sural nerve biopsies, 54-55, 109
Synovial fluid, in Lyme arthritis, 76-77
Synovial pathology, in Lyme arthritis, 77
Synovitis, 55-56
  in children, 212
  treatment of, 80-81
    in refractory disease, 81
Syphilis, 66
  arthritis in, 79
  cardiovascular manifestations of, 86
  ophthalmic manifestations of, 98

T

T cells
  assay for reactivity, 121-125
  response in Lyme disease, 46, 50
Tazobactam therapy, 169
Temporomandibular joint inflammation, differential di-
    agnosis of, 78
Tetracycline, susceptibility of *Borrelia burgdorferi* to,
    151
Ticks. *See also* Ixodes
  animal hosts of, 22-24, 29
  avian hosts and reservoirs of, 24, 29
  classification of, 18
  geographic distribution of, 18-19, 28-30
  life history and seasonal activity of, 19-21
  pathobiology of *Borrelia burgdorferi* in, 21-22
Transmission of disease, 22, 27
  direct contact between animals and humans, 36
  salivary, 21
  transovarial, 22
Traumatic arthritis, differential diagnosis of, 80
Treatment
  in acute and chronic disease, 163-165
  in carditis, 91
  in childhood, 215-216

of early Lyme disease with erythema migrans, 149-
    159
  assessment of response to, 159
  efficacy of, 153-155
  historical aspects of, 149-150
  in pregnancy, 159
  recommendations for, 156-159
of fatigue, 200-202
inadequate, persisting symptoms from, 187
in neurologic disorders, 110-111
persistent fatigue after, 199
in pregnancy, 159, 185-186
of rheumatic manifestations, 80-82
susceptibility of *Borrelia burgdorferi* in, 150-153,
    167-168
of uveitis, 95
vaccine development in, 172-175
Treponema pallidum, 66
Trichinosis, differential diagnosis of, 78
Trigeminal neuralgia, 104
in children, 214
Trimethoprim-sulfamethoxazole, susceptibility of *Borrelia burgdorferi* to, 151
Trochlear nerve palsy, 97, 104
in children, 214
Tumor necrosis factor-alpha levels in Lyme disease, 49
21- to 25-kF protein in *Borrelia burgdorferi*, 13

U

Urticaria, 71
Uveitis, 94-95

V

Vaccine development, 172-175
Vagus nerve palsy, 104
in children, 214
Vasculopathy, 54
arthritis with, 79
and neurologic abnormalities, 108
Vestibulocochlear nerve palsy, 104
in children, 214
Virus infections
arthritis in, differential diagnosis of, 80
myocarditis in, 87
Vitritis, 94-95

W

Weil's disease, 65-66
Western blot test, 117-118